Medical Microbiology *Volume 3*

Medical Microbiology *Volume 3*

*Role of the Envelope in the Survival of
Bacteria in Infection*

edited by

C. S. F. EASMON
*Wright Fleming Institute
St Mary's Hospital Medical School
London*

J. JELJASZEWICZ
*National Institute of Hygiene
Warsaw
Poland*

M. R. W. BROWN
*Department of Pharmacy
University of Aston in Birmingham
Birmingham, UK*

P. A. LAMBERT
*Department of Pharmacy
University of Aston in Birmingham
Birmingham, UK*

ACADEMIC PRESS · 1983

A Subsidiary of Harcourt Brace Jovanovich, Publishers

London · New York · Paris · San Diego · San Francisco
São Paulo · Sydney · Tokyo · Toronto

ACADEMIC PRESS INC. (LONDON) LTD
24/28 Oval Road, London NW1 7DX

United States Edition published by
ACADEMIC PRESS INC.
111 Fifth Avenue, New York, New York 10003

British Library Cataloguing in Publication Data

Medical microbiology.
vol. 3
1. Medical microbiology
I. Easmon, C.S.F.
616′.01   QR46

ISBN 0–12–228003–2

LCCCN 83-71539

Printed in Great Britain at The Pitman Press, Bath

Contributors

M. R. W. Brown
Department of Pharmacy,
University of Aston in Birmingham,
Birmingham, UK

J. W. Costerton
Department of Biology,
University of Calgary, Calgary,
Alberta, Canada

S. B. Formal
Department of Bacterial Diseases,
Division of Communicable Diseases
and Immunology,
Walter Reed Army Institute of Research,
Walter Reed Army Medical Center,
Washington DC, USA

E. Griffiths
National Institute for Biological
Standards and Control,
Hampstead, London, UK

T. L. Hale
Department of Bacterial Diseases,
Division of Communicable Diseases
and Immunology,
Walter Reed Army Institute of Research,
Walter Reed Army Medical Center,
Washington DC, USA

P. Hambleton
Public Health Laboratory Service
Centre for Applied Microbiology and
Research,
Porton Down, Salisbury, Wiltshire,
UK

P. A. Lambert
Department of Pharmacy,
University of Aston in Birmingham,
Birmingham, UK

T. J. Marrie
Department of Medical Microbiology,
Dalhousie University,
Halifax, Nova Scotia, Canada

J. Melling
Public Health Laboratory Service
Centre for Applied Microbiology and
Research,
Porton Down, Salisbury, Wiltshire,
UK

H. Mett
Pharmaceuticals Division,
Research Department, Ciba-Geigy Ltd.,
Basle, Switzerland

C. W. Penn
Department of Microbiology,
University of Birmingham,
Birmingham, UK

P. S. Ringrose
Sandoz Research Institute,
Vienna, Austria

P. A. Schad
Department of Bacterial Diseases,
Division of Communicable Disease
and Immunology,
Walter Reed Army Institute of Research,
Walter Reed Army Medical Center,
Washington DC, USA

O. Stendahl
*Department of Medical Microbiology,
Linköping University, Medical School,
Linköping, Sweden*

K. Vosbeck
*Pharmaceuticals Division,
Research Department, Ciba-Geigy Ltd.,
Basle, Switzerland*

Preface

This book is based on a recent meeting of the same title sponsored by the British Society for Antimicrobial Chemotherapy at Aston University. The surface of bacteria plays a crucial role in determining sensitivity to chemotherapy and to host defence mechanisms and thus forms an integrating theme in discussing the survival of the bacterium in an infection. The distinguished authors have taken a critical look at their subject and, where relevant, considered the possible influence of chemotherapy on the various processes contributing to virulence.

It has long been known that environment plays a significant role in determining important characteristics of the bacterium. What is now much clearer are the consequences of specific nutrient depletion and of growth rate *per se*, especially for envelope structure and function. The contribution of Dr Elwyn Griffiths describes the important effects of iron availability on the capacity of a bacterium to survive in the host. The book ends with chapters which examine ways of exploiting our knowledge of the bacterial envelope in designing antibacterial agents and vaccines.

Michael Brown
August 1983

Contents

Contents of Volume 1

Contents of Volume 2

1 The bacterial surface and drug resistance

PETER A. LAMBERT

I. INTRODUCTION

Bacteria are capable of resisting or avoiding the action of antibiotics in a number of ways, the most important of which are:

(a) production of enzymes which inactivate the antibiotics
(b) modification of the target site so that it is insensitive to the antibiotic
(c) prevention of access of the antibiotic to the target site.

Over the years mechanism (a) has provided the biggest obstacle to the effective chemotherapy of infectious diseases. The most striking example is the production of β-lactamases: enzymes which inactivate penicillins and cephalosporins by hydrolysing their vital β-lactam ring (Sykes and Matthew, 1976). Other important examples are enzymes which inactivate antibiotics by the addition of groups which destroy their antimicrobial activity. Adenylating, phosphorylating and acetylating enzymes are the most important factors responsible for resistance to aminoglycosides (Davies and Smith, 1978).

Resistance by mechanism (b) has been recognized for many years but has not posed a major therapeutic problem. An example is the resistance of pneumococci to sulphonamides, which is due to a decreased affinity of the target enzyme, tetrahydropteroic acid synthetase, for the sulphonamides (Wolf and Hotchkiss, 1963). Mechanism (c) is also familiar: the intrinsic insensitivity of Gram-negative bacteria to antibiotics which are effective against Gram-positive bacteria generally results from the inability

Medical Microbiology, 3
ISBN 0 12 228003 3

of the agents to penetrate the Gram-negative outer membrane (Nikaido, 1976).

In recent years the successful development and introduction of anti-biotics which are resistant to inactivating enzymes has altered the selective pressure for the emergence of resistant strains. Consequently the pattern of antibiotic resistance is beginning to change. Resistance to β-lactams due to altered penicillin binding proteins has been reported in clinical isolates of *Neisseria gonorrhoeae* (Dougherty *et al.*, 1980), *Streptococcus pneumoniae* (Hakenbeck *et al.*, 1980), and *Staphylococcus aureus* (Hayes *et al.*, 1981). Resistance caused by a reduced level of antibiotic uptake has been demonstrated in many laboratory strains of bacteria (Foulds and Chai, 1978; Harder *et al.*, 1981; Sawai *et al.*, 1982) and is now being encountered in clinical isolates (Rodriguez-Tebar *et al.*, 1982). This review is concerned with the mechanisms by which bacteria can prevent or restrict antibiotic uptake and, like an earlier review by Costerton and Cheng (1975), will concentrate upon the role of the cell envelope. It must be emphasized that even small increases in resistance can have an important bearing upon the success or failure of antimicrobial therapy. This may be particularly true in cases such as lung infections in cystic fibrosis patients, where it is difficult to achieve effective concentrations of antibiotics at the site of infection (Govan, 1976; Govan and Fyfe, 1978; Lam *et al.*, 1980; Bergogne-Berezin, 1981; Slack and Nichols, 1982).

With the exception of the β-lactams, the target sites of action of the major groups of antibiotics are intracellular. Aminoglycosides, tetra-cyclines, macrolides, chloramphenicol and fusidic acid all inhibit ribosome function; oxolinic and nalidixic acids inhibit DNA gyrase; rifampicin inhibits DNA-dependent RNA polymerase; trimethoprim and the sul-phonamides interfere with folate metabolism; cycloserine and phosphono-mycin inhibit early, cytoplasmic stages of peptidoglycan biosynthesis (Gale *et al.*, 1981). It follows that all of these agents must penetrate into the cytoplasm in order to exert their inhibitory action. In most cases they are transported across the cytoplasmic membrane by permease systems which are present to transport nutrients. The exploitation of natural transport systems to attain high intracellular concentrations of antimicrobial agents is reviewed separately in this volume by Ringrose (Chapter 8).

The targets for β-lactam antibiotics, the penicillin binding proteins, are located in the cytoplasmic membrane, probably on the outer face (Spratt, 1980). Penicillins and cephalosporins therefore only need to penetrate the cell wall in order to reach their sites of action. Any changes in wall composition which affect the rate of penetration of antibiotics are likely to alter the sensitivity, not only to the β-lactams, but also to antibiotics which act at intra-cellular sites, since they must first pass across the cell wall before reaching the permease systems in the cytoplasmic membrane. The capacity of all bacteria to vary the chemical composition of their walls in response to changes in growth rate and nutritional conditions is well documented (Ellwood and Tempest, 1972) and attention has been drawn to the implications for drug resistance and antimicrobial chemotherapy (Brown, 1977; Dean *et al.*, 1979; Brown *et al.*, 1979). In addition to wall permeability changes resulting from phenotypic variation, many envelope mutants have been shown to possess dramatically altered permeability characteristics which influence their antibiotic susceptibility (Coleman and Leive, 1979; Grundstrom *et al.*, 1980).

II.   THE STRUCTURE OF BACTERIAL CELL WALLS

Figure 1 shows how the structure of the walls of Gram-positive bacteria differs from the envelope of Gram-negative bacteria; a detailed account has been given by Rogers *et al.* (1980). The Gram-positive wall is a relatively simple structure composed of roughly equal proportions of

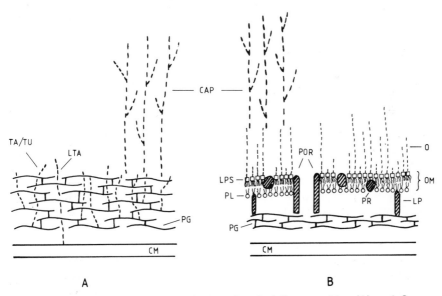

Fig. 1   Cross-section of the envelopes of typical Gram-positive (A) and Gram-negative (B) bacteria. CM, cytoplasmic membrane; PG, peptidoglycan; TA/TU, teichoic or teichuronic acid; LTA, lipoteichoic acid; CAP, capsule; OM, outer membrane; LP, lipoprotein; PR, protein; POR, porin protein; PL, phospholipid; LPS, lipopolysaccharide; O, O antigenic polysaccharide of LPS.

peptidoglycan and an anionic polymer which is usually a teichoic or a teichuronic acid. The peptidoglycan is responsible for the strength and shape of the cell wall. The teichoic and teichuronic acids are long, flexible polymers containing either acidic phosphodiester groups (teichoic acids) or acidic carboxyl groups on uronic acids (teichuronic acids). Both types of polymer are linked covalently at one end to muramic acid residues on the peptidoglycan network. The basic structure of the Gram-positive wall is an open matrix in which the anionic polymers are interwoven with the peptidoglycan (Costerton and Cheng, 1975). The anionic groups have a strong affinity for metal ions, especially magnesium, which is usually tightly bound by the walls. Neutral polysaccharides and proteins are also associated with the walls of some Gram-positive bacteria. The streptococci in particular contain a range of type-specific polymers linked to the wall (Campbell *et al.*, 1978) and some strains of *S. aureus* produce protein A, part of which is released into the medium and part remains linked to peptidoglycan and protrudes from the wall (Sjodahl, 1977). Finally, some Gram-positives produce capsules, normally polysaccharides which are loosely associated with the wall; over 80 different, antigenically-distinct types have been described in *Strep. pneumoniae* (Sutherland, 1977).

The Gram-negative envelope is far more complex. It comprises a thin layer of peptidoglycan accounting for only 10–20% of the weight of the wall. Outside the peptidoglycan layer is the outer membrane (OM) composed of protein, phospholipid and lipopolysaccharide (LPS). One of the interesting features of the OM is the asymmetric distribution of the lipid components. In wild type smooth strains phospholipid is confined to the inner face and LPS to the outer face (Muhlradt and Golecki, 1975), but in certain deep rough strains, where the LPS molecules lack the O antigenic polysaccharide side chains and most of the oligosaccharide core region (Fig. 2) some phospholipid is also located on the outer face (Kamio and Nikaido, 1976). The OM is anchored to the peptidoglycan by covalently-linked low molecular weight lipoproteins originally described by Braun (1975) in *Escherichia coli*. Analogous lipoproteins probably occur in all Gram-negatives but they are not the only means of linkage; several other outer membrane proteins have been shown to be non-covalently associated with peptidoglycan. Additional points of attachment are the zones of adhesion between the outer and cytoplasmic membranes described by Bayer (1979). In *E. coli* the adhesion points number about 300 per cell; they have been implicated in a number of functions including export of LPS to the outer face of the OM, but not in the uptake of nutrients or antibiotics.

Permeability of the OM towards low molecular weight hydrophilic nutrients is due to the presence of a special group of proteins called porins

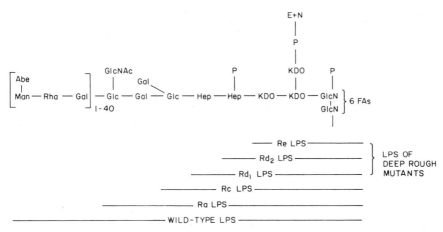

Fig. 2 Structure of the lipoplysaccharide (LPS) in various mutants of *Salmonella typhimurium* and the wild-type strain. Abe, abequose; Man, D-Mannose; Rha, L-rhamnose; Gal, D-galactose; GlcNAc, N-acetyl-D-glucosamine; Glc, D-glucose; Hep, L-glycero-D-mannoheptose; KDO, 2-keto-3-deoxyoctonic acid (3-deoxy-D-mannooctu-losonic acid); GlcN, D-glucosamine; FA, fatty acids; P, phosphate; EtN, ethanolamine.

(Nikaido, 1979; Nikaido and Nakae, 1979). These proteins have molecular weights ranging from 32 000 to 41 000 daltons and are present in large numbers, at least 10^5 per cell. They span the OM forming aqueous channels or pores and are usually associated non-covalently with peptido-glycan. The pores only permit the passage of hydrophilic molecules up to a certain size: the exclusion limit is low in enteric bacteria, of the order of 600–700 daltons in *E. coli* and *Salmonella typhimurium* (Decad and Nikaido, 1976), but is thought to be much higher in other Gram-negatives, the limit in *Pseudomonas aeruginosa* being 4 000–6 000 daltons (Hancock and Nikaido, 1978; Hancock *et al.*, 1979; Benz and Hancock, 1981). Whilst the pore size is a property of the porin proteins themselves, little is yet known about factors which control their functional state. It is possible that other OM proteins and LPS molecules influence the ability of porins to adopt conformations in the OM which enable them to function as pores.

Important advances have been made in recent years on extraction and separation techniques used to study LPS. It has been shown that the LPS from many Gram-negative bacteria is heterogeneous with respect to size (Goldman and Leive, 1980; Palva and Makela, 1980; Munford *et al.*, 1980; Kropinski *et al.*, 1982; Tsai and Frasch, 1982). The total LPS population comprises a range of molecules differing in the number of O antigen subunits from 0 to approximately 40.

The outer surface of the OM is therefore made up from exposed regions of proteins (mainly the porins) surrounded by protruding polysaccharide chains (the O antigens) of varying lengths. Many Gram-negatives also have capsular polysaccharides (the K antigens) loosely associated with the envelope. The polysaccharide chains are often branched and contain negatively charged carboxyl residues (Sutherland, 1977). Capsules provide a highly hydrated gel-like coat around the cell which protects them from phagocytosis *in vivo* and from desiccation in habitats prone to periodic drying (Dudman, 1977). Costerton *et al.* (1981) describe the capsule and other exopolysaccharides as forming a glycocalyx around cells which figures prominently when cells are grown *in vivo* or isolated from natural environments and viewed under the electron microscope. The glycocalyx is presumed to help the cells to adhere, colonize and survive under adverse conditions. Capsular polysaccharides and expolysaccharides probably do not present a physical barrier against the penetration of low molecular weight hydrophilic species, since encapsulated strains have no difficulty in taking up nutrients and are capable of growing as rapidly as unencapsulated strains. In certain cases the negatively charged groups might interfere with the passage of positively charged antibiotics by acting like an ion-exchange resin and immobilizing the antibiotics (Slack and Nichols, 1981). On the other hand, trapping of antibiotics in the capsule would lead to a high local concentration around the cells, which would then be available for transport into the cells if any subsequent dissociation of bound antibiotic occurred (Slack and Nichols, 1982).

III. BARRIER PROPERTIES OF THE GRAM-POSITIVE CELL WALL

The Gram-positive cell wall contains no receptor molecules or permease enzymes to assist the penetration of antibiotics to the underlying cytoplasmic membrane. However, it does not prevent access of antibiotics either; the exclusion limit of the *Bacillus magaterium* wall, which contains a teichuronic acid, is between 30000 and 57000 daltons (Scherrer and Gerhardt, 1971). The strong negative charge of the wall, and of capuslar components when present, might be expected to exert some ion-exchange effect upon the diffusion of charged antibiotics across the wall. In fact Gram-positives are sensitive to anionic, cationic and zwitterionic antibiotics, resistance being generally due to other factors such as inactivation, insensitivity of targets or failure of cytoplasmic membrane transport systems. Take for example *S. aureus* which contains a teichoic acid with a highly crosslinked peptidoglycan and, in some strains, additional components like protein A or a capsule made up of aminosugars. *S. aureus* strains are usually sensitive to fusidic acid (anionic), β-lactamase stable penicillins such as cloxacillin and flucloxacillin (anionic), and the aminoglycosides (cationic).

Attempts have been made to correlate the lipid composition of staphylococci with resistance to agents such as fusidic acid (Chopra, 1976), penicillins (Hugo and Stretton, 1966), and disinfectants which act upon the cytoplasmic membrane (Hugo and Davidson, 1973). Resistance to fusidic acid was related to an increase in the ratio of the phospholipids lysylphosphatidylglycerol : phosphatidylglycerol whilst with penicillin and phenolic disinfectants cells containing high levels of phospholipid were more resistant than cells depleted of lipid by growth under biotin-deficient conditions (Hugo and Davidson, 1973). Lipids are not recognized as components of the Gram-positive wall, they are associated exclusively with the cytoplasmic membrane. Therefore the changes in drug resistance most likely reflect alterations in membrane composition which affect the transport of fusidic acid, accessibility of the penicillin binding proteins to penicillin and susceptibility to damage by phenols.

IV. BARRIER PROPERTIES OF THE GRAM-NEGATIVE CELL WALL

Our current understanding of the diffusion of nutrients and antibiotics across the wall of Gram-negative bacteria has developed rapidly since the recognition, some twelve years ago, of the OM as a vital envelope component. The structure, composition and properties of the OM have been extensively reviewed (Inouye, 1979; Nikaido and Nakae, 1979; Nikaido, 1979). Without doubt, a major contribution has been made by Nikaido and his associates, who introduced the concept of pore-forming proteins and established their fundamental properties (Nakae and Nikaido, 1975). Nikaido has also attempted to distinguish between the uptake of hydrophilic antibiotics by passage through the aqueous porin channels and the uptake of hydrophobic antibiotics by diffusion across hydrophobic regions of the OM.

A. The outer membrane as a permeability barrier

Even before the recognition of the OM as an envelope component it was generally believed that the intrinsic resistance of Gram-negative bacteria towards antimicrobial agents was due to the permeability barrier presented by the cell envelope. In particular, the high lipid content of the envelope was considered to impede access of antimicrobial agents to the cells, although Gram-negatives clearly were able to take up nutrients efficiently. The effectiveness of the barrier was known to depend upon the growth conditions: for example, cells of *P. aeruginosa* grown under conditions of magnesium limitation were shown to be more resistant to agents such as polymyxin and EDTA than cells grown in media containing ample magnesium (for review see Brown, 1975). Leive showed that brief exposure of *Salm. typhimurium* or *E. coli* to EDTA did not kill the cells but released up to 50% of the LPS, together with some protein. The result was a dramatic increase in sensitivity towards agents such as actinomycin D, novobiocin and rifampicin which were ineffective against untreated cells because they could not penetrate the wall (Leive, 1974). As LPS is only found in the OM, it was concluded that the penetration barrier of the OM was impaired by removal of the LPS and that divalent metal ions play an important part in maintaining the integrity of the OM, probably by binding LPS molecules together on the outer face (Nikaido, 1973).

With the discovery of porins the ability of low molecular weight hydrophilic nutrients to penetrate the OM permeability barrier was explained; small hydrophilic antibiotics were presumed to cross the wall by the same route. Nikaido (1976) investigated the uptake mechanisms of a wide range of antimicrobials, including antibiotics, dyes and disinfectants, by considering data on their activity against a series of *Salm. typhimurium* mutants which differed only in the amount of polysaccharide contained in the core and O antigen region of the LPS (Fig. 2). The antimicrobials were chosen to cover a range of molecular weights and hydrophobicities, measured in terms of their partition coefficients between octanol and 0·05 M sodium phosphate buffer, pH 7·0 at 24°C (Table 1). His conclusions are summarized in Fig. 3 (Nikaido, 1979). Firstly, a large group of small, hydrophilic antibiotics, with partition coefficients of 0·02 or less and molecular weights below 650 daltons were equally active against wild type, smooth strains with complete O antigens and the rough mutants containing LPS with varying degrees of truncated polysaccharides. A second group of agents regarded as hydrophobic, with partition coefficients greater than 0·02, were only active against the rough strains. The conclusion reached by Nikaido was that there are two pathways by which agents can cross the OM: a hydrophilic pathway via the aqueous pores, and a hydrophobic pathway involving diffusion across the OM bilayer. The porin-mediated pathway for small hydrophilic molecules is available in rough and smooth strains, the complete LPS O side chains do not impede access of such molecules to the hydrophilic pores. The hydrophobic pathway is not available in wild type smooth strains, either because the LPS O side chains prevent access of the hydrophobic molecules to the outer face of the OM, or because of a lack of hydrophobic patches on the OM which could act as

Table 1 Hydrophobicity, size and activity of some agents against LPS mutants of *Salmonella typhimurium*

Agent	Partition[a] coefficient	Molecular weight	Activity against *Salm. typhimurium*
Actinomycin D	>20	1 255	
Novobiocin	>20	613	
Phenol	>20	94	Active against deep
Crystal violet	14	408	rough mutants. Very
Rifamycin SV	9	698	weak or no activity against
Nafcillin	0·3	414	smooth wild-type
Oxacillin	0·07	418	strain.
Pencillin G	0·02	334	
Ampicillin	<0·01	349	
Cephalothin	<0·01	395	Similar activity
Carbenicillin	<0·01	378	against deep rough
Neomycin	<0·01	615	mutants and smooth
Cycloserine	<0·01	102	wild-type strain.

[a] Octan-1-ol: 0·05 M sodium phosphate buffer, pH 7·0 at 24°C.

receptor surfaces. Only in the deep rough strains can the hydrophobic molecules approach the OM, bind, and cross by a diffusion process. Apart from a lack of protecting O polysaccharide chains on the surface of rough strains, it is thought that phospholipid molecules present on the outer face (Kamio and Nikaido, 1976) might provide sites of access for hydrophobic molecules. The occurrence of phospholipids on the outer surface of rough strains has been questioned (Shales and Chopra, 1982) but it seems likely that excision of 50% of the LPS of smooth strains by EDTA must result in a reorientation of the OM lipids, and that under these conditions the cells become sensitive to the large hydrophobic molecule, actinomycin D (Leive, 1974). Direct measurement of the rate of uptake of the hydrophobic penicillin, nafcillin by the *Salm. typhimurium* mutants (Nikaido, 1976) has shown that it penetrates more rapidly into the deep rough strains (Rd, Rd$_2$ and Re) than into the wild type and rough strains (Ra and Rc).

There are some antibiotics which do not fit in with the general pattern described by Nikaido. Chloramphenicol is extremely hydrophobic but is quite active against smooth Gram-negative strains. Most tetracyclines are also hydrophobic but penetrate smooth strains with little difficulty. Additional factors must be involved in the mechanism by which these agents cross the OM.

The majority of antibiotics used to treat Gram-negative infections are small, hydrophilic molecules which presumably utilize the porin channels

(a)

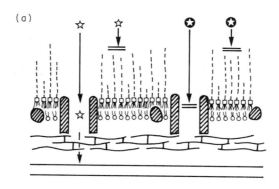

(b)

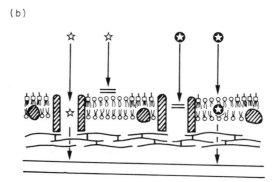

Fig. 3   Pathways for the passage of hydrophilic and hydrophobic antimicrobial agents across the outer membrane of smooth (a) and deep rough strains (b) of Gram-negative bacteria. Hydrophilic agents (☆) penetrate through the aqueous pores; hydrophobic agents (✪) can only penetrate via hydrophobic patches (phospholipid?) on the deep rough outer membrane.

to traverse the OM. Three factors control the rate of passage of molecules through the porin channels: size, hydrophobicity, and charge. The pores of *E. coli* and *Salm. typhimurium* have been 'measured' indirectly by establishing the cut-off point at which a series of oligosaccharides of increasing size are excluded (Decad and Nikaido, 1976). Sucrose and raffinose (342 and 504 daltons) penetrate easily; stachyose (666 daltons) penetrates at less than 25% of the rate of the smaller sugars; and verbascose (828 daltons) and larger oligosaccharides fail to penetrate at all. Hence the exclusion limit is around 650 daltons, which is equivalent to a diameter of about 1·2 nm. Most β-lactam antibiotics have molecular weights between 350 and 400 daltons; aminoglycosides are larger (around 600 daltons), but still appear to be capable of penetrating the pores of *E. coli* (Nakae and Nakae, 1982).

Many of the hydrophobic compounds listed in Table 1 are small enough to pass through the aqueous pores. Their failure to do so suggests that the pores do not permit the passage of hydrophobic species; one explanation is that the water in the pores is highly structured through hydrogen bonding to ionic groups lining the channel. The passage of hydrophobic species would require an energetically unfavourable disturbance of the hydrogen bonding. Nikaido (1979) used the data of Zimmermann and Rosselet (1977) to study the effect of increasing hydrophobicity in a series of monoanionic cephalosporins upon the rate of penetration across the OM of *E. coli*. He found that the most hydrophilic compounds penetrated most rapidly and that the rate decreased with increasing hydrophobicity (Nikaido, 1979). The rates for some familiar cephalosporins were in the order cephacetrile > cefazolin > cefamandole > cephalothin > cephaloram whilst their hydrophobicities, measured in terms of their octanol/water partition coefficients, were in the order cephacetrile < cefazolin < cefamandole < cephalothin < cephaloram (Nikaido, 1981). A similar study was carried out by Murakami and Yoshida (1982) who showed that the 1-oxa congeners of cephalothin, cefamandole, and an unnamed cephalosporin penetrated the OM of *E. coli* and *Proteus morganii* at about twice the rate of the corresponding 1-sulphur cephalosporins and attained a higher periplasmic concentration at a given concentration outside the cells. In each case the 1-oxa congeners were more hydrophilic than the corresponding 1-sulphur cephalosporins, as determined by mobilities on reversed-phase thin layer chromatography. The third factor affecting the rate of penetration through the pores is the charge carried by the molecules. Cephaloridine, a zwitterionic compound, penetrates the OM of *E. coli* faster than the more hydrophilic monoanionic compounds, cephacetrile and cefazolin (Zimmermann and Rosselet, 1977). Perhaps the anionic charges inhibit the passage of the cephalosporins by repulsion from acidic groups lining the pore. Of course, other factors are involved in determining the overall effectiveness of β-lactams, particularly the sensitivity to β-lactamases and the affinity for the target enzymes. The aim is clearly to design compounds with the best characteristics in each respect; unfortunately, molecular features which give a high rate of penetration might also lead to an increased sensitivity to β-lactamase as was the case with the compounds studied by Murakami and Yoshida (1982). The best β-lactams currently available probably represent a compromise between the optimum properties sought in respect of penetration, β-lactamase stability, target activity, spectrum of activity and pharmacokinetic performance.

B. Resistance of Gram-negatives due to changes in the outer membrane permeability barrier

Most of the antibiotics used against Gram-negative bacteria are hydrophilic, low molecular weight compounds; their uptake, and therefore their effectiveness, depends upon the availability of the porin channels. This raises the possibility of resistance, if for any reason the pores are not available to the antibiotics. Fortunately, Gram-negative bacteria cannot dispense entirely with their porins, since they could not sustain an adequate supply of nutrients for growth. However, many viable mutants have been isolated with defective or missing porins (Bavoil *et al.*, 1977; Nikaido *et al.*, 1977). Most bacteria produce multiple species of porins and are capable of altering the relative proportions in response to changes in the growth conditions. For exampte, porin 1a of *E. coli* is repressed by salts (Van Alphen and Lugtenberg, 1977); 1b depends upon the nature of the peptone in the medium (Bassford *et al.*, 1977); in *P. aeruginosa* porin D1 is induced by growth on glucose (Hancock and Carey, 1980) and porin P is induced under conditions of phosphate-limitation (Hancock *et al.*, 1982). Evidence indicating that antibiotic resistance can result directly from mutational loss of porin function has recently been reported. Harder *et al.* (1981) have isolated mutants of *E. coli* K12 and B/r, both rough laboratory strains, in which increased resistance to carbenicillin, ticarcillin and sulbenicillin results from greatly reduced levels of porin 1a (also termed the ompF porin). Sawai *et al.* (1982) have isolated various mutants of *E. coli*, *Proteus mirabilis* and *Enterobacter cloacae* lacking outer membrane proteins which are presumed to be porins. Loss of the proteins correlated closely with a significant decrease in susceptibility to the cephalosporins (cefazolin, cephalothin, cephaloridine and cefoxitin) but did not affect susceptibility to the penicillins (benzylpenicillin, ampicillin, carbenicillin and piperacillin), in direct contrast to the findings of Harder *et al.* (1981). Sawai *et al.* (1982) were unable to explain the different response of their mutants to cephalosporins and penicillins since all the antibiotics were hydrophilic and small enough to pass through the porin channels according to the criteria established by Nikaido (1981). They tentatively suggest that ampicillin might be capable of crossing the OM by passive diffusion in the absence of available pores (Sawai *et al.*, 1982).

The uptake of aminoglycosides is a complex process involving three distinct phases: an extremely rapid initial phase presumed to represent binding to surface components, possibly phosphate groups on the LPS; followed by two energy dependent phases (designated EDPI and EDPII) involving active uptake across the cytoplasmic membrane (Hancock, 1981). The means by which the aminoglycosides pass from their binding sites on the cell surface to the transport system they exploit in the cytoplasmic membrane is not clear. However, Nakae and Nakae (1982) have shown that gentamicin, kanamycin and streptomycin are capable of passing through porin channels in *E. coli* reconstituted vesicles as rapidly as hexoses and disaccharides, even though the aminoglycosides have molecular weights close to, or larger than, the exclusion limits of the porin channels. The susceptibility of *E. coli* mutants possessing only 3 to 4% of the normal porin proteins was not significantly less than that of wild type strains and it was therefore concluded that the reduced level of penetration of these antibiotics through the residual pores was still sufficient to attain the inhibitory action.

It appears then that resistance due to defective or absent porins is more likely to be encountered with β-lactams than aminoglycosides. The possibility of resistance in clinical isolates resulting from phenotypic rather than mutational alterations in porin composition or function must also be considered. Given the established ability of bacteria to vary their porin composition according to the growth conditions, it is clear that strains need to be examined for porin expression, either directly in an *in vivo* infection, without subculture in laboratory media, or after growth *in vitro* under conditions which faithfully represent those which occur in an infection. Perhaps a clearer understanding of the reasons for the success or failure of antibiotic therapy in various infections would be gained from this approach. As an illustration of phenotypic alterations that occur during growth *in vivo* Griffiths *et al.* (1983) have recently shown that OM proteins acting as receptors for the iron-enterochelin complex are strongly expressed by *E. coli* in a mouse infection.

P. aeruginosa provides an interesting example of intrinsic resistance due to the permeability barrier of the OM. The reason for its resistance has not yet been completely explained; although the cells undoubtedly exclude many antimicrobial agents, nutrients are taken up easily and some strains are able to grow on extremely hydrophobic compounds such as long chain paraffins (Chakrabarty *et al.*, 1973). Since the exclusion limit of the pores is large, 4000–6000 daltons (Hancock and Nikaido, 1978), the exclusion of low molecular weight hydrophilic antibiotics is difficult to explain if the pores are continuously open and functioning. One approach which promises to throw some light on the problem is to study the OM of mutants which are hypersensitive to antibiotics. The strain designated Z61 has been produced by extensive mutagenesis of a normal resistant strain of *P. aeruginosa*, K799 (Zimmermann 1979, 1980). Z61 is sensitive to a wide range of antibiotics to which the parent is resistant and it is presumed to be a permeability mutant, having a defective OM which allows antibiotics to penetrate unhindered. In extensive sudies the surprising conclusion was reached that the composition of the OM of Z61 does not differ in any major respect from the OM of K799 (Angus *et al.*, 1982; Kropinski *et al.*, 1982). Protein F, the major porin was present in the same quantity in both cells and its pore size seemed to be the same in both cases. Analysis of the LPS extracted by the standard phenol–water method (Westphal and Jann, 1965) revealed some very minor differences in the fatty acids of lipid A and the neutral sugars in the core region. The extent of phosphorylation of the core and lipid A region in *P. aeruginosa* LPS is usually high, a factor which explains the high OM content of divalent metal ions, its dependence upon them for stability and its unusual sensitivity towards EDTA (Brown, 1975). Only minor differences were found in the degree of phosphorylation of the LPS from either strain, so the high permeability of Z61 was tentatively explained by the minor changes in neutral sugars of the LPS core influencing the functional state of the pores (Kropinski *et al.*, 1982). Recently an improved procedure for isolating LPS has been developed by Darveau *et al.* (1982). The method involves digestion of envelopes with pronase and nuclease, extraction with sodium dodecyl sulphate and EDTA and precipitation with ethanol. When applied to *P. aeruginosa* the yield of LPS is much higher than achieved by the phenol–water method, which, in this organism at least, is now thought to extract a sub-population of the total LPS (Darveau *et al.*, 1982). It is hoped that when applied to Z61 and K799 more dramatic differences in LPS structure will be observed which will explain the nature of the permeability barrier of *P. aeruginosa*.

Although LPS and porin proteins are the major OM components implicated in the barrier properties of the Gram-negative envelope, there are some instances where other components seem to be directly responsible for preventing antibiotic uptake. A non-pore-forming OM protein of *P. aeruginosa* designated H1 is produced in large quantities when cells are grown in magnesium-deficient medium (Nicas and Hancock, 1980). The cells acquire resistance to gentamicin, polymyxin B and EDTA but regain normal sensitivity when transferred to magnesium-sufficient medium for a few generations with a concomitant decrease in the amount of protein H1 in the OM. In addition to the phenotypic change induced by growth in low concentrations of magnesium, certain mutants which are naturally resistant to the agents were found to produce large amounts of H1 regardless of the magnesium concentration (Hancock *et al.*, 1981). Hancock (1981) has interpreted these observations by suggesting that H1 replaces magnesium on the outer face of the OM by binding to the phosphate groups of LPS molecules. These sites are assumed to be the initial points at which polymyxin B and gentamicin bind to the cells; polymyxin then disrupts the OM and the cytoplasmic membrane whilst gentamicin is subsequently transported into the cells in two distinct energy dependent uptake phases and interferes with ribosome function. Masking of the LPS-phosphate binding sites from the antibiotics therefore reduces the sensitivity to the agents. Other mutants which are resistant to polymyxin B do not display elevated levels of H1, so different mechanisms of resistance must be involved (Gilleland and Lyle, 1979; Conrad and Gilleland, 1981; Gilleland and Beckham, 1982).

An example of a change in phospholipid composition which results in enhanced sensitivity to gentamicin is a mutant of *E. coli* K12 which has a temperature sensitive phosphatidylserine synthetase (Raetz and Foulds, 1977). Growth at the restrictive temperature reduces the amount of phosphatidylethanolamine, the major phospholipid present in the whole cells (and presumably in the OM) and increases the sensitivity to gentamicin. Although the decreased phosphatidylethanolamine content might not directly affect the uptake of gentamicin, changes made in the OM composition to compensate for depletion of the phospholipid could affect the initial binding of the antibiotic.

C. Resistance of Gram-negatives due to other permeability barriers

The contribution of the capsule and extracellular slime to the permeability barrier is highly variable. Mucoid isolates of *P. aeruginosa* are generally more resistant to antibiotics than nonmucoid isolates (Govan and Fyfe, 1978) but hypersusceptible mucoid and nonmucoid strains can be isolated from respiratory tract infections with equal frequency (May and Ingold, 1973; Demko and Thomassen, 1980). Irvin *et al.* (1981) have shown that hypersusceptibility is not related to the ability to synthesize alginate, and that hypersusceptible mucoid strains possess two additional OM proteins (32 000 and 25 000 daltons), the larger of which is lost on reversion to normal carbenicillin sensitivity. Since the isolates are hypersusceptible to a range of antibiotics (β-lactams, aminoglycosides, tetracycline and trimethoprim), they are presumably permeability mutants, but the basis of their permeability is not yet known.

Scudamore and Goldner (1982) consider that the OM of *P. aeruginosa* makes only a limited contribution to the intrinsic resistance of the organism. They have compared the action of various antibiotics upon growth curves of normal cells and cells treated with low levels of EDTA to release some LPS and protein from the OM without impairing the viability. They conclude that the organism must have an additional permeability barrier and tentatively suggest that it might consist of periplasmic proteins or a protein-glycoprotein layer covering the outer surface of the cytoplasmic membrane.

The interplay between OM proteins and LPS in determining OM permeability has been explored by Grundstrom *et al.* (1980) using an *envA1* mutant of *E. coli* K12. The *envA1* strain was hypersensitive to hydrophobic and hydrophilic antibiotics; the OM contained less LPS than the parent strain, slightly more protein, but the same amount of phospholipid. Two-phase partitioning studies showed the mutant to have a more hydrophobic surface than the parent strain, giving a possible explanation for the increased sensitivity to hydrophobic compounds. Hypersensitivity to hydrophilic compounds was ascribed to an altered pore function, although no direct evidence was presented. A second mutation, *sefA1*, introduced into the *envA1* strain, restored sensitivity to that of the wild type. Suppression of the *envA1* hypersensitivity phenotype was apparently due to the introduction of more protein into the OM. The OM protein:LPS ratio was 85% higher in the *envA1* double mutant than in the *envA1* mutant, and the rate of penetration of cephalosporin C was decreased from 4·5 times the parent wild type rate in the *envA1* strain to 1·8 times the parent wild type rate in the *envA1 sefA1* double mutant. Grundstrom *et al.* (1980) concluded that either the functional diameter of the pores or their activity were affected by the amount of protein in the OM.

V. CONCLUDING REMARKS

With the emergence of antibiotic resistance due to exclusion by bacteria it is becoming increasingly important to understand the mechanism of exclusion so that drugs with better penetration properties can be designed. Considerable attention is now being paid to the ability of antibiotics to penetrate the Gram-negative OM, the aim being to design an antibiotic possessing optimal properties of penetration, target site activity, resistance to inactivating enzymes and pharmacological performance. In the β-lactams some of the features affecting these different properties are becoming clearer, and, although some may be mutually exclusive, a compromise between the desired properties has produced compounds with excellent performance (Selwyn, 1980).

Deep rough strains of Gram-negative bacteria which are highly sensitive to antibiotics because they present no permeability barrier are valuable tools in research. Firstly, they have been used successfully in screens to detect low levels of novel antibiotics or very weak antibiotics in fermentation products (Kitano *et al.*, 1977; Aoki *et al.*, 1977; Brown, 1981); the monobactams were recently discovered in this way (Sykes *et al.*, 1981). Secondly, they can be used in combination with their parent strains to distinguish between antibiotics with good and poor penetrability (Zimmermann, 1979; Curtis *et al.*, 1979a,b; Ohmori *et al.*, 1977). Finally, the Ames test, used to detect carcinogens, employs deep rough strains of *Salm. typhimurum* to permit uptake of hydrophobic molecules under test (Ames *et al.*, 1973).

REFERENCES

Ames, B. N., Lee, F. D. and Durston, W. E. (1973). *Proc. Natl. Acad. Sci. USA* **70,** 782–786.

Angus, B. L., Carey, A. M., Caron, D. A., Kropinski, A. M. B. and Hancock, R. E. W. (1982). *Antimicrob. Ag. Chemother.* **21,** 299–309.

Aoki, H., Kungita, K., Hosoda, J. and Imanaka, H. (1977). *Jpn. J. Antibiotics* **30** (suppl.), 207–217.

Bassford, P. J., Jr. Diedrich, D. L., Schnaitman, C. A. and Reeves, P. (1977). *J. Bacteriol.* **131,** 608–622.

Bavoil, P., Nikaido, H. and von Meyenburg, K. (1977). *Mol. Gen. Genet.* **158,** 23–33.

Bayer, M. E. (1979). *In* "Bacterial Membranes Biogenesis and Functions" (M. Inouye, ed.) pp. 167–202. John Wiley and Sons, New York.

Benz, R. and Hancock, R. E. W. (1981). *Biochim. Biophys. Acta* **646,** 298–308.

Bergogne-Berezin, E. (1981). *J. Antimicrob. Chemother.* **B,** 171–174.

Braun, V. (1975). *Biochim. Biophys. Acta* **415,** 335–347.

Brown A G. (1981). *J. Antimicrob. Chemother.* **7,** 15–48.

Brown, M. R. W. (1975). *In* "Resistance of *Pseudomonas aeruginosa*" (M. R. W. Brown, ed.) pp. 71–107. John Wiley and Sons, New York.

Brown, M. R. W. (1977). *J. Antimicrob. Chemother.* **3,** 198–201.

Brown, M. R. W., Gilbert, P. and Klemperer, R. M. M. (1979). *In* "Antibiotic Interactions" (J. D. Williams, ed.) pp 69–86. Academic Press, London.

Campbell, L. K., Knox, K. W. and Wicken, A. J. (1978). *Infect. Immun.* **22,** 842–851.

Chakrabarty, A. M., Chou, G. and Gunsalus, I. C. (1973). *Proc. Natl. Acad. Sci. U.S.A.* **70,** 1137–1140.

Chopra, I (1976). *J. Gen. Microbiol.* **96,** 229–238.

Coleman, W. and Leive, L. (1979). *J. Bacteriol.* **139,** 899–910.

Conrad, R. S. and Gilleland, H. E. (1981). *J. Bacteriol.* **148,** 487–497.

Costerton, J. W. and Cheng, K-J. (1975). *J. Antimicrob. Chemother.* **1,** 363–377.

Costerton, J. W., Irvin, R. T. and Cheng, K-J. (1981). *Ann. Rev. Microbiol.* **35,** 299–324.

Curtis, N A. C., Brown, C. Boxall, M. and Boulton, M. G. (1979a). *Antimicrob. Ag. Chemother.* **15,** 332–336.

Curtis, N. A. C., Orr, D., Ross, G. W. and Boulton, M. G. (1979b). *Antimicrob. Ag. Chemother.* **16,** 533–539.

Darveau, R. P., Mutharia, L. M. and Hancock, R. E. W. (1982). XIII Int. Congr. Microbiol. p. 135.*

Davies, J. and Smith, D. I. (1978). *Ann. Rev. Microbiol.* **32,** 469–518.

Dean, A. C. R., Ellwood, D. C., Melling, J. and Robinson, A. (1979). *In* "Continuous Culture 6" (A. C. R. Dean, D. C. Ellwood, C. G. T. Evans and J. Melling, eds) pp 251–261. Ellis Horwood Ltd, Chichester.

* See also Darveau, R. P. and Hancock, R. E. W. (1983). *J. Bacteriol.* **155,** 831–838.

Decad, G. M. and Nikaido, H. (1976). *J. Bacteriol.* **128**, 325–336.

Demko, C. A. and Thomassen, M. J. (1980). *Curr. Microbiol.* **4**, 69–73.

Dougherty, T. J., Koller, A. E. and Tomasz, A. (1980). *Antimicrob. Ag. Chemother.* **18**, 730–737.

Dudman, W. F. (1977). *In* "Surface Carbohydrates of the Prokaryotic Cell" (I. W. Sutherland, ed.) pp. 357–414. Academic Press, London.

Ellwood, D. C. and Tempest, D. W. (1972). *Adv. Microb. Physiol.* **7**, 83–117.

Foulds, J. and Chai, T-J. (1978). *J. Bacteriol.* **133**, 1478–1483.

Gale, E. F., Cundliffe, E., Reynolds, P. E., Richmond, M. H. and Waring, M. J. (1981). "The Molecular Basis of Antibiotic Action," 2nd edition. John Wiley and Sons, London.

Gilleland, H. E. Jr. and Beckham, M. W. (1982). *Curr. Microbiol.* **1**, 235–240.

Gilleland, H. E. and Lyle, R. D. (1979). *J. Bacteriol.* **138**, 839–845.

Goldman, R. C. and Leive, L. (1980). *Eur. J. Biochem.* **107**, 145–153.

Govan, J. R. W. (1976). *J. Antimicrob. Chemother.* **2**, 215–216.

Govan, J. R. and Fyfe, J. A. M. (1978). *J. Antimicrob. Chemother.* **4**, 233–240.

Griffiths, E., Stevenson, P. and Joyce, P. (1983). *FEMS Microbiol. Lett.* **16**, 95–99.

Grundstrom, T., Normark, S. and Magnusson, K-E. (1980). *J. Bacteriol.* **144**, 884–890.

Hakenbeck, R., Tarpay, M. and Tomasz, A. (1980). *Antimicrob. Ag. Chemother.* **17**, 364–371.

Hancock, R. E. W. (1981). *J. Antimicrob. Chemother.* **8**, 249–276.

Hancock, R. E. W. and Carey, A. M. (1980). *FEMS Microbiol. Lett.* **8**, 105–109.

Hancock, R. E. W. and Nikaido, H. (1978). *J. Bacteriol.* **136**, 381–390.

Hancock, R. E. W., Decad, G. and Nikaido, H. (1979). *Biochim. Biophys. Acta* **554**, 323–331.

Hancock, R. E. W., Raffle, V. J. and Nicas, T. I. (1981). *Antimicrob. Ag. Chemother.* **19**, 777–785.

Hancock, R. E. W., Poole, K. and Benz, R. (1982). *J. Bacteriol.* **150**, 730–738.

Harder, K. J., Nikaido, H. and Matsuhashi, M. (1981). *Antimicrob. Ag. Chemother.* **20**, 549–552.

Hayes, M. V., Curtis, N A. C., Wyke, A. W. and Ward, J. B. (1981). *FEMS Microbiol. Lett.* **10**, 119–122.

Hugo, W. B. and Davidson, J. R. (1973). *Microbios* **8**, 43–72.

Hugo, W. B. and Stretton, R. J. (1966). *J. Gen. Microbiol.* **42**, 133–138.

Inouye, M. (1979). "Bacterial Outer Membranes Biogenesis and Functions". John Wiley and Sons, New York.

Irvin, R. T., Govan, J. W. R., Fyfe, J. A. M. and Costerton, J. W. (1981). *Antimicrob. Ag. Chemother.* **19**, 1056–1063.

Kamio, Y. and Nikaido, H. (1976). *Biochemistry* **15**, 2561–2570.

Kitano, K., Nara, K. and Kakao, Y. (1977). *Jpn. J. Antibiotics* **30**, S-239.

Kropinski, A. M. B., Kuzio, J., Angus, B. L. and Hancock, R. E. W. (1982). *Antimicrob. Ag. Chemother.* **21**, 310–319.

Lam, J., Chan, R., Lam, K. and Costerton, J. W. (1980). *Infect. Immun.* **28**, 546–556.

Leive, L. (1974). *Ann. N.Y. Acad. Sci.* **235**, 109–129.

May, J. R. and Ingold, A. (1973). *J. Med. Microbiol.* **6**, 77–82.

Muhlradt, P. F. and Golecki, J. R. (1975). *Eur. J. Biochem.* **51**, 343–352.

Munford, R. S., Hall, C. L. and Rick, P. D. (1980). *J. Bacteriol.* **144**, 630–640.

Murakami, K. and Yoshida, T. (1982). *Antimicrob. Ag. Chemother.* **21**, 254–258.

Nakae, R. and Nakae, T. (1982). *Antimicrob. Ag. Chemother.* **22**, 554–559.
Nakae, T. and Nikaido, H. (1975). *J. Biol. Chem.* **250**, 7359–7365.
Nicas, T. I. and Hancock, R. E. W. (1980). *J. Bacteriol.* **143**, 872–878.
Nikaido, H. (1973). *In* "Bacterial Membranes and Walls" (L. Leive, ed.) pp. 131–208. Marcel Dekker Inc., New York.
Nikaido, H. (1976). *Biochim. Biophys. Acta* **433**, 118–132.
Nikaido, H. (1979). *In* "Bacterial Membranes Biogenesis and Functions" (M. Inouye, ed.) pp. 361–407. John Wiley and Sons, New York.
Nikaido, H. (1981). *In* "β-lactam Antibiotics. Mode of Action, New Developments and Future Prospects" (M. R. J. Salton and G. R. Shockman, eds) pp. 249–260. Academic Press, New York.
Nikaido, H. and Nakae, T. (1979). *Adv. Microb. Physiol.* **20**, 163–250.
Nikaido, H., Song, S. A., Shaltiel. L. and Nurminen, M. (1977). *Biochem. Biophys. Res. Commun.* **76**, 324–330.
Ohmori, H., Azuma, A., Sazuki, Y. and Hashimoto, Y. (1977). *Antimicrob. Ag. Chemother.* **12**, 537–539.
Palva, E. T. and Makela, P. H. (1980). *Eur. J. Biochem.* **107**, 137–143.
Raetz, C. R. and Foulds, J.·(1977) *J. Biol. Chem.* **252**, 5911–5915.
Rodriguez-Tebar, A., Rojo, F., Damaso, D. and Vazquez, D. (1982). *Antimicrob. Ag. Chemother.* **22**, 255–261.
Rogers, H. J., Perkins, H. R. and Ward, J. B. (1980). "Microbial Cell Walls and Membranes." Chapman and Hall, London.
Sawai, T., Hiruma, R., Kawana, N., Kaneko, M., Tanigasu, F. and Inami, A. (1982). *Antimicrob. Ag. Chemother.* **22**, 585–592.
Scherrer, R. and Gerhardt, P. (1971). *J. Bacteriol.* **107**, 718–735.
Scudamore, R. A. and Goldner, M. (1982). *Can. J. Microbiol.* **28**, 169–175.
Selwyn, S. (1980). "The β-lactam Antibiotic: Penicillins and Cephalosporins in Perspective." Hodder and Stoughton, London.
Shales, S. and Chopra, I. (1982). *J. Antimicrob. Chemother.* **9**, 325–327.
Sjodahl, J. (1977). *Eur. J. Biochem.* **73**, 343–351.
Slack, M. P. E. and Nichols, W. W. (1981). *Lancet* **ii**, 502–503.
Slack, M. P. E. and Nichols, W. W. (1982). *J. Antimicrob. Chemother.* **10**, 368–372.
Spratt, B. G. (1980). *Phil. Trans. Roy. Soc. Lond. Series B* **289**, 273–283.
Sutherland, I. W. (1977). *In* "Surface Carbohydrates of the Prokaryotic Cell" (I. W. Sutherland, ed.) pp. 27–96. Academic Press, London.
Sykes, R. B. and Matthew, M. (1976). *J. Antimicrob. Chemother.* **2**, 155–157.
Sykes, R. B., Bonner, D. P., Bush K. Georgopapadakou, N. H. and Wells J. S. (1981). *J. Antimicrob. Chemother.* **8**, suppl. E, 1–16.
Tsai, G. M. and Frasch, C. E. (1982). *Analyt. Biochem.* **119**, 115–119.
Van Alphen, W. and Lugtenberg, B. (1977). *J. Bacteriol.* **131**, 623–630.
Westphal, O. and Jann, K. (1965). *Methods Carbohydr. Chem.* **5**, 83–91.
Wolf, B. and Hotchkiss, R. D. (1963). *Biochemistry* **2**, 145–150.
Zimmermann, W. (1979). *Int. J. Clin. Pharm. Biopharm.* **17**, 131–134.
Zimmermann, W. (1980). *Antimicrob. Ag. Chemother.* **18**, 94–109.
Zimmermann, W. and Rosselet, A. (1977). *Antimicrob. Ag. Chemother.* **12**, 368–372.

2 Bacterial adhesion: influence of drugs*

KLAUS VOSBECK and HELMUT METT

I. INTRODUCTION

Adhesion of bacteria to surfaces is an essential first step in the colonization of microbial habitats, especially in locations where mechanical cleansing mechanisms are operative, as in flowing water and on many surfaces in living organisms. Adhesive interactions between bacteria and epithelial cells are consequently presumed to be crucial events in the colonization of mucosal surfaces by pathogenic as well as by commensal bacteria (Ofek and Beachey, 1980a, b; Savage, 1980; Jones, 1977; Gibbons, 1977). The evolution of specific adhesive mechanisms by a wide spectrum of bacterial species furnishes evidence of the general importance of such interactions and may account, at least in part, for the specific distribution of organisms in different habitats (Gibbons and van Houte, 1975).

The apparent significance of bacterial adhesion in the pathogenesis of different infectious diseases of animals and man suggests alternative possibilities of prophylactic or therapeutic interference with the infectious process. However, these possibilities cannot be investigated systematically until more is known about the biochemical and biological mechanisms of adhesion. A more precise conception of the nature of different adhesive phenomena is slowly emerging from an increasing number of reports dealing with the molecular and genetic basis of bacterial adhesion.

Before practicable modes of pharmacological intervention can be contemplated, it is essential to arrive at an understanding of the relation between the adhesion of commensal and that of pathogenic organisms, on

---

* Dedicated to Dr F. Kradolfer on the occasion of his 65th birthday.

MEDICAL MICROBIOLOGY, 3
ISBN 0 12 228003 3

the one hand, and between harmful adhesion of pathogens to epithelial surfaces and beneficial adhesion to phagocytic cells on the other.

This chapter presents a hypothetical exposition of the sequential, adhesive interactions that may occur between microorganisms and epithelia. Some of the more recent findings relating to functional aspects of adhesion are reviewed, and possibilities of pharmacological intervention discussed on the basis of results obtained in experimental model systems.

II. ADHESIVE INTERACTIONS IN THE PATHOGENESIS OF BACTERIAL INFECTIONS

A. Types of adhesive interaction

Adhesive interactions between eukaryotic organisms and colonizing microorganisms, whether pathogenic or not, are important but also complex phenomena (Jones, 1977). Two main types of interaction, the *process of adhesion* and the *state of adherence*, should be distinguished conceptually and terminologically (Fig. 1). They may occur consecutively in a given pathogenic sequence of events. As a bacterium carrying adhesion factors on its surface comes into close contact with a host epithelial cell, it is thought to recognize the corresponding specific receptors located on the epithelial cell surface. This may result in reversible binding, which in turn may lead to interactions with further receptors. This *process of adhesion* can be defined by its rate and the affinity of the bacteria for the epithelial surface. It can be described by Michaelis–Menten kinetics. The maximum rate of adhesion (v_{max}) and the affinity (K_s) can be determined graphically

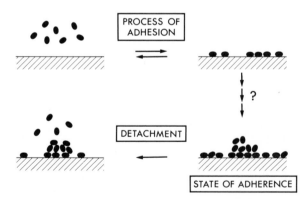

Fig. 1 Hypothetical concept of the adhesive interactions between bacteria and epithelial surfaces. The *process of adhesion* should be differentiated conceptually from the state of being adherent, called *state of adherence* (see text for details).

from Lineweaver–Burk plots in simple model systems (Cohen *et al.*, 1981; Bose and Mudd, 1981).

Adhesion of bacteria to epithelial surfaces may subsequently lead to irreversible attachment of the bacteria and also the formation of adherent microcolonies (Källenius *et al.*, 1980a; Marrie *et al.*, 1980; Cantey *et al.*, 1981; Clausen and Christie, 1982). The *state of adherence* should be differentiated from the actual *process of adhesion*. The rate and affinity of the process of adhesion, and possibly also adhesive specificity, is thought to be solely dependent on the interaction between bacterial adhesion factors and eukaryotic receptor structures. By contrast, the forces contributing to the maintenance of the *state of adherence* of a bacterium or even a microcolony are very ill-defined and may include not only interactions mediated by bacterial adhesion factors and eukaryotic receptors, but also secondary events, like the excretion of polysaccharide material, multiplication of adherent bacteria, shift to a quiescent state, and thus the formation of adherent, encapsulated microcolonies (Costerton and Marrie, this volume ch. 3; Costerton *et al.*, 1981; Lam *et al.*, 1980; Marrie *et al.*, 1980; Cantey *et al.*, 1981).

Adherent bacteria may present a surface different from that of non-adherent bacteria, which may lead to changes in their interaction with the host defense systems. Adherent bacteria appear to be less sensitive to antibiotics (Gwynn *et al.*, 1981) and to the natural host defense systems, such as the bactericidal activity of serum and phagocytosis (Peterson and Quie, 1981; Zimmerli *et al.*, 1982; Costerton and Marrie, this volume ch. 3), and may play a role in chronic, persistent infections.

Most of the existing quantitative or semiquantitative assays measure the rate of adhesion, whereas morphological studies and colonization studies furnish information on the adherent state of bacteria. Quantitative assessments of the state of adherence are technically not feasible in a simple manner (Fowler and McKay, 1981) and to the best of our knowledge none have been made. However, the electron-microscopical study performed by Cantey *et al.* (1981) provides morphological evidence of at least two stages of adhesive interaction, which may correspond to those postulated above. The process of adhesion is certainly one of the initial events in the pathogenesis of infectious diseases, whereas the forces operating in maintaining bacteria in the adherent state may be more relevant for later stages of disease, especially in chronic and persistent infections, but also in the normal colonization of mucosal surfaces.

The detachment of bacteria from an adherent population has so far not been studied in detail (Sugarman and Donta, 1979).

There is ample evidence that the adhesion of Gram-negative bacteria is in most cases mediated by bacterial surface appendages, fimbriae or pili

(Duguid and Old, 1980), although there are some notable exceptions (Jones and Freter, 1976; Jann *et al.*, 1981b; Eshdat *et al.*, 1981b; Chabanon *et al.*, 1982a; Izhar *et al.*, 1982; Pruzzo *et al.*, 1982). The adhesion of Gram-positive bacteria appears to depend upon quite different mechanisms (Beachey, 1981; Ofek and Beachey, 1980a,b; Ellen and Gibbons, 1972).

The following discussion will be restricted in the main to the process of adhesion, as defined above, of Gram-negative bacteria.

B. Bacterial adhesion and pathogencity

The importance of bacterial adhesion in the pathogenesis of infectious diseases has been well established in animal and human diarrhoea caused by enterotoxin-producing strains of *Escherichia coli*, in human urinary-tract infections caused by *E. coli*, in gonorrhoea, and in streptococcal endocarditis.

Enterotoxigenic *E. coli* express a number of different species-specific adhesion factors that can be distinguished serologically. Thus, *E. coli* strains isolated from pigs with diarrhoea frequently carry adhesion factor K88 (Jones and Rutter, 1972). The genetic information for this adhesion factor, as for many others, is usually located on a plasmid, as is the genetic information for the production of entertoxins. Smith and Linggood (1972) have demonstrated that the expression of both the K88 adhesion factor and enterotoxin is required to render an *E. coli* strain pathogenic. They transferred the two plasmids' coding for the K88 adhesion factor (K88) and enterotoxin (Ent) separately to a non-pathogenic *E. coli* strain. The resultant K88+Ent− and K88−Ent+ variants of the strain were apathogenic, although K88+Ent− multiplied profusely in the intestine. A derivative containing both plasmids (K88+Ent−), by contrast, colonized the intestinal tract of the pig and caused diarrhoea.

Sellwood *et al.* (1975) reported that some pigs were genetically resistant to enterotoxigenic *E. coli* expressing K88, and that this trait was inherited in a simple Mendelian fashion. K88 strains failed to adhere *in vitro* to intestinal brush borders of these resistant pigs. The same animals were, however, fully sensitive to strains possessing a different adhesion factor, 987P (Smith and Huggins, 1978). These observations constitute further evidence of the important role of adhesion in the pathogenesis of diarrhoea. The simple pattern of inheritance of resistance strongly suggests the participation of a specific receptor molecule on the host-cell surface. More recently, resistance to adhesion of *E. coli* K88 strains has been related to the absence of a glycolipid fraction in the intestinal mucosa of resistant animals (Kearns and Gibbons, 1979). This glycolipid is thought to represent the specific receptor for the K88 adhesion factor (Table 1).

Similar, but less detailed evidence indicates the presence of specific bacterial adhesion factors in human enterotoxigenic *E. coli* strains. Evans *et al.* (1978) and Evans and Evans (1978) described two adhesion factors, which they called colonization factor antigens (CFA/I and CFA/II), and which have been found in up to 86% of enterotoxigenic clinical isolates in different studies (Evans *et al.*, 1978; Cravioto *et al.*, 1979; Cravioto *et al.*, 1982). An enterotoxigenic CFA/I strain of *E. coli* lost its pathogenicity for human volunteers, when the CFA/I adhesion factor was removed, although the derivative strain still produced enterotoxin (Satterwhite *et al.*, 1978). These results support the notion that the expression of an adhesion factor is an essential determinant of virulence in the pathogenesis of human diarrhoea.

Adhesion factors different from CFA/I and CFA/II have been associated with the ability of *E. coli* strains to cause urinary-tract infections. *E. coli* strains isolated from patients with upper-urinary-tract infections tend to adhere more readily to exfoliated urinary-tract epithelial cells than do strains from asymptomatic bacteriuria, or faecal strains (Svanborg Edén *et al.*, 1976). One type of *E. coli* adhesion factor could be unequivocally associated with pyelonephritis in anatomically normal patients. These P-fimbriae occurred in approximately 90% of *E. coli* strains isolated from upper-urinary-tract infections, in approximately 20% of *E. coli* strains from lower-urinary-tract infections (cystitis and asymptomatic bacteriuria), but in only 7% of normal faecal isolates (Källenius *et al.*, 1981). Extensive work on the binding specificity and the structure of P fimbriae has been done recently because of their apparent clinical importance (see Section II.C).

There is also evidence that uropathogenic *E. coli* strains adhere better to uroepithelial, to periurethral, or vaginal cells of female patients prone to urinary-tract infections than to those of healthy controls (Svanborg Edén and Jodal, 1979; Källenius *et al*, 1980a; Källenius and Winberg, 1978; Schaeffer *et al.*, 1981). Susceptibility to urinary-tract infections therefore appears to depend on the degree of adhesiveness of the infecting bacteria as well as on the receptivity of the host epithelial cells (Lomberg *et al.*, 1981).

Neisseria gonorrhoeae also expresses fimbriae, which serve as adhesion factors (Pearce and Buchanan, 1978), and gonoccocal adhesion is correlated with virulence, although this correlation is less clear than in the case of diarrhoea caused by *E. coli* (Punsalang and Sawyer, 1973; Brinton *et al.*, 1978; Watt *et al.*, 1978; Tramont, 1981).

Certain streptococci adhere to fibrin deposits *in vitro* and *in vivo*. Their adhesion is mediated by streptococcal dextran, and it is augmented by the presence of platelets. The significance of bacterial adhesion in the pathogenesis of streptococcal endocarditis has been well documented by Gould *et al.* (1975), Scheld *et al.* (1978) and Ramirez-Ronda (1978).

Adhesive interactions have also been implicated in the pathogenesis of a large number of other diseases and as virulence factors of other bacterial species. Adhesive properties can be observed, for instance, in many enteric pathogens, such as *Vibrio cholerae* (Srivastava *et al.*, 1980; Jones *et al.*, 1976; Levett and Daniel, 1981), *Vibrio parahaemolyticus* (Iijima *et al.*, 1981), and *Aeromonas hydrophila* (Atkinson and Trust, 1980; Levett and Daniel, 1981), which colonize the small intestine, and in *Yersinia enterocolitica* (Okamoto *et al.*, 1980), and *Shigella flexneri* (Izhar *et al.*, 1982), both pathogens of the large intestine. Urinary-tract pathogens other than *E. coli* also exhibit adhesive properties, and this has been shown in *Proteus mirabilis* (Silverblatt and Ofek, 1978; Svanborg Edén *et al.*, 1980) and in *Klebsiella penumoniae* (Fader *et al.*, 1979). Adhesion of *Pseudomonas aeruginosa* to the epithelium of the respiratory tract has been implicated in the pathogenesis of *P. aeruginosa* lung infections in patients with cystic fibrosis (Woods *et al.*, 1980b; Woods *et al.*, 1981a). A correlation between the adhesiveness of *Bordetella pertussis* and its pathogenicity has been demonstrated in a rabbit and a mouse model (Matsuyama, 1971; Burns and Freer, 1982). Adhesion of Group A streptococci appears to play a role in the pathogenesis of rheumatic fever, but in this case it is the cells of susceptible patients rather than the bacteria that exhibit increased receptivity (Selinger *et al.*, 1978; Reed *et al.*, 1980). Similarly, increased adhesion of Group B streptococci and other Gram-positive cocci to virus-infected tissue-culture cells has been demonstrated, and this may partly account for the clinically known risk of bacterial superinfection in viral diseases (Sanford *et al.*, 1978; Selinger *et al.*, 1981). Bose and Mudd (1981) furnished evidence that the adhesion of *E. coli* and of *Staphylococcus aureus* to cells infected with the intracellular parasite *Chlamydia trachomatis* may be increased.

Although increased bacterial adhesion has in most cases been associated with pathogenicity, there may be cases in which reduced adhesiveness appears to increase pathogenicity. In *Neisseria meningitidis* adhesion appears to mediate asymptomatic colonization of the nasopharynx, but the isolates obtained from meningitis patients seemed to be less adhesive (Craven *et al.*, 1980; Stephens and McGee, 1981). Similar observations have been made with *Haemophilus influenzae* (Lampe *et al.*, 1982).

C. Mechanisms of bacterial adhesion

As mentioned above, bacteria display a bewildering assortment of adhesive surface structures. At present, it appears impossible to classify all the many different mechanisms of bacterial adhesion on the basis of their molecular components, but new structural information is rapidly becoming available. The different mechanistic aspects of bacterial adhesion have recently been reviewed in detail (Beachey, 1981). The most thoroughly investigated, and probably also most important aspect in the pathogenesis of infectious diseases is bacterial adhesion mediated by fimbriae; but adhesion of non-fimbriated organisms, by way of either specific, membrane-associated recognition structures, or physicochemical interaction, has also been described.

1. Adhesion mediated by fimbriae

Table 1 lists some of the properties of the fimbriae of *E. coli* that have so far been isolated and studied in detail. These fimbriae consist of protein subunits and are thought to interact in a lectin-like manner with surface carbohydrate structures of eukaryotic cells. They can be differentiated according to the molecular weights of the subunits, their amino-acid compositions and, most importantly, the specificity of their binding to certain eukaryotic cells, their antigenicity and their receptor specificity (Korhonen *et al.*, 1981; Jann *et al.*, 1981a; Salit and Gotschlich, 1977a,b; Mett *et al.*, 1983a; Wevers *et al.*, 1980; Isaacson and Richter, 1981; Hermodson *et al.*, 1978).

Type 1 fimbriae mediating mannose-sensitive adhesion represent one class of fimbriae distinguished from other fimbriae not so much by structural or mechanistic differences as for historical reasons and possibly because of functional differences. They occur on many different Gram-negative species (Table 2) and their presence appears to be unrelated to the specific pathogenicity of the bacteria, since they seem to occur with equal, high frequency in isolates from normal faeces or from patients with urinary-tract infections (Ørskov *et al.*, 1982; Ofek *et al.*, 1981; Vosbeck, unpublished observations). Serologically, all type 1 fimbriae tested so far appear to be similar, although quantitative differences exist in their cross-reactivity with a particular antiserum, especially between fimbriae isolated from different genera (Klemm *et al.*, 1982; Korhonen *et al.*, 1981). Bacteria possessing type 1 fimbriae may interact indiscriminately with very different eukaryotic cell surface structures containing mannose residues, as shown by the fact that their adhesion *in vitro* may be inhibited by high-molecular-weight yeast mannans as well as by methyl α-D-mannoside (Firon *et al.*, 1982). Mannose-containing structures are common features of

Table 1 Characteristics of some fimbriae mediating adhesion of *Escherichia coli*

Fimbrial type	Origin of strains	Gene localization	Subunit molecular weight $\times 10^3$	Adhesion inhibited by	References
Type 1	Ubiquitous	Chromosome	17.1	D-Mannose and derivatives	Salit and Gotschlich, 1977a,b
K88	Porcine diarrhoea	Plasmid	23.5–25[a]	N-Acetylglucosamine, N-acetyl-galactosamine, β-D-galactose, glycolipids	Sellwood, 1979; Rutter et al., 1975; Kearns and Gibbons, 1979; Stirm et al., 1967; Klemm, 1981; Jones and Rutter, 1974; Gibbons et al., 1975
987P	Procine diarrhoea	Plasmid	23.0	Glycoprotein	Isaacson and Richter, 1981; Dean and Isaacson, 1982
K99	Bovine diarrhoea	Plasmid	18.5	Ganglioside GM_2 (GalNAc-Gal(NeuNAc)-Glc-ceramide)	De Graaf et al., 1981; Faris et al., 1980
F41	Bovine diarrhoea	—	29.5	—	De Graaf and Roorda, 1982
CFA/I	Human diarrhoea	Plasmid	23.8	Ganglioside GM_2 (see K99)	Faris et al., 1980; Evans et al., 1975; Evans et al., 1979
CFA/II	Human diarrhoea	Plasmid	17/21	—	Jann et al., 1981a; Evans and Evans, 1978
018ac	Human diarrhoea	—	19.5	—	Wevers et al., 1980
P	Human urinary-tract infection	Chromosome	17.8	Globotetraosyl ceramide (GalNAc-Gal-Gal-Glc-ceramide)	Korhonen et al., 1980; Leffler and Svanborg Edén, 1981; Hull et al., 1981
X[b]	Human urinary-tract infection				
—SS142		—	18.0	(Galactose-containing structure)	Mett et al., 1983a
—X		—	—	—	Väisänen et al., 1981
—F7		—	22.0	—	Klemm et al., 1982

[a] Different, serologically cross-reacting variants of K88 fimbriae have slightly different subunit molecular weights (Mooi and De Graaf, 1979).
[b] X fimbriae: collective term for fimbriae of human urinary-tract strains mediating mannose-resistant adhesion.

Table 2 Adhesion of various bacterial species other than *Escherichia coli* mediated by fimbriae

Bacterial species	Fimbrial type	Adhesion inhibited by	References
Salmonella typhimurium	Type 1	D-Mannose and derivatives	Korhonen et al., 1981; Duguid et al., 1966
Shigella flexneri	Type 1	D-Mannose and derivatives	Duguid and Gillies, 1957
Klebsiella pneumoniae	Type 1	D-Mannose and derivatives	Fader and Davis, 1980; Fader et al., 1982
Erwinia sp.	Type 1	D-Mannose and derivatives	Christofi et al., 1979
Providentia sp.	Multiple[a]	—[b]	Old and Scott, 1981
Aeromonas hydrophila	Multiple[a]	Fucose, galactose, mannose	Atkinson and Trust, 1980
Proteus sp.	—	—	Silverblatt and Ofek, 1978
Neisseria gonorrhoeae	—	Gal-GalNAc-Gal	Hermodson et al., 1978; Punsalang and Sawyer, 1973; Swanson, 1973
Pseudomonas aeruginosa	—	—	Woods et al., 1980a
Moraxella bovis	—	—	Pedersen et al., 1972
Bordetella pertussis	—	(Sterol?)	Morse and Morse, 1970
Corynebacterium sp.	—	—	Honda and Yanagawa, 1978; Sato et al., 1982
Actinomyces viscosus	—	Lactose	Cisar et al., 1980; Revis et al., 1982

[a] Different strains showed different patterns of receptor specificity.
[b] Not defined.

many glycoproteins, and thus of most eukaryotic cell surfaces, including those of phagocytes (Hughes, 1975; Sharon and Lis, 1972; Bar-Shavit *et al.*, 1977; Nicolson, 1976), which may explain the indiscriminate adhesion of type 1 fimbriated bacteria to various tissues and the lack of correlation with their pathogenicity (see below). Pruzzo *et al.* (1982) recently reported on a membrane-associated, mannose-inhibitable adhesion factor of *Klebsiella pneumoniae*, which exhibited functional characteristics different from those of type 1 fimbriae in its interaction with human polymorphonuclear neutrophils.

Fimbriae mediating mannose-resistant adhesion do not, as is frequently implied, constitute a homogeneous group opposed to those mediating mannose-sensitive adhesion. The collective epithet "mannose-resistant" is applied rather to all the different groups of fimbriae that recognize structures different from mannose. Consequently, adhesion of such bacteria can be inhibited by monosaccharides or oligosaccharides other than mannose and its derivatives. Table 1 lists the inhibition specificities of some *E. coli* adhesion factors that have been associated with pathogenicity. The animal and human intestinal adhesion factors, K88, K99, 987P and CFA/I have been shown to be inhibited by glycolipids (Table 2), but the detailed specificity of the inhibition has not been studied.

The receptor structure of uropathogenic *E. coli* expressing P fimbriae has been firmly established, however. Haemagglutination of human erythrocytes by P-fimbriated *E. coli* strains depends on the presence of the blood group P antigen (Källenius *et al.*, 1980b, 1980c, 1981). Erythrocytes lacking the P antigen become agglutinable after coating with the analogue trihexosyl or tetrahexosyl ceramide (Källenius *et al.*, 1980b; Leffler and Svanborg Edén, 1981). Furthermore, haemagglutination by P-fimbriated *E. coli* as well as their adhesion to epithelial cells is inhibited by low-molecular-weight oligosaccharide analogues of these glycolipids (Leffler and Svanborg Edén, 1981; Korhonen *et al.*, 1982). Of special interest are the observations that these inhibitory glycolipids occur in the epithelium of the human urinary tract, but not in the intestinal epithelium (Leffler and Svanborg Edén, 1980), and that a mouse strain susceptible to urinary-tract infection by P-fimbriated *E. coli* also has these glycolipids in its urinary-tract mucosa (Svanborg Edén *et al.*, 1982a). Although most of the detailed studies of fimbriae have so far been performed in *E. coli*, these structures also occur on many other bacterial species (Table 2; Beachey, 1981).

2. Adhesion of non-fimbriated bacteria

Some Gram-negative bacteria have no fimbriae but nevertheless adhere specifically to human or animal tissues (Table 3). A non-fimbriated strain

Table 3 Bacterial adhesion to host tissues mediated by bacterial surface structures other than fimbriae

Bacterial species	Proposed adhesive bacterial structure	Inhibitors of adhesion	References
Vibrio cholerae	Flagellum-associated	L-Fucose derivatives,	Jones and Freter, 1976; Srivastava and
		D-Mannose derivatives	Srivastava, 1980; Finkelstein and Hanne, 1982
Serratia marcescens	Flagellum	D-Mannose derivatives	Eshdat et al., 1981a
Escherichia coli	Flagellum	D-Mannose derivatives	Eshdat et al., 1978; 1981a
E. coli	Membrane protein	D-Mannose derivatives	Eshdat et al., 1981b; Jann et al., 1981b
Klebsiella pneumoniae	Membrane protein	D-Mannose derivatives	Pruzzo et al., 1982
Mycoplasma pneumoniae	Membrane protein	Sialic acid derivatives	Sobeslavsky et al., 1968; Banai et al., 1980
M. gallisepticum	Unknown	Sialic acid derivatives	Glasgow and Hill, 1980
Chlamydia psittaci	Unknown	Amino sugars, organic amines	Hatch et al., 1981
Erwinia amylovora	Unknown	Polycations	Romeiro et al., 1981
Shigella flexneri	Lipopolysaccharide	Fucose, glucose	Izhar et al., 1982
Agrobacterium tumefaciens	Lipopolysaccharide	N-Acetylgalactosamine, galactose	Banerjee et al., 1981
Rhizobium sp.	Exopolysaccharide, lipopolysaccharide	—	Lippincott and Lipincott, 1980
Actinomyces naeslundii	Mucopolysaccharides	Galactose, lactose	Saunders and Miller, 1980
Streptococcus sanguis	Dextran	Dextran	Scheld et al., 1978; Larsson and Glantz, 1981
Strep. mutans	Glucan	—	Hamada and Slade, 1980
Strep. pyogenes	Lipoteichoic acid	Lipoteichoic acid	Beachey and Ofek, 1976; Beachey, 1981

of *Shigella flexneri* for example has recently been shown to adhere specifically to guinea-pig colonic epithelial cells (Izhar *et al.*, 1982). Its adhesion could be blocked by fucose and glucose, as well as by a lipopolysaccharide preparation from the bacterial strain. Preincubation of the bacteria with these inhibitors did not alter their adhesiveness, but pretreatment of the eukaryotic cells prevented adhesion. This implies that the lectin-like structure is in this case located on the eukaryotic cell surface, and that it recognizes a possibly fucose-containing carbohydrate structure on the bacterial surface (Izhar *et al.*, 1982).

Similarly, the root cells of legumes contain a lectin-like surface component, which specifically interacts with a carbohydrate surface structure of the symbiotic organisms *Agrobacterium tumefaciens* or *Rhizobium* sp., and this interaction is inhibited by galactose and *N*-acetyl galactosamine (Banerjee *et al.*, 1981; Lippincott and Lippincott, 1980).

In *V. cholerae* and some *E. coli* strains adhesive structures associated with flagella have been described (Jones and Freter, 1976; Srivastava and Srivastava, 1980; Eshdat *et al.*, 1981a; Eshdat *et al.*, 1978).

Specific structures corresponding to those usually present on fimbriae may also be incorporated in the outer membrane of *E. coli*, even though no fimbriae can be detected by electron microscopy (Jann *et al.*, 1981b; Chabanon *et al.*, 1982a; Pruzzo *et al.*, 1982). Mycoplasma species possess adhesins that are always incorporated in the membrane and recognize receptor structures containing sialic acid (Sobeslavsky *et al.*, 1968; Banai *et al.*, 1980; Glasgow and Hill, 1980; Razin *et al.*, 1981).

The adhesion of *Streptococcus sanguis* to fibrin mediated by bacterial dextran is another, though probably less specific, example of adhesion in which a bacterial carbohydrate component binds to an organic surface (Scheld *et al.*, 1978).

The adhesion of Group A streptococci to epithelial cells has been closely studied by Beachey and his collaborators and has been shown to be mediated by lipoteichoic acid and M protein (Beachey, 1981; Beachey and Ofek, 1976). The available, fairly detailed evidence suggests that Group A streptococci adhere to an as yet unidentified eukaryotic cell surface receptor by means of the lipid moiety of secreted lipoteichoic acid (LTA) molecules that are linked with LTA molecules inserted into the bacterial cell wall via a network consisting of M protein and more secreted LTA molecules, some of which may be deacylated (Beachey, 1981).

Unspecific, physicochemical factors may also play a role in bacterial adhesion (Ofek and Beachey, 1981). The hydrophobicity and the charge of the bacterial surface have been implicated as important factors in the adhesion of *Strep. sanguis* and *Streptococcus pyogenes* (Larsson and Glantz, 1981; Tylevska *et al.*, 1979). The role of surface charge in bacterial adhesion has also been discussed in relation to *Chlamydia* (Hatch *et al.*, 1981) and *N. gonorrhoeae* (Watt *et al.*, 1978; Heckels *et al.*, 1976; Magnusson *et al.*, 1979a,b). It must be kept in mind, however, that changes in specific adhesion factors may lead to concomitant changes in the physicochemical properties of bacterial surfaces, and that bacterial adhesiveness may not in all cases be directly correlated with physicochemical properties (Jann *et al.*, 1981).

D. Genetics of bacterial adhesion

The genetic regulation, synthesis and assembly of fimbriae is not fully understood. The biosynthesis of fimbriae appears to be readily modulated by a variety of environmental influences, e.g. nutrition, the rate and phase of growth, the temperature at which growth occurs, the presence of various antibiotics and the physical characteristics of the growth conditions (De Graaf and Roorda, 1982; De Graaf *et al.*, 1980). The molecular basis of these phenomena is unknown.

The genetics of bacterial adhesion factors have so far been investigated mainly in *E. coli*. The genetic material coding for fimbriae may be located either on the chromosome or on a plasmid (Table 1). As a general rule, type 1 fimbriae appear to be coded for by chromosomal genes, whereas adhesion factors associated with pathogenicity, especially with intestinal pathogenicity, are frequently coded for by plasmid DNA (Evans *et al.*, 1975), but may also be chromosomal.

The genes coding for the K88 fimbriae have been cloned into a vector plasmid (Mooi *et al.*, 1979). By deletion mapping it was found that several genes arranged in two different operons (Kehoe *et al.*, 1981) are required for the biosynthesis of functional, adhesion-mediating K88 fimbriae. One of the gene products may be a component of the membrane anchorage structure of the fimbriae. Another gene seems to exert a regulatory function on K88 gene expression.

Genes coding for type 1 fimbriae have also been mobilized from the chromosome into various vector plasmids (Hull *et al.*, 1981; Swaney *et al.*, 1977). Swaney *et al.* (1977) have shown by complementation analysis of various mutants that three cistrons are involved in the expression of functional type 1 fimbriae.

The chromosomal genes for P fimbriae (Table 1) were cloned into a vector plasmid by Hull *et al.* (1981). Upon transfer of this plasmid a non-adhesive recipient strain acquired P-specific adhesive properties.

Type 1 fimbriae, gonococcal fimbriae and possibly also other adhesion factors are subject to a phenomenon known as "phase variation" (Ottow,

1975), which may be important in the physiology of the bacteria (see Section V.E). The term derives from the observation that in a culture of fimbriated bacteria one can detect subclones that possess no fimbriae. From this non-fimbriated population of bacteria, individual cells can revert again and acquire fimbriae. Phase variation occurs for type 1 fimbriae of *E. coli* with a frequency of the order of 10^{-3} in either direction and is genetically controlled on the level of transcription (Eisenstein, 1981). Phase variation has so far been demonstrated for the expression of type 1 fimbriae and of 987P fimbriae in *E. coli* (Isaacson and Richter, 1981), as well as for the fimbriae of *N. gonorrhoeae* (Kellogg *et al.*, 1963).

III. MODEL SYSTEMS FOR STUDYING BACTERIAL ADHESION

Several different assay systems have been employed to measure bacterial adhesion. They include qualitative *in vivo* observations (Evans and Evans, 1978; Freter, 1972), quantitative microscopic counts of bound bacteria (Ofek and Beachey, 1978; Cheney *et al.*, 1979; Hartley *et al.*, 1978; Svanborg Edén *et al.*, 1977) or determinations of bound viable bacteria (Scheld *et al.*, 1978), and the quantitative assessment of the rate of adhesion by radiolabelling procedures (Gubish *et al.*, 1979; Lambden *et al.*, 1979; Ramirez-Ronda, 1978; Sugarman and Donta, 1979; Thorne *et al.*, 1979; Vosbeck *et al.*, 1979).

In general, assays employing radiolabelled bacteria are preferable, since they yield more objective and accurate data, if suitable control experiments are conducted. On the other hand, valuable additional qualitative information can frequently be obtained from experiments using classical techniques, such as microscopical examination or counting of viable bacteria.

Seven groups of model systems can be distinguished:

A.   Animal models
B.   Binding to intact human or animal tissues or isolated cells
C.   Tissue-culture cell assays
D.   Binding to mucus components
E.   Agglutination of erythrocytes, yeast cells, or other particles
F.   Physicochemical properties of bacteria
G.   Serological assays

These different assay systems complement each other and the model system to be used should be carefully chosen to meet the particular requirements of the intended investigation.

A. Animal models

Observations made in the intestinal tract of the intact animals have provided an important impetus in the study of bacterial adhesion (Hohmann and Wilson, 1975; Hartley *et al.*, 1979; Cantey *et al.*, 1981). These investigations are usually performed using electron microscopical (Hartley *et al.*, 1979; Cantey *et al.*, 1981), immunofluorescent (Hohmann and Wilson, 1975; Evans and Evans, 1978), or microbiological (Myhal *et al.*, 1982) techniques, and afford important morphological and qualitative information on colonizing bacteria. They do not allow a clear distinction to be drawn between bacterial adhesion and permanent adherence as defined in Section II.A., but they furnish general information on the entire sequence of events leading to bacterial colonization, and confirm the significance of *in vitro* adhesion data for colonization (Cheney *et al.*, 1980).

B. Binding to intact human or animal tissues or isolated cells

Ward *et al.* (1974) and McGee *et al.* (1976; 1982) successfully used organ cultures from intact segments of human fallopian tubes to study the adhesion of *N. gonorrhoeae* and the morphology of the early stages in the pathogenesis of gonorrhoea.

Adhesion to human epithelia is frequently determined by incubating bacteria with a suspension of urinary sediment cells (Svanborg Edén *et al.*, 1977), or buccal or pharyngeal cells obtained from scrapings of the oral mucosa (Beachey and Ofek, 1976; Thorne *et al.*, 1979). The number of adhering bacteria is then either counted under the microscope in stained smears (Svanborg Edén *et al.*, 1977; Hartley *et al.*, 1978) or measured by using radiolabelled bacteria (Thorne *et al.*, 1979). Microscopic counting has the advantage of permitting differentiation between adhesion to different types of cells and to non-cellular material, such as mucus (Svanborg Edén *et al.*, 1977, 1980; Ørskov *et al.*, 1980a; Chick *et al.*, 1981); but it is rather laborious, relatively inaccurate, and prone to subjective errors. By using radiolabelled bacteria and a filtration technique to remove unbound bacteria, the assay can be considerably improved (Thorne *et al.*, 1979).

C. Tissue-culture cell assays

Tissue-culture methods offer an acceptable compromise between the need for technical simplicity, ease of manipulation and high reproducibility, on the one hand, and biological relevance on the other. These methods appear especially useful for mechanistic studies. It is desirable, however, as in any *in vitro* study, to verify the results in a different model, if possible an *in vivo* model system.

We use a modification of the assay described by Hartley *et al.* (1978), which measures the adhesion of radiolabelled *E. coli* to monolayers of the human epithelioid tissue culture cell line, Intestine 407 (Vosbeck *et al.*, 1979; Vosbeck and Huber, 1982). Our standard strain, *E. coli* SS142 (02:H), exhibits linear adhesion with time and bacterial concentration (Vosbeck *et al.*, 1979; Vosbeck and Huber, 1982). Upon prolonged incubation, and especially at high bacterial concentrations, saturation of bacterial binding is seen, and the adhesion of bacteria can be analysed by applying Michaelis–Menten kinetics (Fig. 2; Cohen *et al.*, 1981). It is

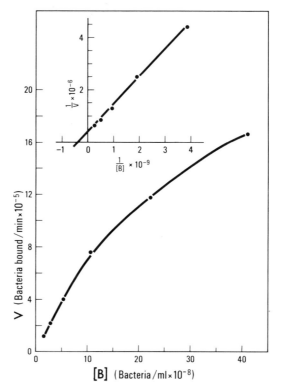

Fig. 2 Michaelis–Menten kinetic analysis of bacterial adhesion to tissue-culture monolayers. Saturation kinetics of the adhesion of *Escherichia coli* SS142 to Intestine 407 monolayers. Insert: Lineweaver–Burk transformation of the curve.
Redrawn with permission from *FEMS* (*Federation of European Microbiological Societies*) *Microbiology Letters* (Cohen *et al.*, 1981).

important to note that the adhesion of bacteria is dependent on the concentration and not on the absolute number of bacteria present in the assay. Therefore, the percentage of bacterial binding in a given assay is only of relative value, and comparisons between different assays on the basis of such percentage values are not meaningful. Comparatively low adhesion rates of between 0·5 and 3·0% per h of the total added bacteria, observed by us (Vosbeck and Huber, 1982) and by others in different assay systems (Scheld *et al.*, 1978; Selinger *et al.*, 1978), are due to the experimental conditions and do not indicate marginal adhesion rates. Conversely, adhesion rates of more than 10% of the total added bacteria can be seen in certain assays within minutes (Cheney *et al.*, 1979; Thorne *et al.*, 1979; Bartelt and Duncan, 1978). Such assays are not ideally suited for determining the rate of adhesion, but the assay conditions could be adapted to give linear kinetics by lowering the bacterial concentration or decreasing the assay time (Svanborg Edén *et al.*, 1977; Thorne *et al.*, 1979).

Adhesion to tissue-culture cells in the described assay takes place by way of binding to specific receptor molecules, and not merely by physico-chemical attachment. This is shown by the observation that *E. coli* SS142 (02:H) binds specifically to Intestine 407 and other human epithelioid tissue culture cell lines, but not to a number of human fibroblast and animal epithelioid or fibroblast cell lines (Fig. 3). Furthermore, different bacterial strains exhibit distinct patterns of adhesion to different cell lines (Jann *et al.*, 1981b). This binding specificity could not be due solely to physicochemical differences in the various cell surfaces. Jann *et al.* (1981b) and Chabanon *et al.* (1982a) also demonstrated that there is a general, but not an absolute, correlation between different assay systems. Vosbeck and Svanborg Edén (1981) arrived at the same general conclusion in a study which compared 32 strains of *E. coli* in seven different assays (Table 4): twelve were adhesive and 8 non-adhesive human urinary strains, and 11 enteropathogenic strains from animals. Their adhesion to exfoliated uroepithelial cells, human buccal epithelial cells, Intestine 407 and PK$_1$ tissue culture monolayers was determined, as well as their behaviour upon hydrophobic interaction chromatography, and their ability to agglutinate human Group A and guinea-pig erythrocytes (Table 4). We found that strains that were adhesive in any one assay system were also more likely to adhere in other assays, but no absolute correlation was detectable either between two different assay systems or between the pathogenic origin of a strain and any positive assay. On the other hand, there was a clear general distinction between the adhesive characteristics of the three groups of strains, and some assays appeared better able to differentiate adhesive from non-adhesive strains. Thus, adhesion to buccal epithelial cells was frequently positive in strains that in most other assays were non-adhesive.

Attempts at studying the characteristics of different adhesion factors by comparing different clinical isolates in a number of assay systems (Jann *et al.*, 1981b; Vosbeck and Svanborg Edén, 1981; Chabanon *et al.*, 1982a) are fraught with difficulties, because the strains employed may express more than one adhesion factor simultaneoulsy (Jann *et al.*, 1981a; Klemm *et al.*, 1982; Hull *et al.*, 1981) and adhesive interactions may be influenced by other bacterial surface components such as O and K antigens. In order to investigate the specific interactions of adhesion factors, it seems necessary to first transfer them individually to a common, genetically defined strain (Hull *et al.*, 1981).

Similar tissue-culture assay techniques have been used successfully by other authors (Clausen and Christie, 1982; Bergman *et al.*, 1981) to demonstrate a correlation between *in vitro* adhesion and bacterial pathogenicity.

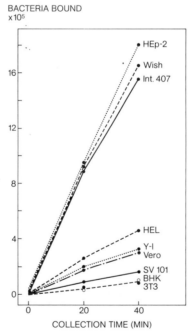

Fig. 3 Specificity of adhesion of *Escherichia coli* SS142 to monolayers of different tissue-culture cell lines. Comparisons were made of adhesion of radiolabelled *E. coli* SS142 to the human epithelioid cell lines HEp-2, Wish, and Intestine 407 (Int. 407), to human embryonic lung (HEL) fibroblasts, to the murine epithelioid cell line Y-1, and to the fibroblastic animal cell lines Vero, SV101, BHK and 3T3. *E. coli* SS142 adhered specifically to three human epithelioid tissue-culture cell lines. Reproduced with permission from *European Journal of Clinical Microbiology* (Vosbeck and Huber, 1982).

Table 4 Adhesion of different *Escherichia coli* strains in various assay systems (Vosbeck and Svanborg Edén, 1981)

Strains	UEC[a]	BEC[b]	407[c]	PK$_1$[d]	HIC[e]	HA$_{hu}$[f] mr	ms	HA$_{GP}$[g] ms
Adhesive human urinary strains[h]								
413	++	++	++	++	+	+	–	+
664	++	+	+	+	+	+	–	+
SS142	++	+	++	+	+	+	–	–
783	+	+	++	++	+	–	–	–
414	+	+	+	+	–	–	+	+
495	++	+	+	–	–	+	–	–
412	+	–	+	++	+	–	–	+
503, 761	++	+	–	–	–	+	–	+
500, 501, 502	++	–	–	–	–	+	–	+
Non-adhesive human urinary strains[i]								
496	–	+	–	–	+	–	–	–
497	–	+	–	–	–	–	–	–
498	–	+	+	–	–	+	–	–
499	–	–	++	++	–	–	–	–
666	–	+	–	–	–	–	+	+
669	–	+	–	+	–	–	–	–
765	–	–	–	–	–	–	–	+
766	–	–	–	+	–	–	–	+
Intestinal pathogenic strains of animal origin								
506 (B$_{am}$)	+	+	++	++	–	–	+	+
527 (K88)	+	+	+	++	+	–	–	–
509 (K99)	+	–	+	–	–	–	–	+
512 (Pig)	+	+	–	+	+	–	–	+
523 (Pig)	–	+	+	+	+	–	–	+
524 (Pig)	–	+	++	++	+	–	–	+
528 (K88)	–	+	+	–	–	–	–	–
530 (Pig)	–	++	–	++	+	–	–	+
507 (K99)	–	–	+	–	+	–	–	+
508 (K99)	–	–	+	–	+	–	–	+
510 (987P)	–	–	+	+	–	–	–	–

mr, Mannose-resistant haemagglutination.
ms, Mannose-sensitive haemagglutination.
[a] Adhesion to uro-epithelial cells (Svanborg Edén *et al.*, 1977).
[b] Adhesion to buccal epithelial cells (Vosbeck *et al.*, 1982).
[c] Adhesion to Intestine 407 tissue-culture monolayers (Vosbeck and Huber, 1982).
[d] Adhesion to PK$_1$ tissue-culture monolayers (Vosbeck and Huber, 1982).
[e] Hydrophobic interaction chromatography (Smyth *et al.*, 1978).
[f] Agglutination of human Group A erythrocytes (Vosbeck *et al.*, 1982).
[g] Agglutination of guinea pig erythrocytes (Vosbeck *et al.*, 1982).
[h] Strains isolated from the urine of patients with pyelonephritis and found to adhere to uro-epithelial cells.
[i] Strains isolated from the urine of patients with asymptomatic bacteriuria and found not to adhere to uro-epithelical cells.

D.   Binding to mucus components

An interesting new way of measuring adhesion of *E. coli* strains has recently been described by Cohen *et al.* (1982). The assay is based on the measurement of the binding of radiolabelled bacteria to isolated mouse colonic mucous gel and thus takes account of the fact that bacteria colonizing the intestine first come into contact with the layer of mucus covering the intestinal epithelium. *E. coli* strains carrying the K88 antigen and human enteropathogenic strains adhere in this model. Adhesion of K88 *E. coli* can be inhibited specifically by antisera directed against K88.

E.   Agglutination of erythrocytes, yeast cells, or other particles

Haemagglutination assays serve as simple and useful screening techniques for adhesive *E. coli* strains causing diarrhoea (Evans and Evans, 1978; DeBoy *et al.*, 1981; Cravioto *et al.*, 1979; Thorne *et al.*, 1979) and urinary-tract infections in man (Källenius *et al.*, 1981). In pyelonephritogenic *E. coli* strains, the agglutination of human P, but not p̄ erythrocytes permits the specific determination of the presence of bacterial P fimbriae (Väisänen *et al.*, 1981; Källenius *et al.*, 1981). The agglutination assay for the detection of P fimbriae has recently been refined by using particles to which the globoside receptor structure was bound (Svenson *et al.*, 1982). Despite the semiquantitative nature of haemagglutination assays and the lack of any absolute correlation with other assays (Jann *et al.*, 1981b; Kehoe *et al.*, 1981; Deneke *et al.*, 1981), they frequently provide data, which corroborate evidence obtained in other assay systems (Mett *et al.*, 1983a; Vosbeck, 1982; Väisänen *et al.*, 1982).

Bacteria carrying mannose-sensitive adhesins bind to the mannan structures of yeast cell walls and agglutinate yeast cells. Yeast cell agglutination permits the measurement of mannose-sensitive adhesion by type 1 fimbriae in a simple and specific way and has been used extensively for this purpose (Ofek *et al.*, 1977; Mirelman *et al.*, 1980; Jann *et al.*, 1981b; Eisenstein *et al.*, 1979, 1980). The methodology has been refined by Ofek and Beachey (1978) by using aggregometry instead of simple titration for quantitation.

F.   Physicochemical properties of bacteria

Fimbriated and non-fimbriated bacteria exhibit different physicochemical properties, and these differences can be measured by hydrophobic interaction chromatography or partitioning in aqueous two-phase systems (for review see Magnusson, 1980). It is, however, difficult to interpret data obtained by such methods and to assess their biological relevance (Magnusson *et al.*, 1979a,b). Smyth *et al.* (1978) reported that porcine enterotoxigenic *E. coli* K88+ strains were consistently more hydrophobic upon hydrophobic interaction chromatography than non-fimbriated strains. Studies performed by a different method, based on salting out of bacterial cells in increasing salt concentrations, indicated that hydrophobicity was associated with the presence of fimbriae causing mannose-resistant haemgglutination, such as CFA/I and II on *E. coli* strains (Lindahl *et al.*, 1981). Similarly, the greater virulence of *Strep. pyogenes* strains expressing M protein on their surfaces has been ascribed to their increased hydrophobicity (Tylewska *et al.*, 1979) as shown by hydrophobic interaction chromatography. Jann *et al.* (1981b), on the other hand, found a negative correlation between the presence of fimbriae causing mannose-resistant haemagglutination and the hydrophobicity of *E. coli* strains. There was, however, a correlation between hydrophobicity and the presence of type 1 fimbriae (Jann *et al.*, 1981b; Öhman *et al.*, 1982).

G. Serological assays

Strictly speaking, serological assays measure not the adhesion of bacteria to surfaces, but the presence of a certain adhesion factor. They are mentioned here only because they are of immense importance in investigating the epidemiology of adhesion factors, a good knowledge of which seems essential to provide a rational basis for the application of certain types of anti-adhesive drugs and vaccinations. Several such studies have been conducted with intestinal pathogenic *E. coli* (Deneke *et al.*, 1981; DeBoy *et al.*, 1981; Evans and Evans, 1978; Bergman *et al.*, 1981; Cravioto *et al.*, 1979, 1982). Serological information on the adhesion factors of uropathogenic *E. coli* has only recently become available (Clegg, 1982; Jann *et al.*, 1981a). It is important to note in this context that the serological identification of bacterial adhesion factors and bacterial haemagglutination patterns do not correlate absolutely (Deneke *et al.*, 1981). Brinton *et al.* (1982) have studied the antigenic relation between fimbriae of *Neisseria* spp. and found that they can classify the fimbriae of *N. gonorrhoeae* and *N. meningitidis* into serological groups based on their antigenic cross-reactivity. Some antigenic determinants occur in all investigated fimbriae, others only in some of them ("seniority" groups).

IV.   INTERFERENCE WITH BACTERIAL ADHESION

A.   Natural inhibitors of bacterial adhesion

Little is known about natural defence mechanisms directed against adhesive properties of bacteria in man. However, there is good evidence that specific antibodies to the adhesion factors of *E. coli* prevent colonization of the small intestine of piglets by enterotoxigenic *E. coli* K88 strains (Rutter *et al.*, 1976; Morgan *et al.*, 1978; Sellwood, 1982). Similarly, Svanborg Edén *et al.* (1979) demonstrated antibodies directed against fimbriae of human enterotoxigenic strains in human milk. It appears likely that protection against colonization by other pathogens can also be acquired by active or passive immunization against adhesion factors (see Section IV.B).

Holmgren *et al.* (1981) described a non-immunoglobulin fraction isolated from human milk, which inhibited the haemagglutination caused by *E. coli* strains carrying different mannose-resistant adhesion factors, whereas the mannose-sensitive adhesion caused by type 1 fimbriae was not affected.

In addition to immunoglobulins directed against adhesive bacterial structures, human urine may also contain less specific anti-adhesive compounds, such as Tamm–Horsfall protein, which was shown to bind type 1 fimbriated bacteria (Ørskov *et al.*, 1980b) and to inhibit mannose-resistant bacterial adhesion to tissue-culture monolayers (Jann, K., unpublished observation; Mett *et al.*, 1983a).

Relatively unspecific mucin layers, able to prevent bacterial adhesion appear to be present on many mucous surfaces. Such an anti-adhesive principle was detected by Parsons *et al.* (1975) in the rabbit bladder. The surface mucin prevented *E. coli, Klebsiella pneumoniae* and *S. aureus* from adhering to the bladder epithelium (Parsons and Mullholland, 1978). The nature of the different adhesion factors involved was, however, not studied. The protective substance could be removed by acid, and it could be replaced by heparin (Parsons *et al.*, 1979).

The upper respiratory tract and oropharyngeal epithelium of humans have been reported to contain a protease sensitive component, that prevented the adhesion of *P. aeruginosa* (Woods *et al.*, 1981a,b).

B.   Immunization against adhesion factors

As mentioned above, suckling piglets, calves and lambs can be protected from *E. coli* diarrhoea by treating the dams with vaccines prepared from

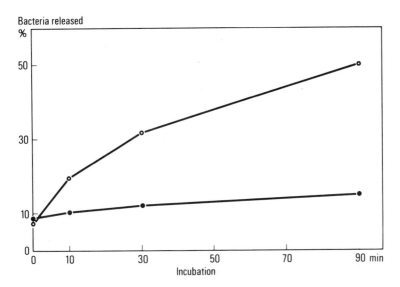

Fig. 4 Release of *Escherichia coli* SS142 bound to intestine 407 tissue-culture monolayers by F(ab) antibody fragments against *E. coli* SS142 fimbriae. Radiolabelled *E. coli* SS142 were allowed to adhere to intestine 407 tissue-culture monolayers for 30 min. Thereafter unbound bacteria were removed, and either buffer alone (●——●) or buffer containing specific F(ab) fragments directed against *E. coli* SS142 fimbriae (○——○) was added. The monolayers were further incubated and after the indicated times the supernatants were analysed for the release of rdiolabelled bacteria from the cell monolayers (Mett *et al.*, 1983b).

the respective adhesive fimbriae. The vaccination raises the anti-adhesive antibody titre in the colostrum, thereby protecting the suckling offspring (Nagy, 1980; Moon, 1981). Such "indirect" vaccinations are administered as a matter of routine in animal husbandry and lead to a significant decrease in the incidence of neonatal diarrhoea caused by enterotoxigenic *E. coli. In vitro*, antibodies directed against the fimbriae of *E. coli* SS142 (02:H) not only prevented adhesion to tissue-culture cells, but were also able to release previously bound bacteria (Fig. 4; Mett *et al.*, 1983b).

Attempts to activate immunization of adult animals or of humans against *E. coli* adhesion factors are faced with a number of difficulties, such as the need to elicit local, secretory immunity at mucosal surfaces and to maintain this secretory immunity for prolonged periods, as well as the high specificity of the immune response on the one hand, and the immunological heterogeneity of adhesion factors on the other, as a result of which protection could only be afforded against a limited bacterial spectrum, unless a mixture of all possible fimbriae were used for vaccinating (see Section V.B).

The most significant advances towards the use of anti-adhesive vaccination in human medicine have been made with *Neisseria*: vaccines against *N. gonorrhoea* and *N. meningitidis* are being tested in man (Brinton *et al.*, 1982). Gonococcal fimbrial vaccines have been developed and shown to be safe for human use by Brinton *et al.* (1982) and Siegel *et al.* (1982). Both vaccines are antigenic, and the elicited antibodies inhibit the adhesion of gonococci to epithelial cells (Tramont *et al.*, 1981) and enhance the phagocytosis of gonococci *in vitro* (Siegel *et al.*, 1982). Gonococcal fimbrial vaccine has also been shown to be protective in human volunteers (Brinton *et al.*, 1982). Tramont *et al.* (1981) demonstrated that their vaccine elicited antibodies inhibiting epithelial cell adhesion not only of the homologous gonococcal strain, but also of several heterologous strains. This possibly implies that different gonococcal fimbriae contain immunologically cross-reactive antigenic determinants, and that the fimbriae employed as vaccine can elicit a response against such common determinants. After parenteral vaccination a good antibody response was observed in genital secretions of volunteers (McChesney *et al.*, 1982).

C.   Competitive inhibitors of bacterial adhesion

Since many adhesive interactions appear to be mediated by protein–carbohydrate binding (Beachey, 1981), it seems reasonable to employ low-molecular-weight analogues of the carbohydrate receptor structures (Tables 1–3) as competitive inhibitors of bacterial adhesion. The adhesion and pathogenicity of an *E. coli* strain carrying mannose-sensitive type 1 fimbriae could be reduced in a mouse model when methyl-α-D-mannopyranoside was used as an inhibitor, although relatively high concentrations were needed (Aronson *et al.*, 1979). Similarly, the adhesion of *E. coli* with P fimbriae to human uroepithelial cells and to erythrocytes can be blocked *in vitro* by receptor analogues (Svanborg Edén *et al.*, 1981), such as globotetraosyl ceramide (Leffler and Svanborg Edén, 1980, 1981) or the α-D-Galp-(1–4)-β-D-Galp-1-*O*-methyl glycoside (Källenius *et al.*, 1980c, 1981; Väisänen, 1981), However, these and other inhibitors have so far not been tested *in vivo*.

Apart from the difficulties inherent in synthetic carbohydrate chemistry, major obstacles to any potential therapeutic or prophylactic use of such monovalent, low-molecular-weight carbohydrate receptor analogues are the need to achieve local concentrations high enough to compete successfully with the co-operative binding of multivalent adhesive bacteria and, possibly, the marked specificity of adhesive structures, which may limit the anti-adhesive spectrum of inhibitors.

D.   Absorption by receptor analogues

Other possibilities for the therapeutic use of receptor analogues have been suggested. On the basis of the reported increased hydrophobicity of enteropathogenic *E. coli*, Wadström *et al.* (1981) suggested the use of orally administered agarose beads substituted with hydrophobic ligands as a means of absorbing the enteropathogen from the intestinal lumen. The treatment was effective in infant rabbits. Svanborg Edén *et al.* (1982b) suggest that potential urinary pathogens might be removed selectively from the intestinal tract, which is thought to be a source of bacteria infecting the urinary tract by adsorption on orally given particles substituted with globoside receptor analogues that bind P-fimbriated strains.

E.   Effects of antibacterial agents on bacterial adhesion

Whether anti-adhesive properties of antibiotics may be clinically useful is an open question. An anti-adhesive antibiotic might conceivably be of advantage in prophylactic treatment and in limiting the spread of a bacterial infection, especially in locations where it is difficult to ensure that sufficiently high bacteriostatic or bactericidal concentrations of antibiotic are sustained for a sufficiently long time.

   A number of antibacterial agents have been shown to affect bacterial adhesion in several different assay systems. Adhesion of *E. coli* strains was usually reduced after growth in subinhibitory concentrations of protein synthesis inhibitors (Beachey *et al.*, 1981). Vosbeck *et al.* (1979, 1982) demonstrated that tetracycline, trimethoprim–sulphametrole, streptomycin, chloramphenicol and clindamycin tended to reduce the adhesion of 10 different *E. coli* strains to Intestine 407 tissue culture cells without concomitantly affecting bacterial viability, when the bacteria were grown overnight in the presence of 1/4 of the minimum inhibitory concentration (MIC) of the antibiotics. The anti-adhesive effect was dependent on the concentration of the antibiotic (Vosbeck *et al.*, 1979) and it was strain-specific in the sense that some strains were affected only by certain antibiotics and not by others (Vosbeck *et al.*, 1982). There was no correlation detectable between the susceptibility of a strain to the anti-adhesive effect of any two antibiotics. A similar trend towards reduced adhesiveness was observed when the same strains were tested for alterations in their haemagglutinating activity after growth in the presence of subinhibitory antibiotic concentrations (Vosbeck *et al.*, 1982). Nalidixic acid caused a consistent increase in both adhesion to Intestine 407 tissue culture cells and haemagglutination. Tetracycline, trimethoprim–sulphametrole, and clindamycin exerted a fairly consistent anti-adhesive effect on *E. coli* SS142 (02:H), when assayed for binding to Intestine 407 tissue-culture cells, human buccal cells, human uroepithelial cells and haemagglutinating activity (Vosbeck, 1982). Streptomycin and chloramphenicol had little effect on this strain in any of these assays, whereas nalidixic acid increased its adhesiveness in all assays. Chabanon *et al.* (1982b) confirmed the anti-adhesive effect of tetracycline on different *E. coli* strains. Similar effects were observed by Eisenstein *et al.* (1980) on the mannose-sensitive adhesiveness of an *E. coli* strain as measured by yeast cell agglutination and buccal cell adhesion. Yeast cell agglutination was reduced in a dose-dependent manner by streptomycin, neomycin, gentamicin, spectinomycin and tetracycline; but chloramphenicol had little effect when the bacteria were grown for 24–48 hours in the presence of subinhibitory concentrations (1/2–1/16 of the MIC) of the antibiotics.

With β-lactam antibiotics some discrepanices between the results of different laboratories exist. These may be due to the different assay systems and conditions employed, and also due to strain differences. Beachey *et al.* (1981) found a decrease in the mannose-sensitive adhesiveness of an *E. coli* strain after growth in sublethal concentrations of penicillin G. A negative effect of ampicillin on the adhesion of many uropathogenic *E. coli* strains to uroepithelial cells was also reported by Sandberg *et al.* (1979) and Svanborg Edén *et al.* (1978). In this study, nitrofurantoin and chloramphenicol did not influence bacterial adhesiveness, when the bacteria were treated at 1/4 of the MIC for 4 hours. Vosbeck *et al.* (1979) did not observe a change of the adhesion of *E. coli* SS142 to tissue culture cells, when the bacteria were grown overnight in the presence of a number of β-lactam antibiotics. With some other β-lactam antibiotics, particularly those that led to the formation of bacterial filaments under the conditions employed, inconsistent results were obtained. An apparent increase of the adhesion to tissue culture cells was in some strains associated with a diminished capability of the bacteria to agglutinate human erythrocytes (Vosbeck *et al.*, unpublished observations). Klein and Opferkuch (personal communication) have similarly observed a divergence in the effect of β-lactam antibiotics on different *E. coli* strains, the type 1 fimbriated ones being more haemagglutinating, and the ones exhibiting mannose-resistant haemagglutination being less haemagglutinating after treatment with subinhibitory concentrations of β-lactam antibiotics. Chabanon *et al.* (1982b) likewise described a divergent effect of subinhibitory concentrations of tetracycline on mannose-sensitive and mannose-resistant haemagglutination and adhesion to uroepithelial cells. The significance of these findings is unclear at present. We believe that these effects cannot yet be interpreted correctly because of their complexity.

Väisänen *et al.* (1982) have recently studied the effect of subinhibitory concentrations of trimethoprim and several sulphonamides on the haemagglutination and epithelial cell adhesion of *E. coli* strains with P fimbriae. Growth of the bacteria for 18 hours on agar plates containing 1/2 to 1/8 of the MIC of the respective antibiotic resulted in a dose-dependent reduction in bacterial adhesiveness.

As expected, the decrease in bacterial adhesiveness after growth in low concentrations of antibiotics could be traced in most cases to a reduction of bacterial fimbriation (Vosbeck *et al.*, 1980; Vosbeck *et al.*, 1982; Väisänen *et al.*, 1982; Beachey *et al.*, 1981; Svanborg Edén *et al.*, 1978). On the other hand, Eisenstein *et al.* (1979) presented evidence that streptomycin at low concentrations might lead to the synthesis of non-functional type 1 fimbriae by translational misreading.

The observation of Eisenstein *et al.* (1979) that a streptomycin-resistant mutant of an *E. coli* strain was no longer affected by streptomycin in its adhesiveness suggests that the anti-adhesive effect was mediated by the classic mechanism of the drug's action at the ribosome. It thus appears that at low concentrations producing no significant effect on bacterial growth, inhibitors of protein synthesis differentially inhibit the synthesis of adhesion factors. β-Lactam antibiotics, by contrast, are known to disturb bacterial cell-wall metabolism at levels below their growth inhibitory concentrations (Lorian, 1980; Atkinson and Amaral, 1982). Their anti-adhesive effect on bacteria is most likely due to ill-defined changes in the architecture of the bacterial cell wall (Beachey, 1981; Sandberg *et al.*, 1979).

Sugarman and Donta (1979) reported that various antibiotics not only inhibited enterobacterial adhesion, but also augmented the release of adherent bacteria.

Penicillin G at low concentrations reduced the adhesiveness of *Strep. pyogenes* to buccal epithelial cells, even in resting bacteria. This was attributed to a penicillin-induced loss of lipoteichoic acid (Alkan and Beachey, 1978; Horne and Tomasz, 1977, 1979) which plays an important role in the adhesion of *Strep. pyogenes* (see Section II.C.; Ofek *et al.*, 1975; Beachey and Ofek, 1976).

Tylewska *et al.* (1981) studied the influence of several antibiotics on the adhesiveness of *Strep. pyogenes* to human pharyngeal cells and on their hydrophobicity as measured by hydrophobic interaction chromatography. Penicillin G, tetracycline and rifampicin decreased bacterial adhesiveness significantly after overnight antibiotic treatment, whereas cephalothin and polymyxin were ineffective. A concomitant reduction in hydrophobicity was detectable after treatment with rifampicin and with penicillin G (Tylewska *et al.*, 1980). The reduction of bacterial adhesiveness to epithelial cells and of hydrophobicity after treatment with rifampicin was, however, much more pronounced.

In an *in vitro* model system simulating the adhesion step in the pathogenesis of endocarditis, Scheld *et al.* (1981) demonstrated that the adhesion of *Strep. sanguis* and *Strep. faecalis* to a fibrin-platelet matrix was significantly reduced after treatment of the bacteria for 4 hours with vancomycin, penicillin G, tetracycline, chloramphenicol or streptomycin at 1/4 of the MIC. Rifampicin decreased adhesion of *Strep. faecalis*, but not of *Strep. sanguis*, and trimethoprim–sulphametrole did not affect bacterial adhesiveness. None of the antibiotic treatments caused any change in bacterial hydrophobicity. The decrease in the adhesiveness of *Strep. sanguis* after pretreatment with 1/4 of the MIC of vancomycin was paralleled by a decrease in the infectivity of the bacteria in a rabbit endocarditis model (Scheld *et al.*, 1978). Similarly, Bernard *et al.* (1981) demonstrated that vancomycin given prophylactically to experimental animals at concentrations below the growth-inhibitory level afforded significant protection against the development of *Strep. sanguis* endocarditis.

Only few clinical studies have been made of the effects of treatment with low doses of antibiotics exhibiting anti-adhesive properties *in vitro*. Ben Redjeb *et al.* (1982) reported successful results of therapy with as little as 10 mg ampicillin daily in women suffering from recurrent urinary-tract infections; and a low-dose regimen of trimethoprim–sulphamethoxazole was found to be effective in severe urinary-tract infections (O'Grady *et al.*, 1969; Pearson *et al.*, 1979) and as prophylaxis against recurrences in urinary-tract infection (Stamey *et al.*, 1977).

The actual local concentrations of antibiotics in these studies and their antibacterial effectiveness at the site of the infection are not known. Therefore neither the results obtained in the animal model of bacterial endocarditis, nor the clinical findings mentioned above can be unequivocally associated with the anti-adhesive properties of the antibiotics used, but it seems possible that these properties may have contributed towards the favourable effects observed in these investigations.

V. FEASIBILITY OF ANTI-ADHESIVE TREATMENT OF INFECTIOUS DISEASES

The pathogenicity of certain bacteria has been ascribed to their ability to adhere specifically to mucosal surfaces (Section II.B). On this premise, the application of anti-adhesive measures would appear *prima facie* to be a logical and practicable approach to the treatment of bacterial infections. However, upon closer inspection a number of complicating aspects emerge: the high tissue specificity of adhesion and the multiplicity of different adhesion factors must be taken into account; and any anti-adhesive treatment should not interfere with normal colonization, beneficial epithelial adhesion, or adhesion to phagocytes.

A. Tissue specificity of adhesion

The highly tissue-specific adhesion of pathogenic bacteria implies that different receptors are exposed on different mucosal surfaces and that competitive receptor analogues will therefore, by definition, have an anti-adhesive spectrum limited to the respective tissues. On the other hand, this restriction represents an important advantage, since it would theoretically permit a very specific treatment directed at a single organ, e.g. the urinary or intestinal tract. At present, the number of relevant receptors in different organ systems cannot be accurately assessed. In the urinary tract, at least two adhesion specificities for *E. coli* have been described (Väisänen *et al.*, 1981), which appear to be responsible for most, but not all adhesive interactions. P-specificity accounted for approximately 90% of the studied uropathogenic strains. X-specificity (Väisänen *et al.*, 1981) has not been characterized in detail and may include several other specificities (Ørskov *et al.*, 1980a; Klemm *et al.*, 1982; Jann *et al.*, 1981a; Mett *et al.*, 1983a). It is not known how many different urinary tract surface receptors are involved in these adhesive interactions. In the intestinal tract, no receptors have been definitely identified so far. Similarly, the molecular nature of receptor structures for other bacterial species, especially for Gram-positive bacteria, or in other tissues has not yet been elucidated.

  The restrictions imposed by tissue specific receptors do not, however, affect treatments that act directly on bacterial adhesion factors. Immunization against common fimbrial antigenic determinants may give protection against colonization by different bacterial species and even different genera, regardless of differences in the receptor structures to which they bind (see Section V.B). Similarly, common structural features suggest common biosynthetic and regulatory pathway of various fimbrial types. Drugs acting on these pathways might have a broad anti-adhesive spectrum.

B. Multiplicity of bacterial adhesion factors

Gram-negative bacteria possess a relatively large number of serologically different adhesion factors and are therefore epidemiologically very flexible. Certain adhesion factors appear to predominate in particular infections, but many others with similar tissue specificity exist, which would seem to make any treatment directed against a specific adhesion factor quite useless. Thus, in enterotoxigenic *E. coli* CFA/I and CFA/II occur frequently (Evans and Evans, 1978; Cravioto *et al.*, 1982), but serologically different adhesion factors continue to be detected (Thomas *et al.*, 1982; Wevers *et al.*, 1980; Thorne *et al.*, 1979; Bergman *et al.*, 1981). In the urinary tract the situation is similar. Serological homogeneity of the frequently occurring P-fimbriated *E. coli* strains has so far not been demonstrated, but a number of adhesion factors serologically different from P fimbriae have been described (Klemm *et al.*, 1982; Jann *et al.*, 1981a; Clegg, 1982). To be of any benefit, immunological measures must therefore be directed not against individual adhesion factors, but against common antigenic sites on different adhesion factors. Such common sites may in fact occur in *N. gonorrhoeae* (Tramont *et al.*, 1981; Brinton *et al.*, 1982). Analysis of the amino acid sequences of different Gram-negative fimbriae revealed distinct homologies, whereupon it was tentatively concluded that all may originate from one, or a few, common, ancestral fimbrial genes (Hermodson *et al.*, 1978; Fader *et al.*, 1982; De Graaf *et al.*, 1981, 1982). It therefore appears possible to detect common antigenic sites on these fimbriae, which could be employed to develop an active or passive immunization.

One great obstacle to immunological protection is the need for the production of mucosal, secretory immunoglobulin. The inability of achieving sustained levels of local, secretory antibodies despite the existence of a good immunological memory in the secretory mucosal immune system may be largely responsible for the failure of vaccinations against cholera and similar diseases to produce lasting protection (Pierce and Koster, 1980, 1982).

C. Interference with normal colonization

The adhesive processes involved in normal colonization and the maintenance of colonization resistance (van der Waaij, 1982) are largely unknown. Pathological colonization by Gram-negatives usually occurs on more or less sterile surfaces, such as those of the small intestine or the urinary tract, and pathogenic strains differ clearly from commensal strains in certain adhesion factors. Bacterial adhesion may therefore be of different specificity in pathological and normal colonization. Moreover, if the hypothesis advanced in Section II.A. is correct, the adhesive interactions of the commensal flora may even be largely restricted to factors involved in maintaining the *state of adherence* rather than to the process of *adhesion* (see Section II.A). The majority of the commensal Gram-negatives can express type 1 fimbriae. The role of these fimbriae in the normal colonization of the intestinal tract is, however, not known. On the basis of the available evidence it is not yet possible to assess the risk of a treatment interfering with adhesion of pathogens also disturbing the normal flora.

D.   Beneficial adhesion to epithelia

Adhesion of pathogenic bacteria to epithelia may not always be a harmful event. Craven *et al.* (1980) and Stephens and McGee (1981) found *N. meningitidis* isolated from asymptomatic carriers to be more adhesive than isolates from patients with meningitis. Similarly, reduced adhesiveness may be a characteristic property of pathogenic *H. influenzae* (Lampe *et al.*, 1982). Type 1 fimbriae mediate attachment of bacteria to urinary mucus, and this may prevent them from causing ascending, upper-urinary-tract infection (Ørskov *et al.*, 1980b; Ofek *et al.*, 1981). Recently, Leunk and Moon (1982) reported that type 1- fimbriated *Salmonella typhimurium* was cleared more rapidly by the liver than non-fimbriated strains. These few observations suggest that in some cases certain epithelial surfaces perform a filtering function and that adhesion of the bacteria to the epithelium prevents them from invading the host organism. Since nothing is known about the mechanism of adhesion in these cases, the implications of these observations in regard to anti-adhesive therapy cannot be assessed at present.

E.   Adhesion to phagocytes

Adhesion of bacteria to phagocytes is essential to the successful function of the phagocytic defence system. Bacteria adhere to polymorphonuclear neutrophils (PMNs) or macrophages after opsonization by complement or specific antibodies by means of specific surface receptors of the phagocyte. Gram-negative bacteria carrying type 1 fimbriae adhere directly to mannose-containing receptor structures on PMNs or macrophages without needing further opsonization (Bar-Shavit *et al.*, 1977; Mangan and Snyder, 1979; Silverblatt *et al.*, 1979; Blumenstock and Jann, 1982). This interaction with phagocytes is, in anthropocentric terms, clearly a beneficial one. Silverblatt and Ofek (1978) have investigated the role of type 1 fimbriae in rat pyelonephritis using type 1-fimbriated and non-fimbriated *Proteus mirabilis*. The fimbriated bacteria, which adhered to rat urinary epithelial cells, as well as to phagocytes, caused an ascending colonization of the urinary tract and pyelonephritis. After intravenous application they were, however, cleared rapidly from the circulation. The non-fimbriated bacteria, by contrast, were unable to colonize the urinary tract, but caused a haematogenous pyelonephritis. It thus appears that type 1 fimbriae on the one hand enabled the bacteria to colonize the urinary tract, but, on the other hand, prevented their survival after invasion of the renal parenchyma, presumably because they mediated their phagocytosis. Thus, type 1 fimbriae appear to be useful to the bacterium during the initial phase of the infectious process, but harmful during later stages. One might speculate therefore that bacteria profit to a certain extent from the phenomenon of phase variation, the regulatory ability to switch from the fimbriated to a non-fimbriated phenotype (Ottow, 1975; Eisenstein, 1981).

Fimbriae mediating mannose-resistant adhesion, by contrast, have been shown to protect *N. gonorrhoeae* (Ofek *et al.*, 1974) from phagocytosis by human PMN. Mannose-resistant fimbriae of *E. coli* also do not mediate adhesion to rat peritoneal macrophages or human peripheral PMNs (Blumenstock and Jann, 1982; Vosbeck, unpublished observation). It is, however, uncertain whether these observations can be generalized.

Bacteria carrying both mannose-sensitive and mannose-resistant fimbriae occur commonly (Jann *et al.*, 1981a; Klemm *et al.*, 1982; Hull *et al.*, 1981) and may adapt to their environment by expressing the most beneficial combination of adhesion factors.

VI. SUMMARY AND CONCLUSIONS

The essential role of bacterial adhesion in the pathogenesis of a number of diseases of animals and man has been well established. The *process of bacterial adhesion*, characterized by the rate and affinity of attachment to a surface, and the *state of adherence*, characterized by complex, irreversible binding interactions, must be clearly distinguished. The process of bacterial adhesion may be especially important in the initial phase of pathogenesis. The association described by the term state of adherence, by contrast, is viewed as the dominant adhesive interaction in normal colonization and, perhaps, chronic, persistent infections.

Different complementary adhesion models yield data that can shed light on different aspects of adhesive interactions. Information on the molecular mechanism, the biochemical and serological specificity, the genetic and metabolic regulation, and the functional role of bacterial adhesion is accumulating rapidly. The complex picture emerging is characterized by a number of fundamentally different types of adhesion in different groups of bacteria. So far, the functionally and structurally most thoroughly investigated mechanism of adhesion is that of Gram-negative bacteria mediated by fimbriae.

Drugs that interfere with bacterial adhesion may be competitive receptor analogues, inhibitors of the synthesis or metabolism of bacterial adhesion factors, specific absorbents, or antibodies. The multiplicity of adhesive interactions constitutes, on the one hand, an obstacle to anti-adhesive pharmacological intervention; on the other hand it may afford an opportunity for selective interference. The existence of common antigenic structures, and perhaps also common metabolic regulatory features of different adhesion factors, may provide a basis for the development of techniques of immunization or inhibition of the synthesis of different, but related adhesion factors. Such an approach appears especially well founded in *N. gonorrhoeae* and possibly also uropathogenic *E. coli*. One or a few types of receptor analogues may be sufficient to cope with the majority of uropathogenic *E. coli* strains. Some antibiotics appear to act as inhibitors of the synthesis of a fairly wide spectrum of bacterial adhesion factors.

Bacterial adhesion and adherent bacteria may not always be undesirable events, and any anti-adhesive treatment must not interfere with either the normal colonization of mucosal surfaces, or the desirable adhesion of bacteria to phagocytes or to certain mucosal surfaces that apparently act as traps for some pathogens. At present, type 1 fimbriae of Gram-negative bacteria appear to be associated with beneficial adhesion of this nature, whereas the various types of fimbriae that cannot be inhibited by mannosides are associated with pathogenic adhesion. Before any systematic evaluation of the feasibility of anti-adhesive therapy against Gram-negative, and even more so against other bacteria, can be attempted, more experimental data will have to be accumulated.

ACKNOWLEDGEMENTS

We wish to thank our colleagues for helpful discussions and for making information on not yet published work available to us. We thank Prof.

V. Lorian and Prof. K. Jann for critical reading of the manuscript, Mr A. Kirkwood and Dr P. James for linguistic support, and Mrs V. Forster for expert secretarial help.

REFERENCES

Alkan, M. L. and Beachey, E. H. (1978). *J. Clin. Invest.* **61,** 671–677.
Aronson, M., Medalia, O., Schori, L., Mirelman, D., Sharon, N. and Ofek, I. (1979). *J. Infect. Dis.* **139,** 329–332.
Atkinson, H. M. and Trust, T. J. (1980). *Infect. Immun.* **27,** 938–946.
Atkinson, B. A. and Amaral, L. (1982). *CRC Crit. Rev. Microbiol.* **9,** 101–138.
Banai, M., Kahane, I., Bredt, W. and Razin, S. (1980). *Israel J. Med. Sci.* **16,** 69.
Banerjee, D., Basu, M., Choudhury, I. and Chatterjee, G. C. (1981). *Biochem. Biophys. Res. Commun.* **100,** 1384–1388.
Bar-Shavit, Z., Ofek, I. and Goldman, R. (1977). *Biochem. Biophys. Res. Commun.* **78,** 455–460.
Bartelt, M. A. and Duncan, J. L. (1978). *Infect. Immun.* **20,** 200–208.
Beachey, E. H. (1981). *J. Infect. Dis.* **143,** 325–345.
Beachey, E. H. and Ofek, I. (1976). *J. Exp. Med.* **143,** 759–771.
Beachey, E. H., Eisenstein, B. I. and Ofek, I. (1981). *In* "Adhesion and Microorganism Pathogenicity" (K. Elliott *et al.*, eds), Ciba Foundation Symposium, Vol. 80, pp. 288–304. Pitman Medical, London.
Ben Redjeb, S., Slim, A., Horchani, A., Zmerilli, S., Boujnah, A. and Lorian, V. (1982). *Antimicrob. Ag. Chemother.* **22,** 1084–1086.
Bergman, M. J., Updike, W. S., Wood, S. J., Brown, S. E. and Guerrant, R. L. (1981). *Infect. Immun.* **32,** 881–888.
Bernard, J.-P., Francioli, P. and Glauser, M. P. (1981). *J. Clin. Invest.* **68,** 1113–1116.
Blumenstock, E. and Jann, K. (1982). *Infect. Immun.* **35,** 264–269.
Bose, S. K. and Mudd, R. L. (1981). *Infect. Immun.* **34,** 154–159.
Brinton, C. C., Bryan, J., Dillon, J.-A., Guerina, N., Jacobson, L. J., Labik, A., Lee, S., Levine, A., Lim, S., McMichael, J., Polen, S., Rogers, K., To, A. C.-C. and To, S. C.-M. (1978). *In* "Immunobiology of *Neisseria gonorrhoeae*" (G. F. Brooks *et al.*, eds) pp. 155–178. American Society for Microbiology, Washington, D.C.
Brinton, C. C., Wood, S. W., Brown, A., Labik, A. M., Bryan, J. R., Lee, S. W. Polen, S. W., Tramont, E. C., Sadoff, J. and Zollinger, W. (1982). *Seminars in Infect. Dis.* **4,** 140–159.
Burns, K. A. and Freer, J. H. (1982). *FEMS Microbiol. Lett.* **13,** 271–274.
Cantey, J. R., Lushbaugh, W. B. and Inman, L. R. (1981). *J. Infect. Dis.* **143,** 219–230.
Chabanon, G., Hartley, C. L. and Richmond, M. H. (1982a). *Annales de Microbiologie (Institut Pasteur)* **133A,** 357–369.
Chabanon, G., Archambaud, M., Marty, N. and Enjalbert, L. (1982b). *Pathologie Biologie* **30,** 543–548.
Cheney, C. P., Boedeker, E. C. and Formal, S. B. (1979). *Infect. Immun.* **26,** 736–743.

Cheney, C. P., Schad, P. A., Formal, S. B. and Boedeker, E. C. (1980). *Infect. Immun.* **28,** 1019–1027.
Chick, S., Harber, M. J., Mackenzie, R. and Asscher, A. W. (1981). *Infect. Immun.* **34,** 256–261.
Christofi, N., Wilson, M. I. and Old, D. C. (1979). *J. Appl. Bacteriol.* **46,** 179–183.
Cisar, J. O., Barsumian, E. L., Curl, S. H., Vatter, A. E., Sandberg, A. L. and Siraganian, R. P. (1980). *J. Reticulo-Endothelial Soc.* **28,** Suppl., 73s–79s.
Clausen, C. R. and Christie, D. L. (1982). *J. Pediatr.* **100,** 358–361.
Clegg, S. (1982). *Infect. Immun.* **35,** 745–748.
Cohen, P. S., Elbein, A. D., Solf, R., Mett, H., Regös, J., Menge, E. B. and Vosbeck, K. (1981). *FEMS Microbiol. Lett.* **12,** 99–103.
Cohen, P. S., Rossoll, R., Cabelli, V. J., Yang, S.-L. and Laux, D. C. (1983). *Infect. Immun.,* **40,** 62–69.
Costerton, J. W., Irvin, R. T. and Cheng, K.-J. (1981). *Ann. Rev. Microbiol.* **35,** 299–324.
Craven, D. E., Peppler, M. S., Frasch, C. E., Mocca, L. F., McGrath, P. P. and Washington, G. (1980). *J. Infect. Dis.* **142,** 556–568.
Cravioto, A., Gross, R. J., Scotland, S. M. and Rowe, B. (1979). *FEMS Microbiol. Lett.* **6,** 41–44.
Cravioto, A., Scotland, S. M. and Rowe, B. (1982). *Infect. Immun.* **36,** 189–197.
Dean, E. A. and Isaacson, R. E. (1982). *Infect. Immun.* **36,** 1192–1198.
DeBoy, J. M., Thorne, G. M., Deneke, C. F. and Wachsmuth, I. K. (1981). *Curr. Microbiol.* **6,** 49–53.
De Graaf, F. K. and Roorda, I. (1982). *Infect. Immun.* **36,** 751–758.
De Graaf, F. K., Klaasen-Boor, P. and van Hees, J. E. (1980). *Infect. Immun.* **30,** 125–128.
De Graaf, F. K., Klemm, K. and Gaastra, W. (1981). *Infect. Immun.* **33,** 877–883.
Deneke, C. F., Thorne, G. M. and Gorbach, S. L. (1979). *Infect. Immun.* **26,** 362–368.
Deneke, C. F., Thorne, G. M. and Gorbach, S. L. (1981). *Infect. Immun.* **32,** 1254–1260.
Duguid, J. P. and Gillies, R. R. (1957). *J. Pathol. Bacteriol.* **74,** 397–411.
Duguid, J. P. and Old, D. C. (1980). *In* "Bacterial Adherence" (Beachey, E. H., ed.), pp. 185–217. Chapman and Hall, London and New York.
Duguid, J. P., Anderson, E. S. and Campbell, I. (1966). *J. Pathol. Bacteriol.* **92,** 107–138.
Eisenstein, B. I. (1981). *Science* **214,** 337–339.
Eisenstein, B. I., Ofek, I. and Beachey, E. H. (1979). *J. Clin. Invest.* **63,** 1219–1228.
Eisenstein, B. I., Beachey, E. H. and Ofek, I. (1980). *Infect. Immun.* **28,** 154–159.
Eisenstein, B. I., Ofek, I. and Beachey, E. H. (1981). *Infect. Immun.* **31,** 792–797.
Ellen, R. P. and Gibbons, R. J. (1972). *Infect. Immun.* **5,** 826–830.
Eshdat, Y., Ofek, I., Yashouv-Gan, Y., Sharon, N. and Mirelman, D. (1978). *Biochem. Biophys. Res. Commun.* **85,** 1551–1559.
Eshdat, Y., Izhar, M., Sharon, N. and Mirelman, D. (1981a). *Israel J. Med. Sci.* **17,** 468.
Eshdat, Y., Speth, V. and Jann, K. (1981b). *Infect. Immun.* **34,** 980–986.
Evans, D. G. and Evans, D. J. (1978). *Infect. Immun.* **21,** 638–647.
Evans, D. G., Silver, R. P., Evans, D. J., Chase, D. G. and Gorbach, S. L. (1975). *Infect. Immun.* **12,** 656–667.

Evans, D. G., Evans, D. J., Tjoa, W. S. and DuPont, H. L. (1978). *Infect. Immun* **19,** 727–736.

Evans, D. G., Evans, D. J., Clegg, S. and Pauley, J. A. (1979). *Infect. Immun.* **25,** 738–748.

Fader, R. C. and Davis, C. P. (1980). *Infect. Immun.* **30,** 554–561.

Fader, R. C., Avots-Avotins, A. E. and Davis, C. P. (1979). *Infect. Immun.* **25,** 729–737.

Fader, R. C., Duffy, L. K., Davis, C. P. and Kurosky, A. (1982). *J. Biol. Chem.* **257,** 3301–3305.

Faris, A., Lindahl, M. and Wadström, T. (1980). *FEMS Microbiol. Lett.* **7,** 265–269.

Finkelstein, R. A. and Hanne, L. F. (1982). *Infect. Immun.* **36,** 1199–1208.

Firon, N., Ofek, I. and Sharon, N. (1982). *Biochem. Biophys. Res. Commun.* **105,** 1426–1432.

Fowler, H. W. and McKay, A. J. (1981). *In* "Microbial Adhesion to Surfaces" (R C. W. Berkeley *et al.*, eds) pp. 143–162. John Wiley & Sons, Somerset, N.J. USA.

Freter, R. (1972). *Infect. Immun.* **6,** 134–141.

Gibbons, R. J. (1977). *In* "Microbiology 1977" (D. Schlessinger, ed.) pp. 395–406 American Society for Microbiology, Washington, D.C.

Gibbons, R. J. and van Houte, J. (1975). *Ann. Rev. Microbiol.* **29,** 19–44.

Gibbons, R. A., Jones, G. W. and Sellwood, R. (1975). *J. Gen. Microbiol.* **86,** 228–240.

Glasgow, L. R. and Hill, R. L. (1980). *Infect. Immun.* **30,** 353–361.

Glorioso, J. C., Jones, G. W., Rush, H. G., Pentler, L. J., Darif, C. A. and Coward, J. E. (1982). *Infect. Immun.* **35,** 1103–1109.

Gould, K., Ramirez-Ronda, C. H., Holmes, R. K. and Sanford, J. P. (1975). *J. Clin. Invest.* **56,** 1364–1370.

Gubish, Jr., E. R., Mace, Jr., M. L., Steiner, S. M. and Williams, R. P. (1979). *Infect. Immun.* **25,** 1043–1050.

Gwynn, M. N., Webb, L. T. and Rolinson, G. N. (1981). *J. Infect. Dis.* **144,** 263–269.

Hagberg, L., Jodal, U., Korhonen, T., Lidin-Janson, G., Lindberg, U. and Svanborg Edén, C. (1981). *Infect. Immun.* **31,** 564–570.

Hamada, S. and Slade, H. D. (1980). *In* "Bacterial Adherence" (E. H. Beachey, ed.) pp. 107–135. Chapman and Hall, London.

Hartley, C. L., Robbins, C. M. and Richmond, M. H. (1978). *J. Bacteriol.* **45,** 91–97.

Hartley, C. L., Neumann, C. S. and Richmond, M. H. (1979). *Infect. Immun.* **23,** 128–132.

Hatch, T. P., Vance, D. W. and Al-Hossainy, E. (1981). *J. Gen. Microbiol.* **125,** 273–283.

Heckels, J. E., Blackett, B., Everson, J. S. and Ward, M. E. (1976). *J. Gen. Microbiol.* **96,** 359–364.

Hermodson, M. A., Chen, K. C. S. and Buchanan, T. M. (1978). *Biochemistry* **17,** 442–445.

Hohmann, A. and Wilson, M. R. (1975). *Infect. Immun.* **12,** 866–880.

Holmgren, J., Svennerholm, A.-M. and Åhrén, C. (1981). *Infect. Immun.* **33,** 136–141.

Honda, E. and Yanagawa, R. (1978). *Amer. J. Vet. Res.* **39,** 155–158.

Horne, D. and Tomasz, A. (1977). *Antimicrob. Ag. Chemother.* **11**, 888–896.
Horne, D. and Tomasz, A. (1979). *J. Bacteriol.* **137**, 1180–1184.
Hughes, R. C. (1975). *Essays Biochem.* **11**, 1–36.
Hull, R. A., Gill, R. E., Hsu, P., Minshew, B. H. and Falkow, S. (1981). *Infect. Immun.* **33**, 933–938.
Iijima, Y., Yamada, H. and Shinoda, S. (1981). *Can. J. Microbiol.* **27**, 1252–1259.
Isaacson, R. E. and Richter, P. (1981). *J. Bacteriol.* **146**, 784–789.
Izhar, M., Nuchamowitz, Y. and Mirelman, D. (1982). *Infect. Immun.* **35**, 1110–1118.
Jann, K., Jann, B. and Schmidt, G. (1981a). *FEMS Microbiol. Lett.* **11**, 21–25.
Jann, K., Schmidt, G., Blumenstock, E. and Vosbeck, K. (1981b). *Infect. Immun.* **32**, 484–489.
Jones, G. W. (1977). *In* "Microbial Interactions" (J. L. Reissig, ed.) pp. 139–176. Chapman and Hall, London and New York.
Jones, G. W. and Rutter, J. M. (1972). *Infect. Immun.* **6**, 918–927.
Jones, G. W. and Rutter, J. M. (1974). *Amer. J. Clin. Nutr.* **27**, 1441–1449.
Jones, G. W. and Freter, R. (1976). *Infect. Immun.* **14**, 240–245.
Jones, G. W., Abrams, G. D. and Freter, R. (1976). *Infect. Immun.* **14**, 232–239.
Källenius, G. and Winberg, J. (1978). *Lancet* **2**, 540–543.
Källenius, G. and Möllby, R. (1979). *FEMS Microbiol. Lett.* **5**, 295–299.
Källenius, G., Möllby, R. and Winberg, J. (1980a). *Infect. Immun.* **28**, 972–980.
Källenius, G., Möllby, R., Svenson, S. B., Winberg, J., Lundblad, A., Svensson, S. and Cedergren, B. (1980b). *FEMS Microbiol. Lett.* **7**, 297–302.
Källenius, G., Möllby, R., Svenson, S. B., Winberg, J. and Hultberg, H. (1980c). *Infection*, Suppl. **3**, 288–293.
Källenius, G., Möllby, R., Svenson, S. B., Helin, I., Hultberg, H., Cedergren, B. and Winberg, J. (1981). *Lancet* **2**, 1369–1372.
Kearns, M. J. and Gibbons, R. A. (1979). *FEMS Microbiol. Lett.* **6**, 165–168.
Kehoe, M., Sellwood, R., Shipley, P. and Dougan, G. (1981). *Nature* **291**, 122–126.
Kellogg, Jr., D. S., Peacock, W. L., Deacon, W. E., Brown, L. and Prikle, C. I. (1963). *J. Bacteriol.* **85**, 1274–1279.
Keusch, G. T. (1979). *Rev. Infect. Dis.* **1**, 517–529.
Klemm, P. (1981). *Eur. J. Biochem.* **117**, 617–627.
Klemm, P., Ørskov, I. and Ørskov, F. (1982). *Infect. Immun.* **36**, 462–468.
Korhonen, T. K., Nurmiaho, E.-L., Ranta, H. and Svanborg Edén, C. (1980). *Infect. Immun.* **27**, 569–575.
Korhonen, T. K., Leffler, H. and Svanborg Edén, C. (1981). *Infect. Immun.* **32**, 796–804.
Korhonen, T. K., Väisänen, V., Saxén, H., Hultberg, H. and Svenson, S. B. (1982). *Infect. Immun.* **37**, 286–291.
Lam, J., Chan, R., Lam, K. and Costerton, J. W. (1980). *Infect. Immun.* **28**, 546–556.
Lambden, P. R., Heckels, J. E., James, L. T. and Watt, P. J. (1979). *J. Gen. Microbiol.* **114**, 305–312.
Lampe, R. M., Mason, Jr., E. O., Kaplan, S. L., Umstead, C. L., Yow, M. D. and Feigin, R. D. (1982). *Infect. Immun.* **35**, 166–172.
Larsson, K. and Glantz, P.-O. (1981). *Acta Odontol. Scand.* **39**, 79–82.
Leffler, H. and Svanborg Edén, C. (1980). *FEMS Microbiol. Lett.* **8**, 127–134.
Leffler, H. and Svanborg Edén, C. (1981). *Infect. Immun.* **34**, 920–929.

Leunk, R. D. and Moon, R. J. (1982). *Infect. Immun.* **36**, 1168–1174.
Levett, P. N. and Daniel, R. R. (1981). *J. Gen. Microbiol.* **125**, 167–172.
Lindahl, M., Faris, A., Wadström, T. and Hjertén, S. (1981). *Biochim. Biophys. Acta* **677**, 471–476.
Lippincott, J. A. and Lippincott, B. B. (1980). *In* "Bacterial Adherence" (E. H. Beachey, ed.) pp. 375–398. Chapman and Hall, London and New York.
Lomberg, H., Jodal, U., Svanborg Edén, C., Leffler, H. and Samuelson, B. (1981). *Lancet* **1**, 551–552.
Lorian, V. (1980). *In* "Antibiotics in Laboratory Medicine" (V. Lorian, ed.) pp. 342–408. Williams and Wilkins, Baltimore and London.
Magnusson, K.-E. (1980). *Scand. J. Infect. Dis.*, Supplement **24**, 131–134.
Magnusson, K.-E., Kihlström, E., Norlander, L., Norqvist, A., Davies, J. and Normark, S. (1979a). *Infect. Immun.* **26**, 397–401.
Magnusson, K.-E., Kihlström, E., Norqvist, A., Davies, J. and Normark, S. (1979b). *Infect. Immun.* **26**, 402–407.
Mangan, D. F. and Snyder, I. S. (1979). *Infect. Immun.* **26**, 520–527.
Matsuyama, T. (1977). *J. Infect. Dis.* **136**, 609–616.
Marrie, T. J., Lam, J. and Costerton, J. W. (1980). *J. Infect. Dis.* **142**, 239–246.
McChesney, D., Tramont, E. C., Boslego, J. W., Ciak, J., Sadoff, J. and Brinton, C. (1982). *Infect. Immun.* **36**, 1006–1012.
McGee, Z. A., Johnson, A. P. and Taylor-Robinson, D. (1976). *Infect. Immun.* **13**, 608–618.
McGee, Z. A., Melly, M. A. and Gregg, C. R. (1982). *Semin. Infect. Dis.* **4**, 133–139.
Mett, H., Kloetzlen, L. and Vosbeck, K. (1983a). *J. Bacteriol.* **153**, 1038–1044
Mett, H., Kloetzlen, L. and Vosbeck, K. (1983b). *Infect. Immun.* **40**, 862–868.
Mirelman, D., Altmann, G. and Eshdat, Y. (1980). *J. Clin. Microbiol.* **11**, 328–331.
Mooi, F. R. and de Graaf, F. K. (1979). *FEMS Microbiol. Lett.* **5**, 17–20.
Mooi, F. R., de Graaf, F. K. and van Embden, J. D. A. (1979). *Nucleic Acids Res.* **6**, 849–865.
Mooi, F. R., Harms, N., Bakker, D. and de Graaf, F. K. (1981). *Infect. Immun.* **32**, 1155–1163.
Moon, H. W. (1981). *Amer. J. Vet. Res.* **42**, 173–177.
Morgan, R. L., Isaacson, R. E., Moon, H. W., Brinton, C. C. and To, C.-C. (1978). *Infect. Immun.* **22**, 771–777.
Morse, J. H. and Morse, S. I. (1970). *J. Exp. Med.* **131**, 1342–1357.
Myhal, M. L., Laux, D. C. and Cohen, P. S. (1982). *Eur. J. Clin. Microbiol.*, **1**, 186–192.
Nagy, B. (1980). *Infect. Immun.* **27**, 21–24.
Nicolson, G. (1976). *In* "Concanavalin A as Tool" (H. Bittiger and H. P. Schnebli, eds) pp. 3–15. John Wiley & Sons, London, New York, Sydney, Toronto.
Ofek, I. and Beachey, E. H. (1978). *Infect. Immun.* **22**, 247–254.
Ofek, I. and Beachey, E. H. (1980a). *In* "Bacterial Adherence" (E. H. Beachey, ed.) pp. 1–30. Chapman and Hall, London and New York.
Ofek, I. and Beachey, E. H. (1980b). *Adv. Intern. Med.* **25**, 503–532.
Ofek, I., Beachey, E. H. and Bisno, A. L. (1974). *J. Infect. Dis.* **129**, 310–316.
Ofek, I., Beachey, E. H., Jefferson, W. and Campbell, G. L. (1975). *J. Exp. Med.* **141**, 990–1003.
Ofek, I., Mirelman, D. and Sharon, N. (1977). *Nature* **265**, 623–625.

Ofek, I., Mosek, A. and Sharon, N. (1981). *Infect. Immun.* **34**, 708–711.
O'Grady, F., Chamberlain, D. A. and Stark, J. E. (1969). *Postgrad. Med. J.* **45**, Suppl., 61–64.
Öhman, L., Magnusson, K.-E. and Stendahl, O. (1982). *FEMS Lett.* **14**, 149–153.
Okamoto, K., Inoue, T., Ichikawa, H., Kawamoto, Y., Hara, S. and Miyama, A. (1980). *Microbiol. Immunol.* **24**, 1013–1022.
Okuda, K., Slots, J. and Genco, R. J. (1981). *Curr. Microbiol.* **6**, 7–12.
Old, D. C. and Scott, S. S. (1981). *J. Bacteriol.* **146**, 404–408.
Ørskov, I., Ørskov, F. and Birch-Andersen, A. (1980a). *Infect. Immun.* **27**, 657–666.
Ørskov, I., Ferenc, A. and Ørskov, F. (1980b). *Lancet* **i**, 887.
Ørskov, I., Ørskov, F., Birch-Andersen, A., Klemm, P. and Svanborg Edén, C. (1982). *Semin. Infect. Dis.* **4**, 97–103.
Ottow, J. C. G. (1975). *Ann. Rev. Microbiol.* **29**, 79–108.
Parsons, C. L. and Mulholland, S. G. (1978). *Amer. J. Pathol.* **93**, 423–432.
Parsons, C. L., Greenspan, C. and Mulholland, S. G. (1975). *Invest. Urology* **13**, 72–76.
Parsons, C. L., Mulholland, S. G. and Anwar, H. (1979). *Infect. Immun.* **24**, 552–557.
Pearce, W. A. and Buchanan, T. M. (1978). *J. Clin. Invest.* **61**, 931–934.
Pearson, N. J., Towner, K. J., McSherry, A. M., Cattell, W. R. and O'Grady, F. (1979). *Lancet* **ii**, 1205–1209.
Pedersen, K. B., Frøholm, L. O. and Bøvre, K. (1972). *Acta Patholog. Microbiolog. Scand. Section B* **80**, 911–918.
Peterson, P. K. and Quie, P. G. (1981). *Ann. Rev. Med.* **32**, 29–43.
Pierce, N. F. and Koster, F. T. (1980). *In* "Cholera and Related Diarrheas" (O. Ouchterlony and J. Holmgren, eds) pp. 185–194. S. Karger, Basel.
Pierce, N. F. and Koster, F. T. (1982). *Semin. Infect. Dis.* **4**, 19–23.
Pruzzo, C., Debbia, E. and Satta, G. (1982). *Infect. Immun.* **36**, 949–957.
Punsalang, Jr., A. P. and Sawyer, W. D. (1973). *Infect. Immun.* **8**, 255–263.
Ramirez-Ronda, C. H. (1978). *J. Clin. Invest.* **62**, 805–814.
Razin, S., Kahane, I., Banai, M. and Bredt, W. (1981). *In* "Adhesion and Microorganism Pathogenicity" (K. Elliott *et al.*, eds) Ciba Foundation Symposium, Vol. 80, pp. 98–118. Pitman Medical, London.
Reed, W. P., Selinger, D. S., Albright, E. L., Abdin, Z. H. and Williams, Jr., R. C. (1980). *J. Infect. Dis.* **142**, 803–810.
Revis, G. J., Vatter, A. E., Crowle, A. J. and Cisar, J. O. (1982). *Infect. Immun.* **36**, 1217–1222.
Romeiro, R., Karr, A. and Goodman, R. (1981). *Plant Physiol.* **68**, 772–777.
Rutter, J. M., Burrows, M. R., Sellwood, R. and Gibbons, R. A. (1975). *Nature* **257**, 135–136.
Rutter, J. M., Jones, G. W., Brown, G. T. H., Burrows, M. R. and Luther, P. D. (1976). *Infect. Immun.* **13**, 667–676.
Salit, I. E. and Gotschlich, E. C. (1977a). *J. Exp. Med.* **146**, 1169–1181.
Salit, I. E. and Gotschlich, E. C. (1977b). *J. Exp. Med.* **146**, 1182–1194.
Sanford, B. A., Shelokov, A. and Ramsay, M. A. (1978). *J. Infect. Dis.* **137**, 176–181.
Sandberg, T., Stenqvist, K. and Svanborg Edén, C. (1979). *Rev. Infect. Dis.* **1**, 838–844.
Sato, H., Yanagawa, R. and Fukuyama, H. (1982). *Infect. Immun.* **36**, 1242–1245.

Satterwhite, T. K., DuPont, H. L., Evans, D. G. and Evans, Jr., D. J. (1978). Lancet 2, 181–184.

Saunders, J. M. and Miller, C. H. (1980). Infect. Immun. 29, 981–989.

Savage, D. C. (1980). In "Bacterial Adherence" (E. H. Beachey, ed.) pp. 31–59, Chapman and Hall, London and New York.

Schaeffer, A. J., Jones, J. M. and Dunn, J. K. (1981). N. Engl. J. Med. 304, 1062–1066.

Scheld, W. M., Valone, J. M. and Sande, M. A. (1978). J. Clin. Invest. 61, 1394–1404.

Scheld, W. M., Zak, O., Vosbeck, K. and Sande, M. A. (1981). J. Clin. Invest. 68, 1381–1384.

Selinger, D. S., Julie, N., Reed, W. P. and Williams, Jr., R. C. (1978). Science 201, 455–457.

Selinger, D. S., Reed, W. P. and McLaren, L. C. (1981). Infect Immun. 32, 941–944.

Sellwood, R. (1979). Vet. Record. 105, 228–230.

Sellwood, R. (1982). Infect. Immun. 35, 396–401.

Sellwood, R., Gibbons, R. A., Jones, G. W. and Rutter, J. M. (1975). J. Med. Microbiol. 8, 405–411.

Sharon, N. and Lis, H. (1972). Science 177, 949–959.

Siegel, M., Olsen, D., Critchlow, C. and Buchanan, T. M. (1982). J. Infect. Dis. 145, 300–310.

Silverblatt, F. J. and Ofek, I. (1978). J. Infect. Dis. 138, 664–667.

Silverblatt, F. J., Dreyer, J. S. and Schauer, S. (1979). Infect. Immun. 24, 218–223.

Smith, H. W. and Linggood, M. A. (1971). J. Med. Microbiol. 4, 467–485.

Smith, H. W. and Huggins, M. B. (1978). J. Med. Microbiol. 11, 471–492.

Smyth, C. J., Jonsson, P., Olsson, E., Söderlind, O., Rosengren, J., Hjertén, S. and Wadström, T. (1978). Infect. Immun. 22, 462–472.

Sobeslavsky, O., Prescott, B. and Chanock, R. M. (1968). J. Bacteriol. 96, 695–705.

Srivastava, R. and Srivastava, B. S. (1980). J. Gen. Microbiol. 117, 275–278.

Srivastava, R., Sinha, V. B. and Srivastava, B. S. (1980). J. Med. Microbiol. 13, 1–9.

Stamey, T. A., Condy, M. and Mihara, G. (1977). N. Engl. J. Med. 296, 780–782.

Stephens, D. S. and McGee, Z. (1981). J. Infect. Dis. 143, 525–532.

Stirm, S., Ørskov, F.. Ørskov, I. and Mansa, B. (1967). J. Bacteriol. 93, 731–739.

Sugarman, B. and Donta, S. T. (1979). J. Infect. Dis. 140, 622–625.

Svanborg Edén, C. and Jodal, U. (1979). Infect. Immun. 26, 837–840.

Svanborg Edén, C. and Leffler, H. (1980). Scand. J. Infect. Dis. Suppl. 24, 144–147.

Svanborg Edén, C., Hanson, L. Å., Jodal, U., Lindberg, U. and Sohl Åkerlund, A. (1976). Lancet ii, 490–492.

Svanborg Edén, C., Eriksson, B. and Hanson, L. Å. (1977). Infect. Immun. 18, 767–774.

Svanborg Edén, C., Sandberg, T., Stenqvist, K. and Ahlstedt, S. (1978). Infection 6, Suppl. 1, S121–S124.

Svanborg Edén, C., Carlsson, B., Hanson, L. Å., Jann, B., Jann, K., Korhonen, T. and Wadström, T. (1979). Lancet ii, 1235.

Svanborg Edén, C., Larsson, P. and Lomberg, H. (1980). Infect. Immun. 27, 804–807.

Svanborg Edén, C., Hagberg, L., Hanson, L. Å., Korhonen, T., Leffler, H. and Olling, S. (1981). *In* "Adhesion and Microorganism Pathogenicity" (K. Elliott *et al.*, eds) pp. 161–187. Pitman Medical, London.

Svanborg Edén, C., Hagberg, L., Hanson, L. Å., Lomberg, H., Ørskov, I. and Ørskov, F. (1982a). *Lancet* **1**, 961–962.

Svanborg Edén, C., Fasth, A., Hagberg, L., Hanson, L. Å., Korhonen, T. and Leffler, H. (1982b). *Semin. Infect. Dis.* **4**, 113–131.

Svenson, S. B., Källenius, G., Möllby, R., Hultberg, H. and Winberg, J. (1982). *Infection* **11**, 209–214

Swaney, L. M., Liu, Y.-P. Ippen-Ihler, K. and Brinton, C. C., Jr. (1977). *J. Bacteriol.* **130**, 506–511.

Swanson, J. (1973). *J. Exp. Med.* **137**, 571–589.

Thomas, L. V., Cravioto, A., Scotland, S. M. and Rowe, B. (1982). *Infect. Immun.* **35**, 1119–1124.

Thorne, G. M., Deneke, C. F. and Gorbach, S. D. (1979). *Infect. Immun.* **23**, 690–699.

Tramont, E. C. (1981). *In* "Adhesion and Microorganism Pathogenicity" (K. Elliott *et al.*, eds) pp. 188–201. Pitman Medical, London.

Tramont, E. C., Sadoff, S. C., Boslego, J. W., Ciak, S., McChesney, D., Brinton, C. C. and Takafuji, E. (1981). *J. Clin. Invest.* **68**, 881–888.

Tylewska, S., Hjertén, S. and Wadström, T. (1979). *FEMS Microbiol. Lett.* **6**, 249–253.

Tylewska, S., Wadström, T. and Hjertén, S. (1980). *J. Antimicrob. Chemother.* **6**, 292–294.

Tylewska, S., Hjertén, S. and Wadström, T. (1981). *Antimicrob. Ag. Chemother.* **20**, 563–566.

Väisänen, V., Elo, J., Tallgren, L. G. Siitonen, A., Mäkelä, P. H., Svanborg Edén, C., Källenius, G., Svenson, S. B., Hultberg, H. and Korhonen, T. (1981). *Lancet* **2**, 1366–1369.

Väisänen, V., Lounatmaa, K. and Korhonen, T. (1982). *Antimicrob. Ag. Chemother.* **22**, 120–127.

van der Waaij, D. (1982). *In* "Action of Antibiotics in Patients" (L. D. Sabath, ed.) pp. 104–118. Hans Huber Publishers, Bern, Switzerland.

Varona, R. M., Perez, P., Cohen, P. S., Mett, H. and Vosbeck, K. (1982). Abstracts of the 82nd Annual Meeting of the American Society for Microbiology, p. 24.

Vosbeck, K. (1982). *In* "The Influence of Antibiotics on the Host–Parasite Relationship" (H. U. Eickenberg, W. Opferkuch and H. Hahn, eds) pp. 183–193. Springer Verlag, Berlin, Heidelberg, New York.

Vosbeck, K. and Svanborg Edén, C. (1981). Abstracts of the Annual Meeting of the American Society for Microbiology 1981, Dallas, Texas, USA, p. 31.

Vosbeck, K. and Huber, U. (1982). *Eur. J. Clin. Microbiol.* **1**, 22–28.

Vosbeck, K., Handschin, H., Menge, E. B. and Zak, O. (1979). *Rev. Infect. Dis.* **1**, 845–851.

Vosbeck, K., Bohn, J. and Huber, U. (1980). *Experientia* **36**, 494.

Vosbeck, K., Mett, H., Huber, U., Bohn, H. and Petignat, M. (1982). *Antimicrob. Ag. Chemother.* **21**, 864–869.

Wadström, T., Faris, A., Lindahl, M., Hjertén, S. and Ågerup, B. (1981). *Scand. J. Infect. Dis.* **13**, 129–132.

Ward, M. E., Watt, P. J. and Robertson, J. N. (1974). *J. Infect. Dis.* **129**, 650–659.

Watt, P. J., Ward, M. E., Heckels, J. E. and Trust, T. J. (1978). *In* "Immuno-biology of *Neisseria gonorrhoeae*" (G. F. Brooks *et al.*, eds) pp. 253–257. American Society for Microbiology, Washington, D.C.

Wevers, P., Picken, R., Schmidt, G., Jann, B., Jann, K., Golecki, J. R. and Kist, M. (1980). *Infect. Immun.* **29**, 685–691.

Woods, D. E., Straus, D. C., Johanson, W. G., Berry, V. K. and Bass, J. A. (1980a). *Infect. Immun* **29**, 1146–1151.

Woods, D. E., Bass, J. A., Johanson, W. G. and Straus, D. C. (1980b). *Infect. Immun.* **30**, 694–699.

Woods, D. E., Straus, D. C., Johanson, W. G. and Bass, J. A. (1981a). *J. Infect. Dis.* **143**, 784–790.

Woods, D. E., Straus, D. C., Johanson, W. G. and Bass, J. A. (1981b). *J. Clin. Invest.* **68**, 1435–1440.

Zimmerli, W., Waldvogel, F. A., Vaudaux, P. and Nydegger, U. E. (1982). *J. Infect. Dis.* **146**, 487–497.

3   The role of the bacterial glycocalyx in resistance to antimicrobial agents

J. W. COSTERTON and T. J. MARRIE

I.   INTRODUCTION

In our very extensive examinations of bacterial growth in natural and industrial aquatic systems we have noted that these organisms grow predominantly in microcolonies that form coherent biofilms adherent to available submerged surfaces. This mode of growth, coupled with the anion ion-exchange capacity of the glycocalyx that envelops cells within these biofilms, has the effect of protecting these organisms from biological antagonists (such as amoebae and bacteriophage) and from chemical antibacterial agents (including commercial antiseptics and biocides). When bacteria forsake their more natural habitats in order to invade the human body they often adopt the same protected adherent mode of growth in glycocalyx-enclosed biofilms to withstand the cellular (phagocytic) and humoral (immunological) defences of the host and to withstand the challenge of specific antibiotics.

This biofilm mode of bacterial growth in pathogenesis is readily demonstrable in osteomyelitis, endocarditis, pneumonia, neonatal diarrhoea, cystitis, and infections that emanate from plastic and metal prostheses that have become colonized by adherent bacteria. As might be expected, growth in a coherent protected biofilm limits the vulnerability of the pathogens to host defence mechanisms but it also limits the release of toxins and of free bacteria that might invade surrounding tissues, so that these protected "cryptic" infections tend to be non-acute, non-disseminating and persistent. The most persistent of these cryptic infections have been shown to continue for as long as 20 years, in spite of a

MEDICAL MICROBIOLOGY, 3
ISBN 0 12 228003 3

vigorous cellular and immune response by the host and in spite of aggressive antibiotic therapy, and the persistence of these bacterial pathogens is directly attributable to their adherent mode of growth in biofilms and their production by extensive anionic glycocalyces. The understanding and eventual control of these increasingly common chronic cryptic bacterial infections hinges on our developing perception of the mechanisms of glycocalyx production by pathogenic bacteria and of their consequent growth in protected microcolonies and in adherent coherent biofilms.

II.   ADHERENT BACTERIAL POPULATIONS IN NATURAL AND INDUSTRIAL SYSTEMS

The tendency of aquatic bacteria to colonize submerged surfaces was noted early in this century, by Hendrici (1933) and Zobell (1943), and preferential growth at these surfaces was attributed to their natural tendency to concentrate organic nutrients. With the advent of specific stains that made exopolysaccharides visible by electron microscopy (Luft, 1971) "acid polysaccharides" were shown to surround cells adherent to surfaces in freshwater (Jones *et al.*, 1969), marine (Fletcher and Floodgate, 1973), and soil systems (Bae *et al.*, 1972), and these "glycocalyces" (Costerton *et al.*, 1981a,b) were subsequently shown to mediate the adhesion of aquatic organisms to surfaces (Geesey *et al.*, 1971) and to form the structural "matrix" of coherent bacterial biofilms that develop on submerged substrates (Wyndham and Costerton, 1981a,b).

This adherent biofilm is seen, then, to be composed of a fibrous anionic exopolysaccharide matrix (Fig. 1) within which bacterial cells live, divide and exert a physiological impact on the passing water (Costerton and Colwell, 1979). Bacterial biofilms in aquatic systems assumed more importance when it was shown that their adherent cells comprise a clear majority of the bacterial populations of these systems (Geesey *et al.*, 1978), and that the cells within these adherent layers have complete and free access to organic substrates in the flowing water (Ladd *et al.*, 1979). The definite numerical and physiological predominance of adherent bacteria was equally clearly seen in industrial aquatic systems (Costerton and Geesey, 1979) and the protective effect of the glycocalyx surrounding cells within thick biofilms was unequivocally demonstrated when Ruseska *et al.* (1982) showed that adherent biofilm bacteria are very significantly more resistant to chemical biocides than are their otherwise equivalent planktonic (floating) counterparts. We have developed a device that allows us to

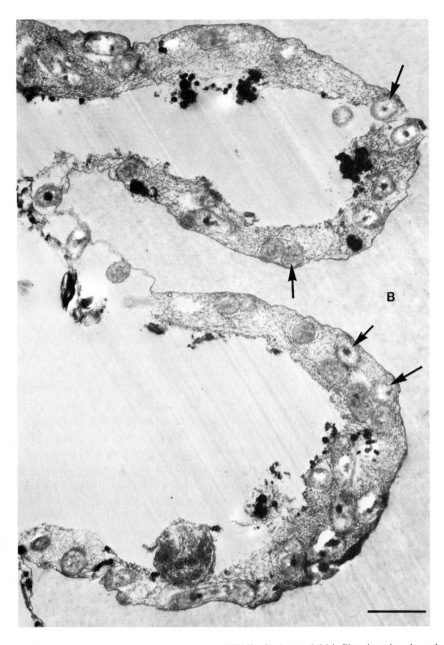

Fig. 1 Transmission electron micrograph (TEM) of a bacterial biofilm that developed when bitumen (B) was exposed in a flowing stream. Note that the biofilm adherent to the bitumen surface is composed of bacteria (arrows) and of a fibrous matrix of anionic exopolysaccharide which is stained with ruthenium red. The bar in this, and all subsequent TEM, indicates $1.0\,\mu m$ and all TEM preparations were stained with ruthenium red.

develop adherent sessile bacterial biofilm populations (Fig. 2) on aseptically-removable metal surfaces (McCoy *et al.*, 1981; McCoy and Costerton, 1982) and this device is now widely used in industry to establish the actual biocide concentration necessary to control the predominant sessile bacterial populations that cause plugging and corrosion in industrial systems.

In summary, when we have eschewed *in vitro* batch cultures and have examined the sessile biofilm populations of bacteria, in natural and industrial aquatic systems, we have been able to generate meaningful and predictive data on real processes such as the actual turnover of nutrients in streams and the actual biocide sensitivity of corrosion-causing microorganisms.

III. AUTOCHTHONOUS BACTERIAL POPULATIONS ADHERENT TO TISSUES

Direct examinations of washed tissues from animal organs that are populated by autochthonous bacteria reveal the development of an adherent biofilm by these native commensal microorganisms (Cheng and Costerton, 1981). Individual bacteria are surrounded by very extensive exopolysaccharide glycocalyces that mediate the formation of microcolonies of morphologically similar cells and ultimately of a coherent biofilm within which the bacterial glycocalyces form a continuous matrix (Fig. 3). Non-secretory squamous epithelia (e.g. human skin, bovine rumen) are often covered by a simple bacterial biofilm (McCowan *et al.*, 1980), within which certain bacterial species have been shown to produce enzymes of vital importance to the host animal (Cheng and Costerton, 1980), and the autochthonous bacterial population has been shown to integrate into the mucous "blanket" covering the surface of secretory gastrointestinal tissues (Rozee *et al.*, 1982). The autochthonous bacterial populations of certain human tissues (e.g. the human female urethra) have been shown to grow in adherent microcolonies (Marrie *et al.*, 1980) within which the bacterial glycocalyx connects cells to each other and to the tissue to form a *de facto* biofilm (Fig. 4). This biofilm of autochthonous bacteria precludes the adhesion of potential pathogens and the adherent native populations of the urethra can be "credited" with the protection of the urinary tract from invasion by fecal pathogens (Marrie *et al.*, 1979). This principle of the "competitive exclusion" of pathogens by the natural or accelerated development of an adherent and protective autochthonous bacterial population has now been used to protect newborn human (Sprunt *et al.*, 1980) and bovine (Cheng and Costerton, unpublished data) infants from severe diarrhoeic disease.

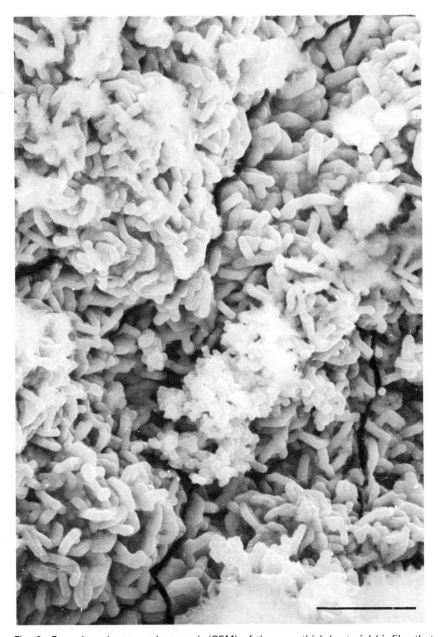

Fig. 2 Scanning electron micrograph (SEM) of the very thick bacterial biofilm that developed on the steel surfaces of an aseptically-removable surface-mounted "stud" in a Robbins Device. Note that the rod-shaped bacterial cells are embedded and partly buried in a very thick amorphous exopolysaccharide matrix of bacterial exopolysaccharide and that the whole thick biofilm has cracked in many places due to the dehydration necessary for SEM preparation. The bar in this, and all subsequent, SEM indicates 5 μm and all preparations were made by thiocarbohydrazide metallization (no metal coating) and all were dried by the critical point method.

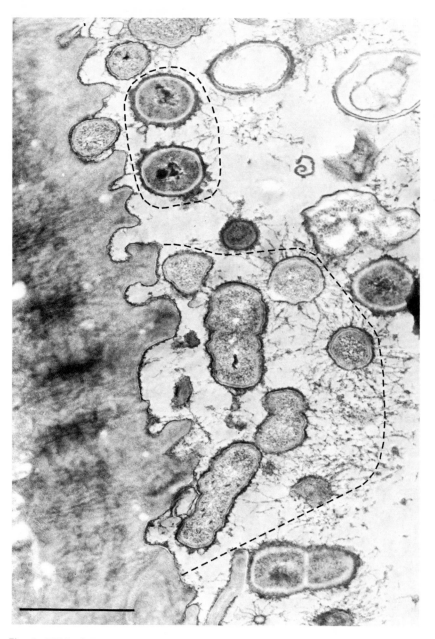

Fig. 3 TEM of the mixed bacterial biofilm composed of beneficial autochthonous bacteria, and their fibrous glycocalyces, on the wall of the bovine rumen. Note that the bacteria adherent to this tissue have formed microcolonies of morphologically similar cells (dotted lines) and that their fibrous glycocalyces have been condensed into thick strands by the dehydration necessary for preparation for TEM.

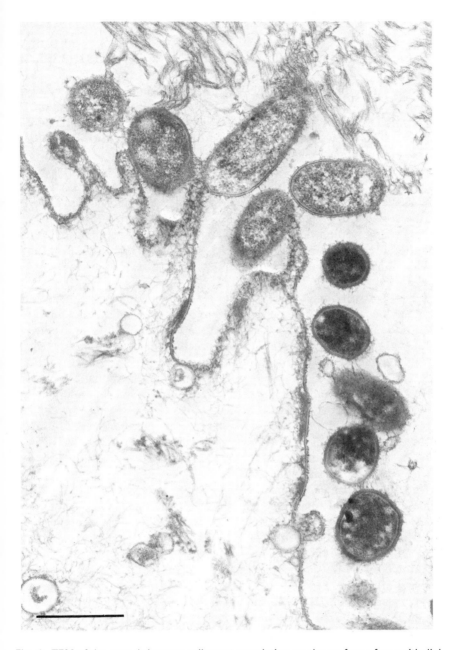

Fig. 4 TEM of the autochthonous adherent population on the surface of an epithelial cell sloughed from the distal urethra of a healthy adult human female. Note that this *de facto* biofilm is composed of a microcolony of Gram-positive cells (lower) and another microcolony of Gram-negative organisms (upper), and that the biofilm is composed of these cells and their fibrous glycocalyces—here condensed by dehydration during processing.

IV. BACTERIAL POPULATIONS ADHERENT TO PROSTHESES

When a plastic or metal prosthesis is introduced into an animal body its biologically inert surface offers a unique substratum for colonization by bacteria, whose preferential mode of growth is the formation of adherent biofilms. This growth stratagem evolved to protect these cells from the depredations of amoebae and bacteriophage in natural environments, and it serves to protect cells of the same species from phagocytic leukocytes and humoral immune factors within the animal body (Costerton et al., 1981a). Specifically, animal phagocytes are less mobile and less avidly phagocytic on the surfaces of biomaterials (Leake et al., 1981) and, once established, adherent microcolonies of bacteria are much less susceptible than their planktonic counterparts to surfactants (Govan, 1975), opsonizing antibodies (Baltimore and Mitchell, 1980), and phagocytosis (Schwarzmann and Boring, 1971).

When a prosthesis spans a "boundary" between naturally colonized and normally uncolonized tissues, such as that between the distal and proximal urethra or that between the vagina and the uterus, it offers an avenue of colonization into normally sterile organs such as the bladder (Marrie et al., 1979) and the upper female reproductive tract (Marrie and Costerton, 1982a). Furthermore, the bacteria that cross these boundaries are subjected to the concerted attack of host defence factors and they adopt a very "defensive" mode of growth in a tightly adherent and coherent biofilm. Examples are seen in the bacterial biofilm formed in the lumen of urinary catheters (Fig. 5), on the surfaces of intrauterine contraceptive devices (Fig. 6), and on the surfaces of a wide variety of prosthetic devices such as intraperitoneal dialysis catheters (Fig. 7).

This adherent and cryptic mode of growth in adherent biofilms limits the release of bacterial toxins and the spread of the colonizing bacteria and many patients whose prostheses are colonized remain asymptomatic for months or years. Routine diagnostic microbiological analysis is generally misleading because these adherent populations shed very few cells that are not immediately phagocytized by activated leukocytes and because, even when the prosthesis is removed, the coherent mode of growth of these biofilm bacteria yields a small number of large coherent aggregates that produce very few colonies on plates, when conventional sampling and plating methods are used. Growth in coherent biofilms has been shown to confer effective resistance to antiseptics such as 2% chlorhexidine (Marrie and Costerton, 1981), and extensive glycocalyx production has been shown to confer resistance to antibiotics such as carbenicillin (Govan and Fyfe, 1978), so that the bacterial cells within biofilms on medical prostheses are seen to be inherently resistant to antibacterial agents, just as the biofilm

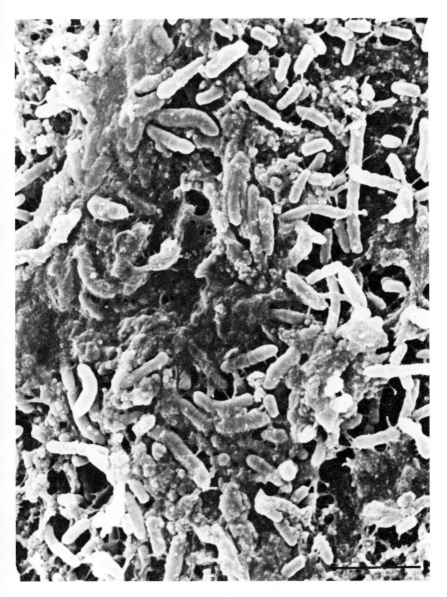

Fig. 5 SEM of a bacterial biofilm that developed on the lumenal surface of a urinary catheter installed in an elderly human male. Note the morphological diversity of this mixed population and the extent to which these cells are buried in the amorphous exopolysaccharide matrix that has condensed during the dehydration steps of processing.

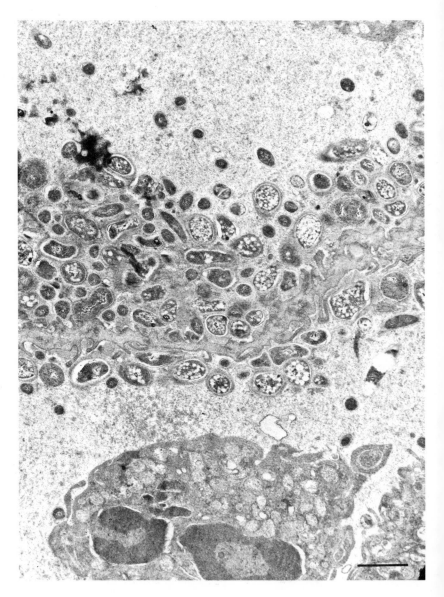

Fig. 6 TEM of the bacterial biofilm found on the surface of an intrauterine contraceptive device removed from an entirely asymptomatic young adult human female. Note the morphologically diverse bacterial population in the central electron-dense band of this biofilm and the small bacteria (*ca.* 0·2 μm) that have produced the very extensive fibrous glycocalyx that constitutes the less electron-dense areas.

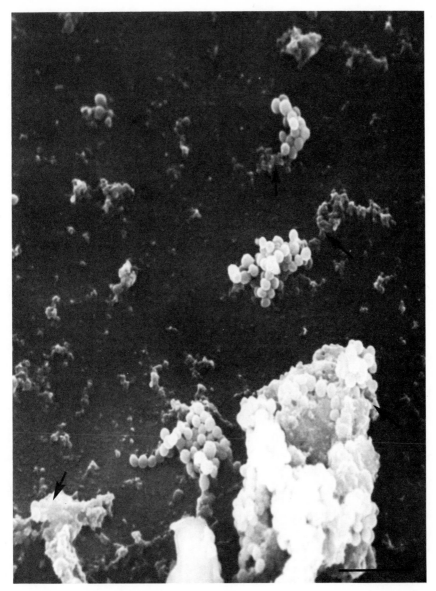

Fig. 7 SEM of the outer surface of an intraperitoneal dialysis catheter removed from a patient in whom it had served as the focus of a peritoneal infection. Note the distinct adherent microcolonies of staphylococci and the extent to which these bacterial aggregates are surrounded by condensed exopolysaccharide material (arrows) that, in the hydrated state, constituted their protective glycocalyx matrix.

population in industrial aquatic systems is inherently resistant to biocides (Ruseska *et al.*, 1982).

Many colonized prostheses become foci of overt bacterial diseases, as when cystitis develops from a colonized catheter or when endocarditis and bacteremia develop from a colonized heart valve, and it is characteristic of these infections that the pathogenic bacterial cells produce large amounts of glycocalyx exopolysaccharide and grow in enormous microcolonies that may even attain macroscopic proportions. Figure 8 shows the microcolonial mode of growth of cells of *Pseudomonas aeruginosa* from a bladder infection that developed from a colonized urinary catheter and Fig. 9 shows the confluent growth of cells of *Staphylococcus aureus* on endocardial tissue adjacent to a very heavily colonized porcine heart valve that had become the focus of an acute bacteremia. In another well-documented clinical case (Marrie and Costerton, 1982b), a staphylococcal bacteremia originating from a traumatic bursitis was seen to lead to colonization of both the plastic and metal components of a cardiac pacemaker and, while the original infection and bacteremia were quickly controlled by conventional antibiotic therapy (cloxacillin and rifampin), the very extensive coherent bacterial biofilm on this colonized prosthesis (Fig. 10) persisted throughout several weeks of very aggressive antibacterial chemotherapy (12 g of cloxacillin per day) until the prosthesis was eventually removed (Marrie and Costerton, 1982b).

Conventional clinical wisdom suggests that colonized prostheses must be removed before any attempt is made chemotherapeutically to resolve the infection for which they have served as a focus, and this consensus reflects a general concern that Minimal Inhibitory Concentration (MIC) data developed against derived planktonic cells growing *in vitro* is not predictive of the antibiotic concentrations required actually to kill pathogens growing *in vivo* in very extensive glycocalyx-protected adherent microcolonies. Similar inherent resistance to host clearance mechanisms and to conventional antibiotic chemotherapy were earlier noted in the extensive microcolonies of *P. aeruginosa* that develop in the lungs in cystic fibrosis (Lam *et al.*, 1980) and it is especially interesting to note that cells of this species can even cause chronic pulmonary infections of normal rats if they are introduced into the lung in large agar-enclosed beads that constitute artificial microcolonies (Cash *et al.*, 1979).

Perhaps the pivotal role of prostheses in bacterial infections is their provision of an inert surface on which phagocytes do not function optimally and colonizing bacteria can replicate and produce large amounts of glycocalyx material until their adherent microcolonies are too large and well-protected to be removed by cellular host defence mechanisms or to be killed by humoral immune factors or by antibiotics.

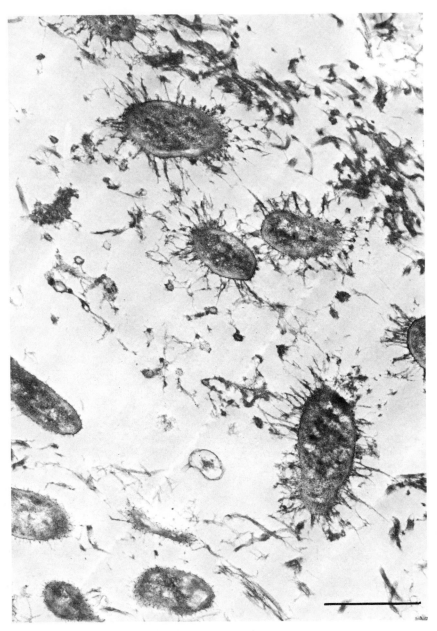

Fig. 8 TEM of a portion of a large (macroscopic) microcolony of cells of *Pseudomonas aeruginosa* recovered from the urine of an elderly male with a catheter-associated cystitis. Note the phenomenal amount of strand-like condensed material surrounding these cells which, in its hydrated state, constituted the matrix that made this huge microcolony coherent.

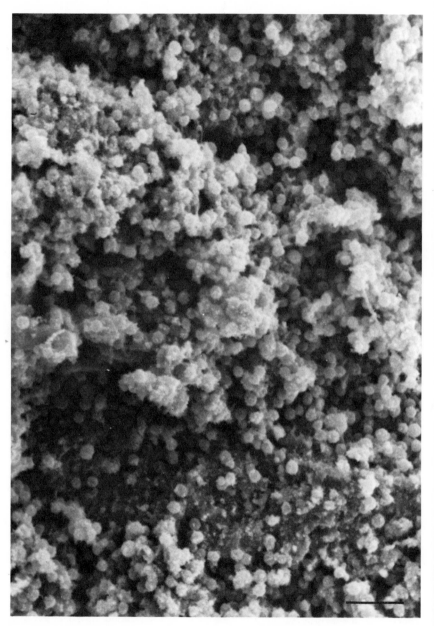

Fig. 9 SEM of the very thick biofilm formed by cells of *Staphylococcus aureus* on the tissue adjacent to a heavily-colonized porcine heart valve that had become the focus of endocarditis and bacteremia in an elderly female patient. Note the enormous thickness of this biofilm which is composed of the pathogenic bacteria and their condensed exopolysaccharide matrix.

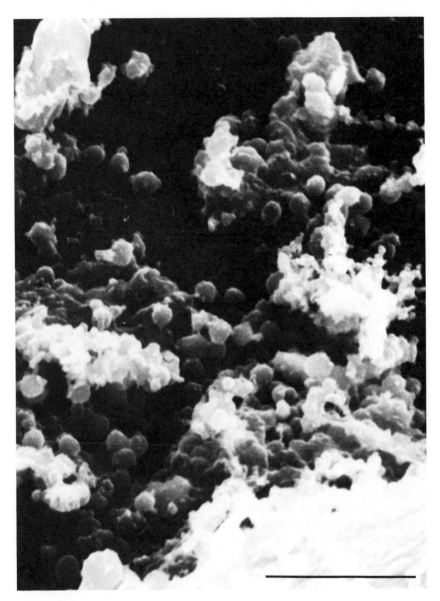

Fig. 10 SEM of the bacterial biofilm that developed on the plastic surface of a cardiac pacemaker following the onset of a bacteremia that developed from a staphylococcal bursitis. Note the extent to which these bacteria, which persisted in spite of very aggressive antibiotic therapy, are buried in the condensed residue of their enveloping glycocalyx matrix.

V. PATHOGENIC BACTERIAL POPULATIONS ADHERENT TO TISSUES

Perhaps the archetype of a cryptic and persistent bacterial infection, in which the pathogens adhere to a tissue in large microcolonies, is bacterial endocarditis. These adherent pathogens routinely produce macroscopic "vegetations" on the endocardium and the cells within these huge dextran-enclosed microcolonies are inherently resistant to conventional therapy even though they are fully and directly exposed to circulating blood levels of these agents. Direct observations of developing vegetations in the rabbit animal model of this disease show clearly that these viridans group *Streptococci* are protected by their dextran glycocalyces (Fig. 11) which form an anionic ion-exchange material that constitutes the basic structural matrix of the vegetation. Recent experiments have shown (Mills and Costerton, unpublished data) that the ability of viridans group *Streptococci* to produce vegetations on the rabbit endocardium, and the ability of cells within these vegetations to resist antibiotic chemotherapy, are related to their ability to produce large amounts of extracellular dextran. Direct examinations of material from human osteomyelitis, and from experimental osteomyelitis induced by the instillation of pathogenic bacteria into the marrow cavity of the femur of the rabbit, show that the bacteria that cause this notoriously chronic disease, which are notably resistant to antimicrobial chemotherapy, also grow in very extensive glycocalyx-enclosed microcolonies.

When we examined the mode of bacterial growth in acute diseases, which often terminate in death within 24 hours, we did not expect to see extensive microcolonies or the production of large amounts of glycocalyx exopolysaccharides. However, exhaustive examination of the growth of enterotoxigenic *Escherichia coli* on the ileal epithelium of experimentally infected newborn calves (Chan *et al.*, 1982) showed that K99 pili mediate the adhesion of K99 pilus-bearing strains to the tissue surface (Fig. 12), and that very extensive glycocalyces composed of the K30 exopolysaccharide surround these adherent cells and mediate further adhesion to the tissue (Fig. 13) and the formation of microcolonies. These relatively small microcolonies are sometimes seen to be approximately as large as phago-cytes on the same tissue (Fig. 14) and it is not known whether micro-colonies of these dimensions are formed and resolved in the small proportion of these infected calves that eventually recover from this acute diarrhoeic disease.

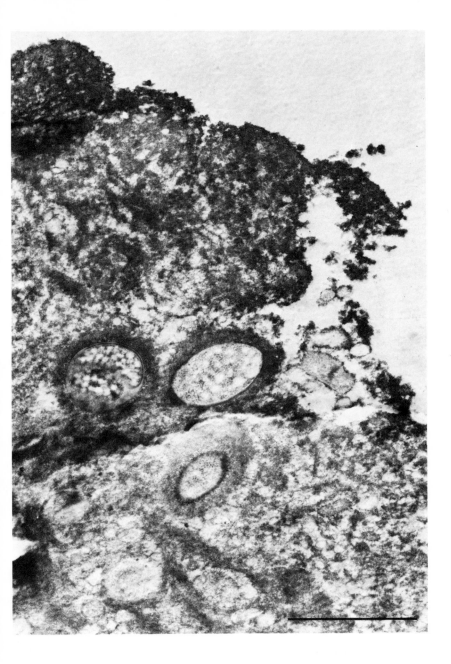

Fig. 11 TEM of part of a macroscopic "vegetation" that developed on the endo-cardium of a rabbit following catheterization and challenge with a dextran-producing strain of a viridans group *Streptococcus.* Specific antibodies were used to stabilize the glycocalyx that surrounds these cells and constitutes the "fabric" of the vegetation.

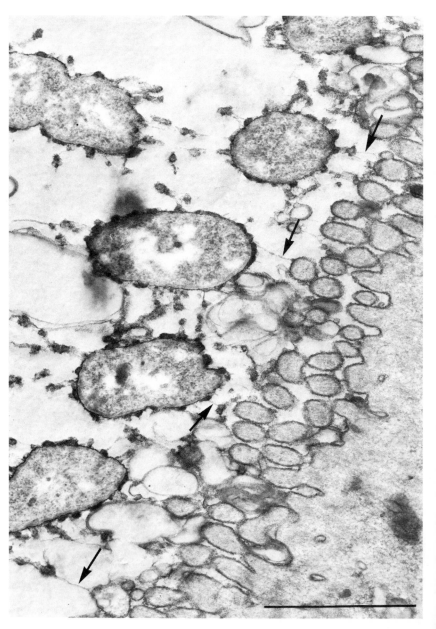

Fig. 12 TEM of the biofilm produced by cells of K99 pilus-bearing strain of entero-toxigenic *Escherichia coli* on the ileum of a newborn calf challenged with this very pathogenic organism. This preparation was treated with monoclonal antibodies specific for the K99 pilus and these structures are thickened by the antibiodies to the extent that they can be resolved (arrows) in TEM of sectioned material and shown to mediate adhesion to the infected tissue.

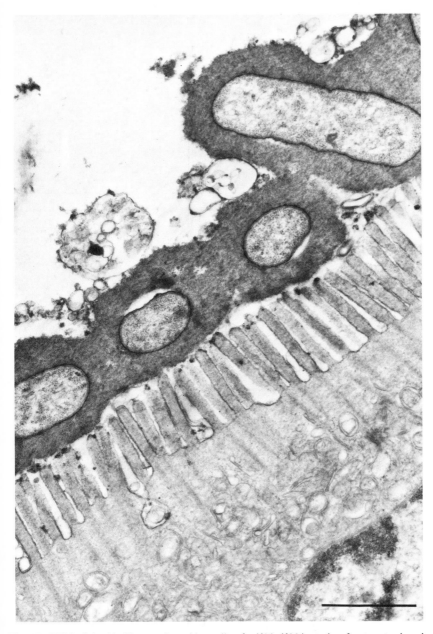

Fig. 13 TEM of the biofilm produced by cells of a K99⁻K30⁺ strain of enterotoxigenic
Escherichia coli on the ileum of a newborn calf. This preparation was treated with
specific antibodies to prevent the collapse of the bacterial glycocalyx during the
dehydration steps of preparation for TEM and these thick anionic polysaccharide
glycocalyces are seen in their true dimensions. They are seen to mediate both bacterial
adhesion to the intestinal tissue and the development of a continuous bacterial biofilm
on the ileal surface.

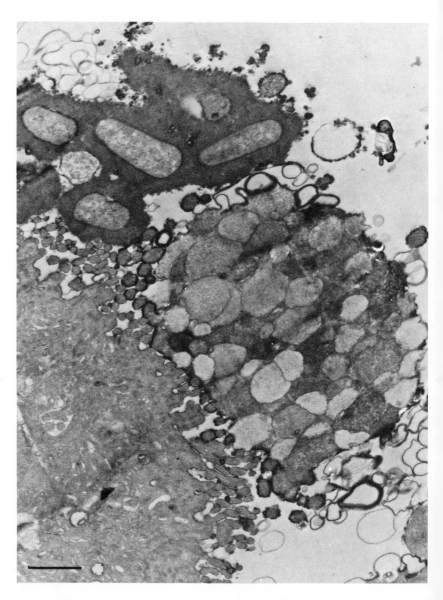

Fig. 14 TEM of the biofilm produced by cells of a K99+K30+ strain of enterotoxigenic *Escherchia coli* on the ileum of a new born calf. This preparation was "stabilized" with specific antibody to prevent the collapse of the bacterial glycocalyx during dehydration and the true dimensions of an adherent bacterial microcolony can be seen. This microcolony is almost as large, in this section, as a phagocytic white blood cell also seen at the tissue surface.

VI. EPILOGUE

Extrapolation is vital to scientific progress and, since the days of Koch, microbiologists have extrapolated from data developed in *in vitro* batch cultures of single organisms in order to describe and control bacterial infections. But, as Professor Brown so clearly explains in the introduction to this volume, batch cultures are not representative of the natural growth of bacteria and true physiological equivalence to the natural is only approached in chemostats with specific nutrient limitations. Our own simple-minded approach to the study of the bacterial surface has included a resolve to use the advanced techniques of modern electron microscopy to examine bacterial growth in natural and pathogenic environments and we can now conclude that the surfaces of bacteria growing in *in vitro* batch cultures differ profoundly from those of the same cells growing in nature.

We speculate (Costerton *et al.*, 1981a,b) that the absence of antagonistic factors in *in vitro* cultures allows the phenotypically plastic bacterial cells to jettison many of its protective cell surface components (viz. the glycocalyx), but that these surface structures are required for survival in natural and pathogenic systems. Direct observation of bacterial growth in natural and pathogenic situations shows a clear predominance of the sessile adherent microcolonial mode of growth and strong preliminary evidence suggests that bacteria growing in the resultant biofilms differ radically from their planktonic counterparts, and especially radically from their naked planktonic counterparts grown *in vitro*. In particular, they are significantly more resistant to phagocytes, bacteriophage, humoral antibacterial factors, and chemical antibacterial agents such as biocides antiseptics and antibiotics.

Antibiotics have been designed and assessed against naked planktonic bacterial cells in *in vitro* cultures, and have been selected on the basis of their efficacy against pure culture of pathogenic bacteria derived from individual infected patients, and these antibiotics have been moderately effective against pathogenic bacteria in acute disseminating disease. However, current infectious disease concerns are dominated by chronic and/or cryptic diseases in which a vigorous host immune response and aggressive antibiotic chemotherapy does not resolve the infection, but the bacteria often persist for months or years even though *in vitro* culture data indicates that they should be susceptible. Our direct observations have shown unequivocally that these cryptic pathogens live in glycocalyx-protected microcolonies and we contend that *in vitro* data is poorly predictive because the mode of bacterial growth in the culture differs so very radically from that in the infected patient.

We have begun to develop a series of antagonist-containing cultures

(Govan, 1975; Govan and Fyfe, 1978) and whole animal experiments within which we are developing data that is predictive of clinical efficacy because the bacterial mode of growth in these systems is similar to that in the infected individual. We take some intellectual comfort from the developing perception that the basic strategies of bacterial survival and persistence are very similar in natural, industrial and pathogenic systems. We are delighted to note that commercial biocides are now tested against adherent mixed biofilm populations, right on the colonized metal surfaces, and we look forward to the development of equally perceptive systems in the assessment of antibiotic efficacy to support chemotherapy in human medicine.

ACKNOWLEDGEMENTS

This work is supported by a special collaborative grant from the Natural Sciences and Engineering Research Council and the Medical Research Council of Canada.

The very competent technical assistance of Joyce Nelligan, Liz Middlemiss and Sheila Costerton is deeply appreciated.

REFERENCES

Bae, H. C., Cota-Robles, E. H. and Casida, L. E. (1972) *Appl. Microbiol.* **23**, 637–648.

Baltimore, R. S. and Mitchell, M. (1980). *J. Infect. Dis.* **141**, 238–247.

Cash, H. A., Woods, D. E., McCullough, B. Johanson, W. G., Jr. and Bass, J. A. (1979). *Amer. Rev. Respir. Dis.* **119**, 453–459.

Chan, R., Acers, S. C. and Costerton, J. W. (1982). *Infect. Immun.* **37**, 1170–1180.

Cheng, K.-J. and Costerton, J. W. (1980). *In* "Digestive Physiology and Metabolism in Ruminants" (Y. Ruckebush and P. Thivend, eds) pp. 227–250. MTP Press, Lancaster, U.K.

Cheng, K.-J. and Costerton, J. W. (1981). *Can. J. Microbiol.* **27**, 461–490.

Costerton, J. W. and Colwell, G. G. (1979). "Native Aquatic Bacteria: Enumeration, Activity and Ecology". ASTM Press, Philadelphia.

Costerton, J. W. and Geesey, G. G. (1979). *In* "Surface Contamination" (K. L. Mittal, ed.) pp. 211–221. Plenum Press, New York.

Costerton, J. W., Irvin, R. T. and Cheng, K.-J. (1981a). *Ann. Rev. Microbiol.* **35**, 299–324.

Costerton, J. W., Irvin, R. T. and Cheng, K.-J. (1981b). *Crit. Rev. Microbiol.* **8**, 303–308.

Fletcher, M. and Floodgate, G. D. (1973). *J. Gen. Microbiol.* **74**, 325–334.

Geesey, G. G., Richardson, W. T., Yeomans, H. G., Irvin, R. T. and Costerton, J. W. (1977). *Can. J. Microbiol.* **23**, 1214–1223.

Geesey, G. G., Mutch, R., Costerton, J. W. and Green, R. B. (1978). *Limnol. Oceanogr.* **23**, 1214–1223.

Govan, J. R. W. (1975). *J. Med. Microbiol.* **8,** 513–522.

Govan, J. R. W. and Fyfe, J. A. M. (1978). *J. Antimicrob. Chemother.* **4,** 233–240.

Henrici, A. T. (1933). *J. Bacteriol.* **25,** 277–286.

Jones, H. C., Roth, I. L. and Sanders, W. M., III. (1969). *J. Bacteriol.* **99,** 316–325.

Ladd, T. I., Costerton, J. W. and Geesey, G. G. (1979). *In* "Native Aquatic Bacteria: Enumeration, Activity and Ecology" (J. W. Costerton and R. R. Colwell, eds) pp. 180–195. ASTM Press, Philadelphia.

Lam, J., Chan, R., Lam, K. and Costerton, J. W. (1980). *Infect. Immun.* **28,** 546–556.

Leake, E. S., Wright, M. J. and Gristina, A. G. (1981). *J. Reticuloendothel. Soc.* **30,** 403–414.

Luft, J. H. (1971). *Anat. Rec.* **171,** 369–416.

Marrie, T. J. and Costerton, J. W. (1981). *Appl. Environ. Microbiol.* **42,** 1093–1102.

Marrie, T. J. and Costerton, J. W. (1982a). *Am. J. Obstet. Gynecol.* **146,** 384–394.

Marrie, T. J. and Costerton, J. W. (1982b). *Circulation* **66,** 1339–1341.

Marrie, T. J., Harding, G. K. M., Ronald, A. R., Dikkema, J., Lam, J., Hoban, S. and Costerton, J. W. (1979). *J. Infect. Dis.* **139,** 357–361.

Marrie, T. J., Lam, J. and Costerton, J. W. (1980). *J. Infect. Dis.* **142,** 239–246.

McCowan, R. P., Cheng, K.-J. and Costerton, J. W. (1980). *Appl. Environ. Microbiol.* **39,** 233–241.

McCoy, W. F. and Costerton, J. W. (1982). *Rev. Indust. Microbiol.* Chapter 53, pp. 551–558.

McCoy, W. F., Bryers, J. D., Robbins, J. and Costerton, J. W. (1981). *Can. J. Microbiol.* **27,** 910–917.

Rozee, K. R., Cooper, D., Lam, K. and Costerton, J. W. (1982). *Appl. Environ. Microbiol.* **43,** 1451–1459.

Ruseska, I., Robbins, J. and Costerton, J. W. (1982). *Oil and Gas Journal*, March 8, pp. 253–264.

Schwarzmann, S. and Boring, J. R. (1971). *Infect. Immun.* **3,** 762–767.

Sprung, K., Leidy, G. and Redman, W. (1980). *Pediatr. Res.* **14,** 308–313.

Wyndham, R. C. and Costerton, J. W. (1981a). *Appl. Environ. Microbiol.* **41,** 783–790.

Wyndham, R. C. and Costerton, J. W. (1981b). *Appl. Environ. Microbiol.* **41,** 791–800.

Zobell, C. E. (1943). *J. Bacteriol.* **46,** 39–56.

4 The envelope and tissue invasion

THOMAS LARRY HALE, PETER A. SCHAD and SAMUEL B. FORMAL

I. INTRODUCTION

The term "tissue invasion" will be used in this discussion to describe infection of mammalian cells when the result is the propagation of an infectious agent. The general outline of the process of tissue invasion contains recurrent themes even though the complexity of invasive agents varies greatly. These themes include adherence of the parasite to the potential host cell, endocytosis triggered by the adherent parasite, and multiplication of the internalized parasite within the intracellular milieu. It must be admitted that the molecular basis of tissue invasion is incompletely understood, but the basic process appears to be analogous, in some respects, to the phagocytosis of foreign particles by professional phagocytes such as macrophages. These cells possess plasma membrane receptors which bind the cleaved third component of complement (C3b) or the Fc portion of IgG. Foreign particles opsonized with either of these immunological ligands are bound to macrophages and ingested by sequential ligand binding. This process is aptly called the "zipper mechanism" of phagocytosis (Griffin *et al.*, 1975). Cytoplasmic contractile proteins such as actin and myosin provide the motive force for the interiorization of bound particles (Stossel and Hartwig, 1976), and they may also be involved in the redistribution of ligand-binding receptors into the psuedopodes which circumscribe ingested particles (Sheterline and Hopkins, 1981). Phagocytosis requires the consumption of energy by a functional microfilament system, thus the process is interrupted by various metabolic inhibitors (Owen *et al.*, 1963) and by cytochalasin B (Axline and Reaven, 1974), a drug which interferes with actin gelatin (Hartwig and Stossel, 1979).

MEDICAL MICROBIOLOGY, 3
ISBN 0 12 228003 3

The infection of normally nonphagocytic mammalian cells by invasive parasites is by no means identical to immune phagocytosis by macrophages. Obviously immunological ligands are not involved in the former process, so the nature of surface receptors involved in attachment and internalization of invasive agents must differ significantly from those involved in immune phagocytosis. There may be even more fundamental differences because some parasites must be metabolically active in order to induce phagocytosis. These organisms seem to actively induce their own endocytosis. None the less, it is instructive to analyse tissue invasion in the context of the more familiar process of immune phagocytosis. Since the latter process is initiated by interactions at the cell surface, particular emphasis will be given to host cell–parasite surface interactions.

II. SURVEY OF INVASIVE AGENTS

A. Obligate intracellular parasites

1. *Virus*
A thorough treatment of viral penetration is beyond the scope of this discussion; however, it should be noted that the recurrent themes of adherence and endocytosis are first encountered at the viral level. For example, enveloped viruses, such as orthomyxovirus and paramyxovirus, modify the host cell envelope by inserting viral glycoproteins while virions are budding from infected host cells. These glycoproteins on the viral envelope bind to sialic acid-containing determinants on the plasma membrane of susceptible host cells. Attached viruses are subsequently taken up by an endocytic process.

2. *Chlamydia*
Bacteria of the genus *Chlamydia* have a unique developmental cycle. Elementary bodies (metabolically quiescent extracellular chlamydiae) are internalized by host cells, and they subsequently reorganize into intracellular reticulate bodies. The latter forms are metabolically active, synthesizing macromolecules and multiplying by binary fission. Eventually reticulate bodies undergo another reorganization, condensing into elementary bodies which are then released from infected host cells.

Tissue invasion by elementary bodies has been studied morphologically in cultured mammalian cells, and it was concluded that infection of these cells involves a phagocytic process (Friis, 1972). This was confirmed by additional experiments which showed that uptake of *Chlamydia psittaci* by mouse L cells is inhibited by low temperature and by 2–4 dinitrophenol, an inhibitor of oxidative phosphorylation (Friis, 1972). However, endocytosis of chlamydiae by fibroblasts and macrophages is not inhibited by cytochalasin B (Gregory et al., 1979), so the process differs somewhat from immune phagocytosis by macrophages. Heat-labile elementary body surface components (perhaps proteins) and trypsin-sensitive host cell receptors are required for ingestion of C. psittaci by L cells (Byrne, 1976). Wheat germ agglutinin, a lectin which binds to N-acetyl-D-glucosamine, inhibits L cell uptake of both C. psittaci and a lymphogranuloma venereum (LGV) strain of Chlamydia trachomatis (Levy, 1979). This indicates that the trypsin-sensitive host cell receptor is a glycoprotein. Pretreatment of HeLa cells with neuraminidase inhibits uptake of a trachoma-inclusion conjunctivitis (TRIC) strain of C. trachomatis (Kuo et al., 1973) indicating that LGV and TRIC strains probably bind to different glycoprotein receptors. Furthermore, LGV strains are more hydrophobic and less negatively charged than TRIC strains (Soderlund and Kihlstrom, 1982). This difference in surface properties may contribute to the enhanced infectivity of LGV strains.

C. trachomatis express a major outer membrane polypeptide (MOMP) of 42000 daltons. In addition, minor polypeptides of 155000 (a species-specific antigen) and 24000 (a type-specific antigen) are detected in chlamydial cell walls. These three polypeptides are radiolabelled with ^{125}I-lactoperoxidase-catalysed oxidation, so they are probably exposed on the surface of intact cells. In LGV strains, some polypeptides of approximately 118000 are also iodinated (Salari and Ward, 1981). One or more of these polypeptides is probably a component of the heat-labile surface structure which induces uptake of chlamydiae by host cells (Byrne, 1976). The MOMP of various C. trachomatis strains have recently been isolated, and antiserum has been raised against these constituents (Caldwell and Schachter, 1982). This polyclonal antiserum, and perhaps monoclonal antibody in the future, should be useful in identifying virulence determinants in the chlamydial envelope.

In addition to triggering an endocytic response which results in parasitization of host cells, the chlamydial envelope also contributes to the survival of internalized organisms (Friis, 1972). In L cells, infectious C. psittaci are segregated into phagocytic vacuoles which do not fuse with lysosomes. Elementary bodies inactivated by heat or coated with antiserum do not inhibit lysosomal fusion. When development of intracellular chlamydiae is inhibited by chloramphenicol, the cells still avoid lysosomal digestion. Thus an intrinsic component of the chlamydial envelope inhibits the normal lysosomal response in infected host cells.

In summary, the data indicate that hydrophobic elementary bodies expressing lectin-like proteins bind to glycoprotein receptors on mammalian host cells. Bound chlamydiae are probably ingested by circumferential ligand binding which requires no metabolic activity by the parasite and minimal host cell microfilament contraction. Once internalized, an unknown chlamydial surface component inhibits lysosomal fusion and allows the completion of the intracellular growth cycle.

3. *Rickettsia*

Rickettsiae are small coccobacillary Gram-negative bacteria which exist in a single fragile form. Transmission of rickettsiae depends on arthropod vectors and survival depends upon the milieu supplied by the host cell cytoplasm. They fall into three basic groups on the basis of pathogenesis and arthropod vector: (1) the typhus group which includes *Rickettsia prowazeksii, R. typhi*, and others; (2) the scrub typhus group represented by *R. tsutsugamushi*; and (3) the Q fever group represented by *Coxiella burnettii*.

The process of host cell infection by rickettsiae was first systematically analysed by Cohn *et al.* (1959). These investigators studied the infection of cultured mouse lymphoblasts or mouse L cell fibroblasts by *R. tsutsugamushi* and concluded that active participation of both the parasites and the host cells is required for invasion. For example, rickettsiae which had been inactivated by mild heat, ultraviolet irradiation, formalin fixation, or exposure to aureomycin were unable to invade mouse cells *in vitro*. Culture medium containing glutamate facilitated lymphoblast infection by stimulating oxidative phosphorylation in invading parasites, and this process was interdicted by the addition of metabolic inhibitors or by cooling of the medium to 4°C. More recently Walker and Winkler (1978) have studied the infection of L cells by *R. prowazeki*. They found that adherence of rickettsiae to L cells is temperature dependent and is a linear function of both time and concentration of parasites; however, the adherence step was less sensitive to low temperature than was the process of internalization. The latter process was interdicted by treatment of L cells with metabolic inhibitors, thio reagents, or cytochalasin B. These data indicate that the host cell plays an active role in rickettsial internalization and that these organisms actively induce a phagocytic event.

Unlike chlamydiae, internalized rickettsiae are not found within phagosomes. Viable *R. tsutsugamusci* escape phagosomes even in professional phagocytes such as polymorphonuclear leukocytes (Rikihisa and Ito, 1980), and *R. prowazeki* are found free in the cytoplasm of L cells (Walker and Winkler, 1978). It has been proposed by the latter investigators that the process of escape from phagosomes may be analogous to the process of haemolysis of sheep erythrocytes by *R. prowazeki*. Rickettsial haemolysis requires attachment of rickettsiae and metabolic activity on the part of both the parasites and the erythrocytes (Ramm and Winkler, 1973). The erythrocyte receptor for haemolytic rickettsiae includes a cholesterol moiety (Ramm and Winkler, 1976), so a similar membrane component may be involved in the dissolution of phagosomes containing viable rickettsiae.

Polyclonal rabbit antiserum will inhibit uptake of *R. prowazekii* by L929 mouse fibroblasts but not by the RAW:264·7 mouse macrophage-like cell line (Turco and Winkler, 1982). These data indicate that rickettsial surface components which can be masked by antibody are essential for the induction of endocytosis in non-professional phagocytes. Some progress has been made in identifying these components. *R. prowazekii* and *R. rickettsii* have a thick slime layer (Silverman *et al.*, 1978), but the composition and function of this capsule remain uncertain. In addition to the slime layer the rickettsial envelope contains peptidoglycan, lipopolysaccharide, and an array of membrane proteins. For example, six major polypeptides are located in the envelope of *R. prowazekii* (Eisemann and Osterman, 1976), and polypeptides with molecular weights of 138000, 31000 and 20000 daltons are accessible to surface iodination (Smith and Winkler, 1980). Recently six mouse lymphocyte clones which produce antibody recognizing various regions of the 138000 outer membrane polypeptide of *R. prowazekii* have been developed (Oaks, E. V., Smith, J. F., and Wissman, C. L., manuscript in preparation). These monoclonal antibodies were used as probes to analyse the biological activity of the 138000 polypeptide, and three antigenic domains were identified. These regions were designated the epidemic typhus "ET-specific" region, the "conserved region", and the "attachment region". The "ET-specific" region contains antigenic determinants specific for *R. prowazekii*, and antibody recognizing this region partially inhibits the haemolytic reaction but has no effect on uptake of rickettsiae by chicken embryo fibroblasts. The "conserved region" of the 138000 polypeptide is recognized in both *R. prowazekii* and *R. mooseri* by group-specific antibody. This antibody has no effect on uptake of rickettsiae by host cells or on haemolysis of sheep erythrocytes, but, like ET-specific antibody, it partially inhibits growth of rickettsiae in macrophages. Finally, antibody recognizing the "attachment region" inhibits uptake of rickettsiae by chicken embryo fibroblasts but has no effect on haemolysis or survival in macrophages. These observations indicate that the 138000 outer membrane polypeptide is involved in both haemolysis and invasion.

Wisseman *et al.* (1976) found that the presence of host cell membrane fragments inhibits the invasion of chicken embryo fibroblasts by *R. prowazekii*. This implies that rickettsiae adhere to receptors on fibroblast membranes. Although the nature of the putative rickettsial receptor on these membranes is unknown, it is possible that the "attachment region" of the 138 000 outer membrane polypeptide is involved in its recognition. It could also be speculated that metabolic activity on the part of isolated rickettsiae is an indicator of cell wall integrity and that, in the absence of such integrity, the "attachment region" is denatured or digested. Alternatively, a specific conformational state may be required for "attachment region" function, and energy expenditure on the part of the parasite may be necessary for the maintenance of the proper configuration. In either manner, the attachment region of the 138 000 outer membrane polypeptide could induce the energy-dependent uptake of rickettsiae by sequentially binding to receptors on the host cell membrane.

4. Protozoans

(a) Trypanosoma

Many protozoan parasites have an obligate intracellular phase in their normal life cycle. Trypomastigotes of *Trypanosoma cruzi*, the organisms responsible for Chagas' disease, are inoculated into man by the bite of the tsetse fly, and they invade the lymph node and brain. Trypomastigotes are able to infect mammalian cells *in vitro* by a process which resembles phagocytosis (Nogueira and Cohen, 1976). Cytochalasin B inhibits the uptake of trypomastigotes by Vero cells, and drugs such as colchicine and vinblastine, which disrupt the cytoskeleton, also inhibit infection of these cells (Henriquez *et al.*, 1981). Crane and Dvorak (1982) attempted to identify carbohydrates which might be involved in trypamastigote uptake, and they found that, of nine monosaccarhide moities commonly found in mammalian membrane carbohydrates, only *N*-acetylglucosamine specifically inhibits infection. This effect was elicited by preincubation of parasites with *N*-acetylglucosamine. Henriquez *et al.* (1981) found that pretreatment of Vero cells with wheat germ agglutinin diminished interiorization of *T. cruzi* as did pretreatment with trypsin and periodate. On the basis of these observations, Crane and Dvorak (1982) concluded that a wheat germ agglutin-like lectin on the trypomastigote surface recognizes and attaches to an *N*-acetylglucosamine-containing receptor on the vertebrate cell surface prior to infection. This lectin-like activity could conceivably be determined by the variant antigen (VA), a glycoprotein of approximately 55 000 daltons which is the primary surface coat component of pathogenic trypanosomes (Cross and Johnson, 1976). Although the precise relationship between attachment and uptake of trypomastigotes remains undefined, thus far the data are consistent with a hypothesis of induced phagocytosis through sequential ligand binding.

(b) Toxoplasma
Protozoan parasites of the genus *Toxoplasma* are capable of invading virtually any tissue encountered in the human host. Electron microscope studies have established that *Toxoplasma gondii* invade mouse L cells and HeLa cells by a phagocytic process (Jones *et al.*, 1972). Since tachyzoites which have been killed by heating or by glutaraldehyde fixation are not taken up by host cells, it appears that these organisms actively induce the phagocytic event (Jones *et al.*, 1972). Synchronized HeLa cell cultures are particularly susceptible to *T. gondii* invasion during the S phase of their growth cycle, so Dvorak and Crane (1981) have suggested that a toxoplasma receptor is present on host cells during this phase. However, these investigators have been unable to inhibit uptake of tachyzoites by treatment with monosaccharides commonly found on mammalian cell surfaces (Crane and Dvorak, 1982), so the nature of the putative toxoplasma receptor remains unknown.

It should be noted that Lycke *et al.* (1975) contend that *T. gondii* mechanically penetrates the cytoplasmic membrane of host cells by excreting an enzyme-like protein called penetration-enhancing factor (PEF). Although the evidence for mechanical penetration of the plasma membrane is unconvincing, it is possible the PEF locally modifies the membrane surface and enhances sequential ligand binding by exposing a previously masked toxoplasma receptor.

(c) Leishmania
Trypanosomatid flagellates of the genus *Leishmania* exist in the alimentary canal of insect vectors as extracellular, motile promastigote forms and an intracellular amastigate forms within the reticuloendothelial system of infected mammalian hosts. Chang (1978) showed that promastigotes of *Leishmania donovani* can invade human skin fibroblasts by a phagocytic process, and he has proposed that promastigotes convert into amastigote forms while growing in such non-professional phagocytes. He also suggested that uptake of the promastigote form by macrophages is by "facilitated phagocytosis" (Chang, 1979), a process which depends upon parasite motility and may involve carbohydrate determinants on the surface of these organisms (Chang, 1981).

(d) Plasmodium
Protozoan parasites of the genus *Plasmodium* exist in two forms in the vertebrate host. Sporozoites, which are induced into the blood stream by infected mosquitoes, invade parenchymal cells of the liver. These intracellular forms multiply as merozoites which are released into the blood stream. In the circulatory system, merozoites invade erythrocytes and

multiply asexually, lysing the host cell and producing the fever-chill cycle characteristic of malarial infections. The accessible form of malarial parasite is the merozoite, so *in vitro* studies have been limited to the interactions of merozoites with erythrocytes (reviewed in Sherman, 1979).

Miller *et al.* (1979) have shown that invasion of erythrocytes from humans and monkeys by the simian strain *Plasmodium knowlesi* occurs through a sequence of events that starts with temperature-sensitive and species-specific attachment of merozoites to the erythrocyte membrane. Chymotrypsin treatment of human erythrocytes or merozoites inhibits the attachment stage. *P. knowlesi* can attach to Duffy blood group-negative erythrocytes, but only Duffy-positive erythrocytes can support the subsequent steps of invasion. At the point of attachment, merozoites form a junction, which is a deformed and thickened area in the erythrocyte membrane. If the erythrocyte is Duffy-positive, the junction migrates parallel to the long axis of the parasite until the merozoite is internalized in a vacuolar membrane. The migrating membrane junction is thought to represent the anchorage site of cytoplasmic contractile proteins (Aikawa *et al.*, 1981). Thus it appears that *P. knowlesi* (and *P. vivax*) attach to human erythrocytes by a chymotrypsin-sensitive plasma membrane protein or glycoprotein and that subsequent internalization of the attached merozoites occurs by sequential ligand binding involving Duffy blood group antigens of unknown chemical composition. In contrast to *P. knowlesi* and *P. vivax*, *P. falciparum* merozoites do not recognize Duffy blood group antigens. These parasites require receptors which can be removed by treatment of human erythrocytes with trypsin or neuraminidase, enzymes which cleave a major membrane sialoglycoprotein called glycophorin A. Extracts of glycophorin A, as well as antibody directed against this glycoprotein, inhibit invasion by *P. falciparum* (Perkins, 1981). Thus, it appears that glycophorin A is a constituent of the erythrocyte receptor for a human species of malarial parasite.

Passive transfer of immune serum can confer protection from infection with *P. knowlesi* or *P. falciparum*, indicating that antibodies recognizing some merozoite antigens could be expected to interdict invasion of erythrocytes *in vitro*. As was discussed previously in regard to rickettsiae, monoclonal antibodies can be used to identify surface antigens which are necessary for the invasion of host cells. Epstein *et al.* (1981) have produced two monoclonal antibodies which block invasion of monkey erythrocytes by *P. knowlesi*. Both of these antibodies precipitate a single merozoite outer membrane protein of approximately 250000 daltons. Although Epstein *et al.* (1981) feel that these antibodies inhibit infection by agglutinating merozoites rather than by blocking receptors, similar experiments employing monoclonal technology should eventually prove useful in identifying the receptors which are necessary for merozoite invasion.

B. Facultative intracellular parasites

1. *Non-enteric bacteria*

(a) Mycobacterium
As early as 1928 it was observed that tubercle bacilli could be grown in primary tissue cultures, and later Shepard (1957) showed that the growth rate of mycobacteria in HeLa cell monolayers was more rapid for virulent than for avirulent strains. He characterized HeLa cell invasion as a phagocytic event; however, he attributed the initiation of endocytic activity not the presence of virulent *Mycobacterium tuberculosis* but to the presence of an undefined substance in certain lots of horse serum which were used to prepare tissue culture medium (Shepard, 1955). Thus the role of the tubercle bacillus in tissue invasion is obscure, and, since the primary host cell of this organism *in vivo* is the macrophage, the biological relevance of HeLa cell infection is unclear. This can also be said of a number of other bacterial species which have been reported to invade HeLa cells or other non-professional phagocytes but are not known to invade parenchymal cells *in vivo* (reviewed in Bovallius and Nilsson, 1975).

(b) Neisseria
A critical determinant of gonococcal virulence may be the ability to invade the mucosal lining of the genital and urinary tract. The process of invasion by *Neisseria gonorrhoeae* has been studied in perfused human fallopian tubes and in HeLa cell monolayers. Thayer *et al.* (1957) and Kenny and Arils (1969) reported the uptake of gonococci by HeLa cells. The latter investigators found that invasion was inhibited by hyperimmune rabbit serum and that avirulent colonial types III and IV were converted to virulent type I colonies by growth in HeLa cells. In contrast, Waitkins and Flynn (1973) found no reversion of type IV to type I in neisseriae grown in 3T3 mouse fibroblast cells, but they did show by transmission electron microscopy that HeLa cells are infected by an endocytic process.

Ward *et al.* (1975) characterized the invasion of the mucosa of perfused human fallopian tubes using transmission electron microscopy. The initial attachment of gonococci was at the tips of microvilli projecting from the columnar epithelium. A small proportion of adherent gonococci were enveloped by microvilli, and it appeared that these microvilli were

subsequently resorbed, internalizing the enveloped bacteria within phagocytic vacuoles. Piliated gonococci adsorb to cultured epithelial cells
more avidly than do nonpiliated organisms (Swanson, 1973), but pili do not
appear to mediate the endocytic uptake of gonococci seen by Ward *et al.*
(1975) or Waitkins and Flynn (1973). Swanson *et al.* (1975) also showed
that "leukocyte association factor", a nonpilus surface protein of approximately 29 000 daltons (King and Swanson, 1978), has no effect of the
association of gonococci with HeLa cells. Thus the role of the gonococcal
envelope in the invasion process remains unknown.

2. *Enteric bacteria*

The invasive genera of enteric bacteria offer opportunities for study of the
process of host cell infection which are not presented by any of the other
invasive agents thus far discussed. The most important opportunity is the
possibility of mapping the genetic loci necessary for invasion. Progress is
being made in this area; however, in some instances more is known about
invasion by some obligate intracellular parasites than is understood about
invasion by enteric bacteria.

(a) Salmonella

Bacteria of the genus *Salmonella* invade the ileal epithelium of the
susceptible mammalian host producing either localized enteritis or spread-
ing to the mesenteric lymphnodes, spleen, and liver in a systemic infection.
Employing electron microscopy, Takeuchi (1967) observed the invasion of
the guinea pig intestinal epithelium by *Salmonella typhimurium*. These
studies showed that microvilli on ileal mucosa cells degenerate when
salmonellae are in close apposition. Invaginations were found in the apical
cytoplasm of some epithelial cells, and bacteria were sometimes observed
within these pits. Finally, some intact epithelial cells were found to harbour
bacteria within membrane-bound vacuoles which resemble phagosomes.

The above observations indicate that salmonellae invade intestinal
epithelial cells by an endocytic process. Subsequent studies of the process
of invasion have employed cultured mammalian cells as models of the
intestinal epithelium. Giannella *et al.* (1973) found that the ability of
S. typhimurium to invade HeLa cells and to invade the rabbit ileal mucosa
are correlated. Jones and Richardson (1981) have differentiated the
interaction of salmonella with HeLa cells into three consecutive but
overlapping stages: (1) accumulation and adsorption, (2) adhesion, and (3)
invasion. Accumulation of *S. typhimurium* in the vicinity of HeLa cells is
facilitated by the motility of these organisms (Jones *et al.*, 1981), and there
is a chemotactic attraction to HeLa cells damaged by exposure to low pH

(Uhlman and Jones, 1982). The attractant released from these damaged cells has been tentatively identified as glycine.

Adsorption, a readily reversible adherence to HeLa cells, is initiated when virulent *S. typhimurium* are influenced by weak London–van der Waals' forces of attraction which occur at the secondary minimum (10–100 nm from the plasma membrane). Since both the bacterium and the host cell are enveloped in positive ionic clouds which are attracted to the fixed negative charges on their respective surfaces, there is an interposing energy barrier which separates the secondary minimum from the primary minimum. At the primary minimum, the close apposition of two negatively charged particles generates an attraction which is stronger than the mutual electrical repulsion of these particles (Jones, 1977). The thickness of the energy barrier of the host cell is dependent upon the ionic strength of the surrounding medium. Thus decreasing the ionic strength increases the electrical repulsion of the bacterium and the host cell. Medium of low ionic strength allows reversible adsorption of *S. typhimurium* to HeLa cells but inhibits irreversible attachment which is essential for invasion (Jones *et al.*, 1981). Under ionic conditions which allow irreversible attachment, i.e. when the energy barrier is less than 15 nm thick, *S. typhimurium* employ a mannose-resistant haemogglutinin (MRHA) to establish a primary minimum (Jones and Richardson, 1981).

Strains of *S. typhimurium* which have incomplete polysaccharide side chains on the lipopolysaccharide (LPS) component of the envelope, probably overcome the energy barrier by a hydrophobic interaction with the surface of host cells. This hydrophobic interface produces favourable changes in free energy by displacing water from the interacting surfaces. Thus Kihlstrom (1977) has found that a rough strain of *S. typhimurium* is much more invasive in the HeLa cell model than is an isogenic smooth strain. The invasiveness of the rough strain probably reflects the extent to which hydrophobic interactions overcome the energy barrier and allow the MRHA to establish adherence.

The nature of bacterial attachment as mediated by the MRHA is unclear. None of the monosaccharides which commonly occur on mammalian cell surfaces inhibits the agglutination of fixed sheep erythrocytes by salmonellae which express the MRHA (Jones, G. W., personal communication). Thus the chemical nature of the mammalian receptor for this ligand can not be predicted. The role of the MRHA in invasion is also undefined; however, the observations of Kihlstrom (reviewed in 1980) suggest that a bacterial lectin (such as the MRHA) might facilitate uptake of salmonellae by promoting sequential ligand binding. He found that scanning electron microscopy of HeLa cells exposed to virulent *S. typhimurium* reveals adherent salmonellae which are embedded in membrane folds similar to those found around opsonized erythrocytes which are being phagocytosed by macrophages. No evidence of plasma membrane damage during invasion is seen, and, with few exceptions, intercellular organisms are found in membrane-bound vacuoles. Thus Kihlstrom and Latkovic (1978) concluded that infection of HeLa cells by salmonellae shares many morphological similarities with the uptake of bacteria by professional phagocytes.

The role of the bacterium in the invasion process was analysed by killing *S. typhimurium* with heat (56°C for 60 min) or ultraviolet radiation. These treatments greatly reduce, but do not totally abolish, the association of bacteria with HeLa cells (Kihlstrom and Edebo, 1976). Glycolytic inhibitors such as iodoacetic acid or *N*-ethylmaleimide, which reduce endocytosis of particles by phagocytic cells, have little effect upon attachment of *S. typhimurium* but significantly inhibite uptake of these organisms. Cytochalasin B also inhibits invasion of HeLa cells. These experiments indicate that HeLa cells internalize salmonellae by an energy-requiring process that depends on microfilament function (Kihlstrom and Nilsson, 1977).

The role of the bacterial envelope in triggering uptake by host cells is unknown; however, the myriad secondary and tertiary configurations of proteins make them prime candidates for informational molecules which induce phagocytosis. The outer membrane of *S. typhimurium* contains 18 to 20 polypeptides, and between 11 and 13 of these are exposed to the external environment (Kamio and Nikaido, 1977). Proteins exposed on the bacterial surface should be antigenic (Dankert and Hofstra, 1978), but hyperimmune polyclonal rabbit antiserum raised against rough or smooth strains of *S. typhimurium* has no statistically significant effect on uptake of these organisms by HeLa cells (Kihlstrom, 1979). As was the case with rickettsiae, monoclonal antibody may be necessary for identification of outer membrane proteins which are involved in invasion.

In addition to proteins, lipopolysaccharides are potential informational molecules which may induce phagocytosis. However, the enhanced uptake of rough *S. typhimurium* strains by HeLa cells (Kihlstrom and Edebo, 1976) indicates that, at least in this experimental model, O-polysaccharide side chains are not necessary for invasion. Rough *S. typhimurium* mutants can colonize the intestines of rats and penetrate the intestinal mucosa, but isogenic smooth strains are at least 10-fold more virulent than rough mutants (Tannock *et al.*, 1975). Much experimental data indicates that very specific polysaccharide configurations are necessary for resistance to host defence mechanisms and for stability of outer membrane proteins (reviewed in Lindberg, 1980), but the proteins are probably the key determinants of the invasive phenotype.

(b) Yersinia

Two species of the genus *Yersinia* are able to invade the intestinal mucosa and to evoke a variety of disease syndromes. *Yersinia pseudotuberculosis* may cause acute septicaemia or chronic mesenteric lymphadenitis while *Yersinia enterocolitica* has been implicated in cases of acute gastroenteritis, enterocolitis, and terminal ileitis. The virulence of these organisms has been studied in cultured human epithelial (HEp-2) cells (Maki *et al.*, 1978), and both species have been shown by electron microscopy to be ingested by phagocytosis and vacuole formation (Bovallius and Nilsson, 1975; Lee *et al.*, 1977). In apparent contrast to other invasive agents, non-viable *Y. enterocolitica* may induce phagocytosis by HeLa cells. Pedersen *et al.* (1979) report that organisms which have been inactivated by 0·3% formalin or irradiated with ultraviolet light for 15 min still interact with HeLa cells, while heating bacteria at 100°C for 30 min completely inhibits invasion. These data imply that heat-labile components (perhaps proteins) on the *yersinia* envelope trigger uptake of these organisms.

Zink *et al.* (1980) found that a 41 Mdal plasmid is associated with the ability of *Y. enterocolitica* to evoke keratoconjunctivitis in the guinea pig eye (Sereny test), and a similar-sized plasmid is associated with virulence in *Y. pseudotuberculosis* (Gemski *et al.*, 1980b). *Y. enterocolitica* virulence plasmids are necessary for production of keratoconjunctivis, for translocation of organisms from the intestinal tract to the blood stream in mice (Gemski *et al.*, 1980a), for autoagglutination (Vesikari *et al.*, 1981), for gerbil lethality (Portnoy *et al.*, 1981), and for a cytotoxic effect in HEp-2 monolayers (Portnoy *et al*, 1981; Vesikari *et al.*, 1981). Obviously these plasmids encode crucial virulence determinants, but both Portnoy *et al.* (1981) and Vesikari *et al.* (1981) have conclusively shown that tissue culture cells are readily invaded by plasmid-free *Y. enterocolitica.* Thus the three polypeptides which appear in the outer membrane of plasmid-bearing yersiniae grown at 37°C have no apparent relationship to the invasive phenotype (Portnoy *et al.*, 1981).

(c) Shigella

The pathogenic potential of the etiological agent of bacillary dysentery is directly correlated with the ability to invade the colonic mucosa. This was established by LaBrec *et al.* (1964) who found that virulent *Shigella flexneri* elicit ulcerative lesions in the ileal mucosa of infected guinea pigs by invading epithelial cells. Takeuchi *et al.* (1965) used the guinea pig model to study shigella invasion by electron microscopy. They observed shigellae which were either free in the cytoplasm of ileal epithelial cells or were enclosed in membrane-bound vacuoles. These studies were extended to orally challenged rhesus monkeys which are natural hosts for *S. flexneri* 2a.

In the simian model intracellular organisms were found within colonic epithelial cells (Takeuchi *et al.*, 1968). As in the guinea pig, intracellular shigellae were found either enclosed in membrane-bound vacuoles or free in the cytoplasm. The presence of membrane-bound organisms implies an endocytic mode of entry, but the actual process of penetration was not observed in these studies.

Gerber and Watkins (1961), LaBrec *et al.* (1964), and Ogawa *et al.* (1967) have employed tissue culture monolayers as models of the intestinal epithelium, and they found that virulent strains of shigella readily invade these monolayers while avirulent strains do not. Ogawa *et al.* (1968) studied the process of invasion using phase-contrast time-lapse cinemicrography. They found that *S. flexneri* 2a attach to the surface of HeLa cells and evoke ruffling in the plasma membrane. Some of the attached shigellae are enfolded by the ruffles and incorporated into the host cell cytoplasm. Hale *et al.* (1979) studied the invasion of Henle 407 cells by *S. flexneri* 2a using electron microscopy and found shigellae either free in the cytoplasm or within membrane-bound vacuoles. Recently centrifugation has been employed to enhance the contact of shigellae with the host cell monolayer (Hale and Formal, 1981). Because most cells are infected at approximately the same time, the opportunity to observe the invasion process is greatly enhanced by this procedure. Figure 1 shows the invasion of a HeLa cell by *S. flexneri* 5. An *en bloc* procedure has been employed to label the acid mucosaccharides of the fixed HeLa cell membrane with colloidal thorium dioxide (Hale *et al.*, 1979). This process allows the demonstration of areas of close apposition between the invading bacterium and the host cell plasma membrane. These areas exclude the smallest thorotrast particles indicating that there is a gap of less than 13 nm (Ward *et al.*, 1975). The points of close contact between the surface of the bacterium and the host cell may represent areas of sequential ligand binding which induce uptake of the bacterium by a "zipper mechanism" (Griffin *et al.*, 1975).

The invasion of epithelial cells *in vitro* is inhibited by cytochalasin B, iodoacetate, and dinitrophenol (Hale *et al.*, 1979). Thus host cell microfilament function, glycolysis, and oxidative phosphorylation are required for uptake of shigellae. This process is also inhibited by elevated intracellular levels of cyclic adenosine monophosphate (Hale *et al.*, 1979), a condition which inhibits phagocytic activity in professional phagocytes. Since infection of HeLa cells which have been prelabelled with [3H] uridine does not cause leakage of labelled cytoplasmic constituents (Hale and Formal, 1980), the integrity of the plasma membrane is maintained throughout the invasion process. Thus both morphological and physiological evidence indicates that shigellae invade cultured epithelial cells by an endocytic process.

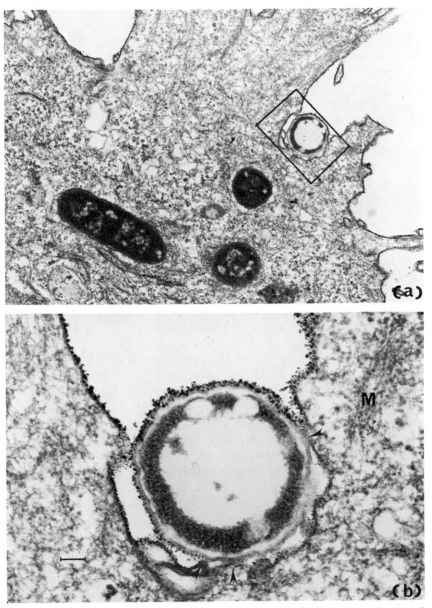

Fig. 1. Electron micrograph of HeLa cell infected with *Shigella flexneri* serotype 5, strain M90T. (a) Three intracellular shigellae are seen in the cytoplasma and one extracellular organism is in the process of invasion. (b) Higher magnification of the area outlined in (a). Arrows indicate areas of close apposition between the bacterium and the host cell. These areas exclude thorotrast particles which were added after fixation. The structure designated M is a microfilament bundle, and the clear areas within the bacterial cell appears to be a vesicular mesosome.

The role of shigellae in the induction of endocytic activity in normally non-phagocytic cells has been studied by Hale and Bonventre (1979). It was found that ultraviolet irradiation, kanamycin treatment, and mild heating (56°C for 3 min) substantially reduces the colony-forming ability and the infectivity of suspensions of *S. flexneri* 2a. These inactivated shigellae were overlaid on monolayers of Henle 407 cells and allowed to settle by gravity—a process which requires at least 1 hr (Hale and Bonventre, 1979). Recently these experiments were repeated using centrifugation to enhance the contact of inactivated *S. dysenteriae* 1 with HeLa cells, and it was found that lethal doses of ultraviolet radiation or kanamycin do not immediately destroy the ability of shigellae to infect host cells. Indeed, there was significant uptake of shigellae if the organisms were centrifuged onto host cells within 30 min of irradiation or kanamycin treatment (Hale, T. L., unpublished data). These observations indicate that shigellae are able to induce phagocytosis for a short period of time after incurring lethal damage to vital synthetic machinery. Pedersen *et al.* (1979) came to a similar conclusion using ultraviolet- or formalin-treated *Y. enterocolitica*. It could be speculated that there are heat-labile virulence determinants on the surface of invasive enteric pathogens which are degraded by endogenous proteases in non-viable cells.

In addition to proteins, there are LPS constituents on the surface of invasive Gram-negative pathogens. However, rough *S. flexneri* 2a mutants lacking O-polysaccharide repeat units readily invade HeLa cells (Okamura and Nakaya, 1977), and antiserum recognizing LPS does not inhibit uptake of smooth *S. flexneri* 2a (Hale and Bonventre, 1979). Apparently LPS O antigens are not necessary for the initiation of infection, but they are necessary for resistance to host defence mechanism. This is evident from the work of Okamura and Nakaya (1977), who found that a rough *S. flexneri* 2a strain which was invasive for HeLa cells did not evoke a positive Sereny test. Gemski *et al.* (1972) have constructed intergeneric hybrids of *S. flexneri* which express either *E. coli* O-25 or O-8 somatic antigen. Only hybrids which express O-25 are Sereny positive, so the chemical composition of the O-repeat unit may be a determining factor for survival of shigellae *in vivo*. However, it should be noted that these hybrids were constructed by conjugation, so genetic loci in addition to those which encode the enzymes necessary for O-8 somatic antigen synthesis may have been transferred to avirulent strains.

Osada *et al.* (1974 and 1975) reported that exogenous divalent cations are necessary for invasion of HeLa cells or the guinea pig corneal epithelium. They also found that *S. flexneri* 2a lost its virulence when grown in medium with reduced levels of divalent actions and suggested that such cations stabilized enzymes in the bacterial envelope which are involved in invasion (Osada *et al.*, 1975). The requirements for divalent cations may be strain specific because we have been unable to demonstrate it using different *S. flexneri* 2a strains (Hale, T. L., unpublished observations). Osada and Ogawa (1977a,b) have also reported that a glycolipid fraction can be extracted from culture medium in which virulent *S. flexneri* 2a have grown. This glycolipid fraction enhanced uptake of homologous formalin-killed shigellae by HeLa cells.

Izhar *et al.* (1982) have studied the adherence of *S. flexneri* to isolated intestinal epithelial cells *in vitro*. They found that shigellae have a definite affinity for colonic epithelial cells from the guinea pig. Colonic cells from rats, rabbits, and hamsters do not bind shigellae, and these animals are also resistant to oral challenge with shigellae. Adherence of these organisms was inhibited by pretreatment of guinea pig colonic epithelial cells with fucose, glucose, *S. flexneri* LPS, and proteolytic enzymes. These investigators concluded that *S. flexneri* adhere to a lectin-like protein on the surface of colonic epithelial cells via an LPS moiety. The specificity of fucose inhibition is puzzling because fucose has not been reported in *S. flexneri* 2a LPS (Simmons, 1971). The role of the colonic adhesion in the uptake of shigellae is uncertain, especially since the adhesin may be a constitutent of the extracellular mucin layer (Izhar *et al.*, 1982). There is also evidence that *S. flexneri* 4b produce extracellular glycosidases or proteases which modify the surface of colonic epithelium in a way which enhances shigella adherence (Prizont and Reed, 1980).

It has recently become apparent that shigellae harbour plasmids which are necessary for virulence. Sansonetti *et al.* (1981) have shown that the spontaneous transition of *S. sonnei* from the virulent form I serotype to the avirulent form II is associated with the loss of a large unstable plasmid. Reintroduction of this plasmid by conjugal mobilization into form II recipients restores lipopolysaccharide synthesis and the virulent phenotype. A plasmid of similar size (approximately 140000 daltons) has also been found in *S. flexneri* and in an invasive strain of *Escherchia coli*. These plasmids are not associated with O-antigen synthesis, but they are necessary for invasiveness in both the HeLa cell assay and the Sereny test (Sansonetti *et al.*, 1982a). The plasmid from *S. flexneri* serotype 5 will restore virulence in *S. flexneri* serotypes 1 and 3 and in an invasive *E. coli* strain (Sansonetti *et al.*, 1982b).

The products of these plasmids have been studied in anucleate minicells isolated from virulent strains of *S. flexneri, S. sonnei* and invasive *E. coli* (Hale, T. L., Sansonetti, P. J., Schad, P.A., Austin, S., and Formal, S. B., submitted for publication). Since *de novo* protein synthesis in minicells is encoded by plasmid DNA (Frazer and Curtiss, 1975, minicell proteins which label with [35S] methionine are assumed to be plasmid-encoded. A number of similar polypeptides are encoded by the virulence-associated plasmids of each species, and some of these polypeptides are probably key virulence determinants in the envelope. For example, three labelled polypeptides of 22 000, 24 000, and 25 000 are missing in the outer membrane of an avirulent *S. flexneri* 5 strain which has sustained a deletion in the 140 Mdal plasmid. It could be speculated that one or more of these polypeptides is a constituent of the putative receptor which induces the endocytic process seen in Fig. 1.

III. CONCLUDING REMARKS

The essence of this survey of invasive agents is presented in Tables 1 and 2. Perhaps the most striking feature of these tables is the frequent occurrence of the word "unknown". This reflects the great difficulty encountered when

Table 1 Invasion: role of the parasite

Agent	Surface ligand	Metabolic requirement	Inhibition by antibody	Exogenous products
Chlamydia	Heat-labile protein (?)	None	Yes	None
Rickettsia	138 000 protein	Oxidative phosphorylation	Yes	Unknown
Trypanosoma	Lectin-like protein	Unknown	Unknown	Unknown
Toxoplasma	Heat-labile protein (?)	Viability	Unknown	Enzymatic "penetration enhancing factor"
Leishmania	Carbohydrate (?)	Unknown	Unknown	Unknown
Plasmodium	Chymotrypsin-sensitive protein or glycoprotein	Unknown[a]	Yes	Unknown
Mycobacterium	Unknown	Unknown	Unknown	Unknown
Neisseria	Unknown	Unknown	Yes	Unknown
Salmonella	Mannose-resistant haemagglutinin (?)	Viability	None	Unknown
Yersinia	Heat-labile protein (?)	None[b]	Unknown	Unknown
Shigella	Heat-liable protein (?)[c]	None (?)[d]	None	Glycolipid (?)

[a] Cytobalasin B treatment inhibits invasiveness.
[b] Ultraviolet irradiation and formalin fixation does not inhibit invasiveness.
[c] May attach to colonic epithelial cells by glucose or frucose residues.
[d] Virulent shigellae remain invasive for a short period after exposure to ultraviolet radiation or kanomycin.

the interactions of two highly evolved biological entities must be understood. The morphological studies of invasion consistently indicate that an endocytic event is involved. Beyond this, the physiological and biochemical aspects of invasion have largely been defined using metabolic inhibitors and steric competitors.

Perhaps the most critical goal for future studies is the identification of ligands in the envelope of invasive parasites which induce endocytosis in the non-professional phagocyte. Neutralization or blocking of these ligands by antibody or by competitive inhibitors should provide protection against infection. Genetic analysis and monoclonal antibodies are two tools which should aid in the identification of these envelope components. Hopefully, these techniques will allow further definition of the process of tissue invasion on a molecular basis.

Table 2 Invasion: role of the host cell

Agent	Morphology of invasion	Receptors	Metabolic req.	Inhibition by cytochalasin B[a]
Chlamydia	Endocytosis	Glycoproteins (N-acetyl-D-glucosamine, N-acetylineuramic acid)	Oxidative phosphorylation	None
Rickettsia	Unknown	Cholesterol[b]	Glycolysis	Yes
Trypanosoma	Endocytosis	Glycoproteins (N-acetyl-D-glucosamine)	Unknown	Yes
Toxoplasma	Endocytosis	Unknown	Unknown	Yes
Leishmania	Endocytosis	Unknown	Unknown	Unknown
Plasmodium[c]	Endocytosis	Duffy blood group antigens; glycophorin A	Unknown	Unknown
Mycobacterium	Unknown	Unknown	Unknown	Unknown
Neisseria	Endocytosis	Unknown	Unknown	Unknown
Salmonella	Endocytosis	Unknown	Glycolysis; oxidative phosphorylation	Yes
Yersinia	Endocytosis	Unknown	Unknown	Unknown
Shigella	Endocytosis	Lectin-like protein (?)[d]	Oxidative phosphorylation; glycolysis	Yes

[a] Indicator of microfilament function (also inhibits glucose transport).
[b] Erythrocyte receptor for rickettsiae (other receptors unknown).
[c] Merozoite form (erythrocyte host cell).
[d] Mediates adherence to colonial epithelial cells (may be mucin and not directly involved in invasion).

IV. REFERENCES

Aikawa, M., Miller, L. H., Rabbege, J. R. and Epstein, N. (1981). *J. Cell Biol.* **91**, 55–62.

Axline, S. G. and Reaven, E. P. (1974). *J. Cell. Biol.* **62**, 647–659.
Bovallius, A. and Nilsson, G. (1975). *Can. J. Microbiol.* **21**, 1997–2007.
Byrne, G. I. (1976). *Infect. Immun.* **14**, 645–651.
Caldwell, H. D. and Schachter, J. (1982). *Infect. Immun.* **35**, 1024–1031.
Chang, K. P. (1978). *Amer. J. Trop. Med. Hyg.* **27**, 1084–1096.
Chang, K. P. (1979). *Exp. Parasitol.* **48**, 175–189.
Chang, K. P. (1981). *Mol. Biochem. Parasitol.* **4**, 67–76.
Cohn, Z. A., Bozeman, F. M., Campbell, J. M., Humphries, J. W. and Sawyer, T. K. (1959). *J. Exp. Med.* **109**, 271–292.
Crane, M. St. J. and Dvorak, J. A. (1982). *Mol. Biochem. Parasitol.* **5**, 333–341.
Cross, G. A. M. and Johnson, J. G. (1976). *In* "Biochemistry of Parasites and Host-parasite Relationships" (H. Von Den Bossche, ed.) pp. 413–421. North-Holland Publishing Co., New York.
Dankert, J. and Hofstra, H. (1978). *J. Gen. Microbiol.* **104**, 311–320.
Dvorak, J. A. and Crane, M. St. J. (1981). *Science* **214**, 1034–1036.
Eisemann, C. S. and Osterman, J. V. (1976). *Infect. Immun.* **14**, 155–162.
Epstein, N., Miller, L. H., Kaushel, D. C., Udeinya, I. J., Rener, J., Howard, R. J., Asofksy, R., Alkawa, M. and Hess, R. L. (1981). *J. Immunol.* **127**, 212–217.
Frazer, A. C. and Curtiss, R. (1975). *Curr. Top. Microbiol. Immunol.* **69**, 1–84.
Friis, R. R. (1972). *J. Bacteriol.* **110**, 706–721.
Gemski, P., Sheahan, D. G., Washington, O. and Formal, S. B. (1972). *Infect. Immun.* **6**, 104–111.
Gemski, P., Lazere, J. R. and Casey, T. (1980a). *Infect. Immun.* **27**, 682–685.
Gemski, P., Lazere, J. R., Casey T. and Wohlhieter, J. A. (1980b). *Infect. Immun.* **28**, 1044–1047.
Gerber, D. F. and Watkins, H. M. S. (1961). *J. Bacteriol.* **82**, 815–822.
Giannella, R. A., Washington, O., Gemski, P. and Formal, S. B. (1973). *J. Infect. Dis.* **128**, 69–75.
Gregory, W. W., Byrne, G., Gardner, M. and Moulder, J. W. (1979). *Infect. Immun.* **25**, 463–466.
Griffin, F. M., Jr., Griffin, J. A., Leider, J. E. and Silverstein, S. C. (1975). *J. Exp. Med.* **142**, 1263–1282.
Hale, T. J. and Bonventre, P. F. (1979). *Infect. Immun.* **24**, 879–886.
Hale, T. L. and Formal, S. B. (1980). *Amer. J. Clin. Nutr.* **33**, 2485–2490.
Hale, T. L. and Formal, S. B. (1981). *Infect. Immun.* **32**, 137–144.
Hale, T. L., Morris, R. E. and Bonventre, P. F. (1979). *Infect. Immun.* **24**, 887–894.
Hartwig, J. H. and Stossel, T. P. (1979). *J. Mol. Biol.* **134**, 539–554.
Henriquez, D., Piras, R. and Piras, M. M. (1981). *Mol. Biochem. Parasitol.* **2**, 359–366.
Izhar, M., Nuchamowitz, Y. and Mirelman, D. (1982). *Infect. Immun.* **35**, 1110–1118.
Jones, G. W. (1977). *In* "*Microbiol Interactions*, Receptors and Recognition" (J. L. Reissig, ed.) Series B, Vol. 3, pp. 141–176. Chapman and Hall, London.
Jones, G. W. and Richardson, L. A. (1981). *J. Gen. Microbiol.* **127**, 36–37.
Jones, G. W., Richardson, L. A. and Uhlman, D. (1981). *J. Gen. Microbiol.* **127**, 351–360.
Jones, T. C., Yeh, S. and Hirsh, J. G. (1972). *J. Exp. Med.* **136**, 1157–1172.
Kamio, Y. and Nikaido, H. (1977). *Biochem. Biophys. Acta* **404**, 589–601.
Kenny, C. P. and Aris, B. J. (1969). *Can J. Public Health* **60**, 34.

Kihlstrom, E. (1977). *Infect. Immun.* **17**, 290–295.

Kihlstrom, E. (1979). *FEMS Lett.* **5**, 439–441.

Kihlstrom, E. (1980). *Am. J. Clin. Nutr.* **33**, 2491–2501.

Kihlstrom, E. and Edebo, L. (1976). *Infect. Immun.* **14**, 851–857.

Kihlstrom, E. and Latkovic, S. (1978). *Infect. Immun.* **22**, 804–809.

Kihlstrom, E. and Nilsson, L. (1977). *Acta Path. Microbiol. Scand. Sect. B* **85**, 322–328.

King, G. J and Swanson, J. (1978). *Infect. Immun.* **21**, 575–584.

Kuo, C., Wang, S. and Grayston, J. T. (1973). *Infect. Immun.* **8**, 74–79.

LaBrec, E. H., Schneider, H., Magnani, T. J. and Formal, S. B. (1964). *J. Bacteriol.* **88**, 1503–1518.

Levy, N. J. (1979). *Infect. Immun.* **25**, 946–953.

Lee, W. H., McGrath, P. P., Carter, P. H. and Eido, E. L. (1977). *Can. J. Microbiol.* **23**, 1714–1722.

Lindberg, A. A. (1980). *Scand. J. Infect. Dis.* Suppl. 24, 86–92.

Lycke, E., Carlberg, K. and Norrby, R. (1975). *Infect. Immun.* **11**, 853–861.

Maki, M., Gronroos, P. and Vesikari, T. (1978). *J. Infect. Dis.* **138**, 677–680.

Miller, L. H., Aikawa, M., Johnson, J. G. and Shiroishi, T. (1979). *J. Exp. Med.* **149**, 172–184.

Nogueira, N. and Cohn, Z. (1976). *J. Exp. Med.* **143**, 1402–1420.

Okamura, N. and Nakaya, R. (1977). *Infect. Immun.,* **17**, 4–8.

Ogawa, H., Nakamura, A., Nakaya, R., Mise, K., Honjo, S., Takasaka, M., Fijuwara, T. and Imaizumi, K. (1967). *Jpn. J. Med. Sci. Biol.* **20**, 315–328.

Ogawa, H., Nakamura, A. and Nakaya, R. (1968). *Jpn. J. Med. Sci. Biol.* **21**, 259–273.

Osada, Y. and Ogawa, H. (1977a). *Microbiol. Immunol.* **21**, 49–55.

Osada, Y. and Ogawa, H. (1977b). *Microbiol. Immunol.* **21**, 405–410.

Osada, Y., Une, T. Ikeuchi, T. and Ogawa, H. (1974). *Jpn. J. Microbiol.* **18**, 321–326.

Osada, Y., Une, T., Ikeuchi, T. and Ogawa, H. (1975). *Jpn. J. Microbiol.* **19**, 163–166.

Owen, R., Farnham, A. E., Saito, K., Milofksy, E. and Karnovsky, M. L. (1963). *J. Cell. Biol.* **17**, 487–501.

Pedersen, K. B., Winblod, S. and Bitsch, V. (1979). *Acta Path. Microbiol. Scand. Sect. B* **87**, 141–145.

Perkins, M. (1981). *J. Cell Biol.* **90**, 563–567.

Prizont, R. and Reed, W. P. (1980). *Infect. Immun.* **29**, 1197–1199.

Portnoy, D. A., Moseley, S. L. and Falkow, S. (1981). *Infect. Immun.* **31**, 775–782.

Ramm, L. E. and Winkler, H. H. (1973). *Infect. Immun.* **7**, 550–555.

Ramm, L. E. and Winkler, H. H. (1976). *Infect. Immun.* **13**, 120–126.

Rikihisa, Y. and Ito, S. (1980). *Infect. Immun.* **30**, 231–243.

Salari, S. H. and Ward, M. E. (1981). *J. Gen. Microbiol.* **123**, 197–207.

Sansonetti, P. J., Kopecko, D. J. and Formal, S. B. (1981). *Infect. Immun.* **34**, 75–83.

Sansonetti, P. J., Kopecko, D. J. and Formal, S. B. (1982a). *Infect. Immun.* **35**, 852–860.

Sansonetti, P. J., D'Hauteville, H., Formal, S. B. and Toucas, M. (1982b). *Inst. Pasteur* **132A**, 351–355.

Shepard, C. C. (1955). *Proc. Soc. Exp. Biol. Med.* **90**, 392–396.

Shepard, C. C. (1957). *J. Exp. Med.* **105**, 39–47.

Sherman, I. W. (1979). *Microbiol. Rev.* **43**, 453–495.
Sheterline, P. and Hopkins, C. R. (1981). *J. Cell Biol.* **90**, 743–754.
Silverman, D. J., Wisseman, C. L., Waddell, A. D. and Jones, M. (1978). *Infect. Immun.* **22**, 233–246.
Simmons, D. A. R. (1971). *Bacteriol. Rev.* **35**, 117–148.
Smith, D. K. and Winkler, H. H. (1980). *Infect. Immun.* **29**, 831–834.
Soderlund, G. and Kihlstrom, E. (1982). *Infect. Immun.* **36**, 893–899.
Stossel, T. P. and Hartwig, J. H. (1976). *J. Cell Biol.* **83**, 602–619.
Swanson, J. (1973). *J. Exp. Med.* **137**, 571–589.
Swanson, J., Sparks, E., Young, D. and King, G. (1975). *Infect. Immun.* **11**, 1352–1361.
Takeuchi, A. (1967). *Am. J. Pathol.* **50**, 109–136.
Takeuchi, A., Spring, H., LaBrec, E. H. and Formal, S. B. (1965). *Amer. J. Pathol.* **47**, 1011–1044.
Takeuchi, A., Formal, S. B. and Spring, H. (1968). *Amer. J. Pathol.* **52**, 503–520.
Tannock, G. W., Blumershine, R. V. H. and Savage, D. C. (1975). *Infect. Immun.* **11**, 365–370.
Thayer, J. D., Perry, M. I., Field, F. W. and Garson, W. (1957). *Antibiol. Ann.* 513–517.
Turco, J. and Winkler, H. H. (1982). *Infect. Immun.* **35**, 783–791.
Uhlman, D. L. and Jones, G. W. (1982). *J. Gen. Microbiol.* **128**, 415–418.
Vesikari, T., Nurmii, T., Maki, M., Skurnik, M., Sundqvist, C., Granfors, K. and Gronroos, P. (1981). *Infect. Immun.* **33**, 870–876.
Waitkins, S. A. and Flynn, J. (1973). *J. Med. Microbiol.* **6**, 399–403.
Walker, S. T. and Winkler, H. H. (1978). *Infect. Immun.* **22**, 200–208.
Ward, M. E., Robertson, J. N., Englefield, P. M. and Watt, P. J. (1975). *In* "Microbiology 1975" (D. Schlessinger, ed.) pp. 188–199. Amer. Soc. for Micro., Washington, DC.
Wisseman, C. L., Jr., Waddell, A. D. and Silverman, D. J. (1976). *Infect. Immun.* **13**, 1749–1760.
Zink, D. L., Feelery, J. C., Wells, J. G., Vanderzant, C., Vickery, J. C., Roof, W. D. and O'Donovan, G. A. (1980). *Nature,* **283**, 224–226.

5 Bacterial envelope and humoral defences

C. W. PENN

I. INTRODUCTION

In order to succeed in infection, most bacteria produce outer layers or envelope components in addition to those strictly necessary for their survival in non-selective environments *in vitro*. It is essentially the exposed outer surface of the bacterial cell, as presented for interaction with host defence systems, which will affect the survival of bacteria in infection, and those surface components which interact with humoral defences to enhance survival in infection are the main concern of this review. Clearly the envelope components which are the targets for host defences in the unsuccessful bacterial invader must also be considered and understood. It is assumed that infection will in general take place only in the non-immune host, and so it is the non-specific host defences with which we are mainly concerned, but the essential role of natural antibody in host defence and the ability of a successful pathogen to counteract early specific immune responses require that antibody should be considered an essential part of the normal humoral defences.

The humoral, i.e. soluble, factors of the host defences are of fundamental importance in determining the outcome of confrontation between the bacterium and the host, not only in humoral bacterial killing but also because reactions with humoral factors often precede subsequent processes such as adhesion to host tissues or phagocytosis which depend on contact between bacteria and host cell surfaces. The interaction of bacteria with humoral factors leading to bacterial death cannot be considered in isolation, since the same factors are involved in opsonization before phagocytosis, and these two effectors of bacterial elimination often cannot

MEDICAL MICROBIOLOGY, 3
ISBN 0 12 228003 3

be distinguished *in vivo*. Opsonizing effects of humoral interactions will therefore be included in this review. It appears helpful first to review current knowledge of the humoral factors of the host, and then to consider the interaction of these with bacterial surface components.

II. HOST FACTORS

A. Antibody

Historically blood serum antibodies, with complement, were the first of the serum proteins to be investigated in detail in relation to their specific antibacterial actions, and the science of immunology was founded largely on the serological study of antibodies and their reactions with bacterial antigens, especially toxins.

Modern immunochemistry has defined five major classes of antibody, IgA, IgD, IgE, IgG and IgM. The first, IgA, has only been recognized as a major host defence during the past 20 years, following its recognition as gamma A immunoglobulin by Heremans *et al.* (1959). The secretory form sIgA, an 11S dimer containing secretory component (SC) is now known to be a major component of antibody found in mucosal secretions (Tomasi and Bienenstock, 1968; Tomasi, 1976), a conceptual advance in view of the commitment to serology of the previous half century. The antibacterial potential of IgA appears limited however. Many reports of its failure to fix complement (e.g. Adinolfi *et al.*, 1966a; Steele *et al.*, 1974; Heddle and Rowley, 1975) were countered only by those of Gotze and Muller-Eberhard (1971) and Burritt *et al.* (1977). The opsonizing activity of IgA has been similarly controversial. Some of these contradictions may have resulted from contamination of IgA preparations by IgM (Rogers and Synge, 1978). Undoubtedly IgA has a greatly reduced activity in bactericidal or opsonic mechanisms compared with IgG or IgM, and the major antibacterial function of IgA appears to be its ability to inhibit the adhesion of bacteria to mucosal surfaces (Williams and Gibbons, 1972; Tomasi, 1976) which is considered elsewhere in this symposium. In addition, a combination of IgA, complement and lysozyme is reported to be bactericidal (Adinolfi *et al.*, 1966b; Hill and Porter, 1971). It should be emphasized, though, that complement is sparse in external secretions (Jonas and Broad, 1972), and conditions on many mucosal surfaces would not favour its activity. A more recent development in the study of IgA has been the observation that, at least in the rat, it is preferentially transported from serum into bile, so that it is available in high concentration in intestinal secretions (Jackson *et al.*, 1978; Orlans *et al.*, 1978; Hall and Andrew, 1980). Serum IgA is a 7S monomer or 10S dimer without SC, and is largely derived from lymphatic drainage of the intestinal lamina propria and mesenteric lymph nodes where many IgA forming plasma cells are found. The transepithelial transport of IgA probably involves its interaction with SC (Brandtzaeg and Baklien, 1977), so that it is complexed with SC in the secretions. It should be emphasized that by far the greatest number of bacteria with which the host comes into intimate contact is in the gut—the major site of encounter with foreign antigens in the normal, intact animal. Thus a shift of attention of students of the immunoglobulins from the serum to the external secretions has led to important advances in our understanding of natural antigenic stimuli: the passage of antigens across the mucosa, probably via specialized cuboidal epithelium overlying the Peyer's patches and lymphoid nodules, to stimulate this extensive gut-associated lymphoid tissue—GALT (Perey and Milne, 1975).

Immunoglobulins D and E are quantitatively minor components of the total serum immunoglobulin, and have not been shown to have any antibacterial activity. IgD has been implicated as a B lymphocyte surface immunoglobulin, probably functioning as an antigen receptor, and IgE is known principally for mediating atopic allergy (type I hypersensitivity) and is thought to function in immunity to enteric parasitic infections.

Immunoglobulin G is the principle immunoglobulin in the bloodstream. Owing to its small size it also diffuses rapidly into the tissues following injury or damage and is the only immunoglobulin able to cross the placenta in those species in which such transfer to the fetus occurs. In these situations, then, IgG is clearly a vital element of host defence, and it is functional in the major antibacterial mechanisms of opsonization (both by direct interaction of the Fc portion of antigen-bound IgG to Fc receptors on phagocytes, and indirectly by fixation of complement which also opsonizes), and complement-mediated bacterial killing. Subclasses of IgG have been described which differ in their biological properties (Spiegelberg, 1974). In the human, IgG4 (the least abundant) does not fix complement efficiently and is the only subclass able to block IgE binding to mast cells. IgG2 does not cross the placenta, and is often the dominant subclass of specific IgG antibody to polysaccharide antigens such as dextran. As yet no differences in the antibacterial activity of these subclasses appear to have been described, although only IgG1 and IgG3 are able to opsonize by binding to Fc receptors on phagocytes (Griffin, 1977). In the bovine, IgG1 is preferentially transported across the mammary epithelium into milk (Tomasi, 1976).

Immunoglobulin M is of particular interest to the bacteriologist for its occurrence as natural antibody. Much knowledge of the course of the serum antibody response, especially to protein antigens, is derived from experiments in which discrete antigenic stimuli are given parenterally, leading after a few days to a rapid early (primary) rise in specific antibody, which is initially IgM. A few days later specific IgG also appears. If a second dose of antigen is given a few weeks later, a rapid rise in specific antibody again results, which is predominantly IgG and of greater magnitude and duration—the secondary response resulting from "memory" of the primary response. However, most natural contact with external antigenic stimuli is more continuous and is with the intestinal contents. The most stimulatory antigens appear to be bacterial, and these are thought to be responsible for the large repertoire of "natural" antibody specificities present in low titre in the blood of normal individuals and occurring particularly in the IgM class (Michael and Rosen, 1963; Schoolnik *et al.*, 1979). It is possible that the predominance of the IgM class in natural antibody results from a constant turnover of indigenous microflora as each antigenic type is eliminated by immune mechanisms (Shedlofsky and Freter, 1974) leading to exposure to a succession of new antigens each causing a primary IgM antibody response. (Whether such "priming" would impart an element of memory to the response to the "first" contact with cross-reacting antigens is not clear.) However, many of the bacterial antigens responsible, such as lipopolysaccharide (LPS) are thymus-independent and preferentially stimulate IgM antibody responses; they may also be non-specific B-lymphocyte mitogens (Coutinho and Moller, 1975). In any event, the wide range of antibody specificities produced are capable of reacting at low titre, with low affinity and presumably often by cross-reactions, with many of the antigens of potential bacterial pathogens. It should be remembered that IgG and IgA fractions may also contain significant amounts of natural antibody and that the concepts of the role of IgM as natural antibody and as the main component of the primary response are generalizations (Cohen and Norins, 1966). However, the high efficiency of IgM in fixing complement, coupled with its frequent presence as natural antibody and early synthesis after specific stimulation, make it an important first line of defence, particularly against bacteremia, as it is too large to diffuse readily from the bloodstream into the tissues. The intrinsic opsonizing activity of IgM by virtue of its interaction with Fc receptors on phagocytes has not been shown. It has been reported (Brandtzaeg, 1975) that IgM may complex with SC to form a secretory immunoglobulin, and in IgA-deficient individuals IgM may take over the role of major secretory immunoglobulin.

B. Complement

Since the discovery by Bordet at the end of the last century that a heat-labile component, present in normal as well as in immune serum (i.e. immunologically non-specific) was required in addition to a heat-stable specific component (antibody) for serum killing of *Vibrio cholerae,* much has been learned about the complement system. This cascade sequence of enzymic reactions controlled by a complex set of inhibition and amplification factors is now known to comprise three main sectors: the classical and alternative pathways of activation of the crucial C3 component, and the terminal "lytic" sequence from C5 to C9—the late components—common to both pathways.

The classical pathway of complement activation (Porter, 1977) in conjunction with antibody has until quite recently been more thoroughly investigated than the alternate pathway. The first component in the sequence is C1q, which is part of the C1 complex (requiring Ca^{2+} and Mg^{2+} for its integrity). C1q has six spatially separated binding sites, and binds to Fc portions of antigen-complexed antibody, and more than one Fc must bind before activation of C1r and C1s takes place. This accounts for the far greater efficiency of pentamer IgM over monomer IgG (only one Fc portion) in activating complement: two molecules of the latter would have to be bound to antigen in close proximity, whereas every molecule of bound IgM would be effective on its own. Fixed C1 then activates C4 and C2 which complex together to form C42, a C3 convertase which mediates the activation of C3 to C3b, central to both the classical and alternative pathways and responsible, with the other fragment C3a, for many of the biological effects of complement activation, as well as leading to activation of the terminal sequence.

Recent interest by bacteriologists has focused particularly on activation of complement by the alternative pathway, initiated by some bacterial components in the absence of specific antibody (Fearson and Austen, 1980). A factor originally designated properdin by Pillemer in the 1950s and now known to be a group of proteins, was subsequently almost ignored for a decade until their role in the activation of complement by endotoxin in the absence of antibody was demonstrated (Mergenhagen *et al.*, 1969). Major components of the alternative pathway are factors B and D, properdin and C3 which itself takes part in a feedback loop resulting in its own further activation. Mg^{2+}, but not Ca^{2+}, is required. This is the rationale for the use of the chelator ethyleneglycol-bis-(β-aminoethyl-ether)-tetra-acetic acid (EGTA) which has a higher affinity for Ca^{2+} than for Mg^{2+} in the inhibition of complement reactions: the classical pathway should be preferentially inhibited due to its requirement for both divalent cations. Initiation of the alternative pathway depends on amplification (in the presence of suitable surfaces provided by activating substances) of the slow spontaneous activation of C3. This amplification, resulting from reaction of spontaneously formed C3b with Bb (produced from B by the action of D) to form the amplification C3 convertase C3bBb, is normally held in check by the control proteins β1H and C3b inactivator, but on binding of spontaneously formed C3b to an activating substance, the action of the inhibitors is retarded. Properdin stabilizes C3bBb by retarding its dissociation. Again the crucial step is the formation of C3b, leading to biological activity and activation of the terminal sequence. It should be noted that action of the inhibitory protein β1H on surface-bound C3b is aided by sialic acid, often absent from efficient alternative pathway activators but often present on mammalian cell surfaces (Fearon and Austen, 1980).

In the terminal sequence, C3b with either C42 or C3bBb coordinates with and activates C5 to give C5a, a small biologically active peptide, and C5b. The latter is critical for initiation of the lytic sequence, forming initially C5b67 by complexing with C6 and C7. This complex can insert into the lipid portion of a membrane under attack, and subsequently bind C8 and C9 to form the complete lytic complex.

The exact nature of the lesion formed, and its physiological effect on bacterial cells, are unknown. Electron microscopy of negatively stained red cells or bacterial membranes after interaction with antibody and complement shows the appearance of characteristic "pits" or holes of uniform (9 nm diameter) in the membrane (Bladen et al., 1967; Humphrey and Dourmashkin, 1970; Gewurz et al., 1971). It is debatable though whether these are actual holes: they are more likely the images of doughnut-shaped terminal complexes and may be at least partly protruding from the membrane rather than embedded in it (Opferkuch and Segerling, 1977). It appears that membrane damage is the primary lesion, perhaps from insertion of modified lipids into the membrane by the complement complex (Dourmashkin et al., 1972). An early biochemical event in the killing of bacteria by complement seems to be inhibition of RNA synthesis (Griffiths, 1971; Melching and Vas, 1971), and respiration is also rapidly inhibited (Pruul and Reynolds, 1972). The actual location of the lethal lesion of complement is also unclear. (Since Gram-positive bacteria are generally resistant to the action of complement, this discussion applies to the Gram-negatives.) Clearly the outer membrane can be severely damaged (see below), but outer membrane integrity should not be essential for bacterial survival, since spheroplasts and L-forms survive in appropriate media (Guze, 1968). Outer membrane damage may be critical in allowing access to internal targets, for example to the peptidoglycan layer for attack by lysozyme and thence to the cytoplasmic membrane for further attack by complement (Freer and Salton, 1971; Reynolds and Pruul, 1971). Certainly the cytoplasmic membrane of spheroplasts of both Gram-positive and Gram-negative bacteria (Muschel and Jackson, 1966; Muschel, 1968) and L-forms (McGee et al., 1972) is liable to attack by complement, and damage to the cytoplasmic membrane of unmodified Gram-negative bacteria following complement killing has also been reported (Wilson and Spitznagel, 1968; Wright and Levine, 1981). It also appears likely that complement damage to the outer membrane, alone or in combination with the effects of lysozyme on the peptidoglycan layer, may often be lethal because of resulting osmotic disruption, perhaps without complement-mediated damage to the cytoplasmic membrane (Wardlaw, 1962; Swanson and Goldschneider, 1969; Olling, 1977). These questions have long been considered (Glynn and Milne, 1967; Freer and Salton, 1971; Muschel and Fong, 1977) but have not yet been fully answered; it is likely that there are several possible sites for damage, and bacterial killing may result from combined attack by variable and multiple factors.

The biological activities of some of the cleavage products of complement proteins, generated during activation of the pathway, are important in activation of other aspects of the host defence system (Opferkuch and Segerling, 1977; Taussig, 1980). C2 generates a C2 kinin which leads to vasodilation and increased vascular permeability. The smaller fragments C3a and C5a are important mediators of the inflammatory response through anaphylatoxic activity, releasing histamine from mast cells. C5 is chemotactic for neutrophils. In addition, the large opsonic fragment C3b is also capable of binding to receptors on platelets leading to their aggregation and the release from them of other inflammatory mediators. The diverse activities of complement products must affect the outcome of bacterial infection if complement is activated and it may well be to the advantage of pathogenic bacteria to avoid setting these effects in motion. This avoidance could result either from presentation of an inert surface layer, such as appears to exist on *Treponema pallidum* (Fitzgerald, 1981; Penn and Lichfield, 1982; Penn and Rhodes, 1982), or by the elaboration of substances able to inhibit the complement pathway, for example an elastase produced by *Pseudomonas aeruginosa* which was shown to destroy several of the components (Schultz and Miller, 1974). It may also be postulated that the release of large amounts of material able to consume complement, for example lipopolysaccharide (LPS), into the surrounding medium might inactivate the pathway before it could reach its target. In this case, the ability to activate complement by the alternative pathway non-specifically would be advantageous to the organism.

Although killing of bacteria by complement has often been shown *in vitro*, its significance *in vivo* is difficult to assess because of the complexity of the host defence system (Davis *et al.*, 1972; Muschel and Fong, 1977; Frank, 1980). It is difficult to distinguish the effects of opsonization by early complement components leading to bacterial killing *in vivo* from those of purely humoral killing following attack by the late sequence. Some indications have come from observations of complement deficiency in animals and humans, but these are often inconsistent. In general, increases in susceptibility to infection resulting from deficiencies are not highly lethal (Gigli, 1977), especially if early components are involved, probably because of the existence of the two convergent early pathways. A patient with C3 deficiency was, however, liable to frequent Gram-negative infection (Alper et al., 1970), and deficiencies of later components C6, C7 and C8 are associated with increased risk of disseminated gonococcal and meningococcal infections (Leddy et al., 1974; Petersen et al., 1976; Lee et al., 1978; Braude, 1981).

In comparison with antibody, we have much to learn about the complement system and its interactions with bacteria. Differences in methodology of workers on in vitro aspects—bacterial species and strains, growth phase and growth conditions (Melching and Vas, 1971; Taylor, 1978), bacterial concentration, serum sources and concentrations for both complement and antibody—have often made the interpretation and correlation of results difficult (Muschel and Fong, 1977). The presence of natural antibody in sera used as complement source is an obvious example which may lead to erroneous definition of antibody specificity required for killing a certain strain, avoidable by the use of agammaglobulinaemic sera (Brooks et al., 1976) or purified complement components (Leist-Welsh and Bjornson, 1982).

As well as the well-defined classical, antibody-dependent and alternative, antibody-independent pathways described above, the classical components may also be activated by bacteria in the absence of antibody (Betz and Isliker, 1981; Clas and Loos, 1981; Baker et al., 1982; Leist-Welsh and Bjornson, 1982), and there may be antibody involvement in the alternate pathway (Winkelstein and Shin, 1974; Tarr et al., 1982). Thus generalization and extrapolation about the mechanism of action of complement upon bacteria, from one antigen on one bacterial species to another situation, is likely to be misleading.

C.   Enzymes and other factors

Heat stable bactericidal substances distinct from the antibody-complement system were originally termed β-lysin (Donaldson and Tew, 1977; Carroll and Martinez, 1979) and were the principle humoral components active against Gram-positive bacteria. Their activity was greater in, for example, rat and rabbit sera than in guinea-pig or human sera. Subsequently, the action of lysozyme was distinguished from that of other heat-stable factors by either adsorption with bentonite, which preferentially removed lysozyme but may have affected other serum proteins as well, or neutralization of lysozyme by specific anti-lysozyme immunoglobulin. Antibacterial action of both lysozyme and additional substances was shown, although lysozyme was unable to attack Gram-negative bacteria in the absence of antibody and complement (Glynn and Milne, 1967; Selsted and Martinez, 1978). Lysozyme is active in the lysis (i.e. conversion to ghosts) of *Escherichia coli* after killing by other serum factors (Martinez and Carroll, 1980), and it has been implicated in bactericidal activity of IgA in conjunction with complement by some workers (Adinolfi *et al.*, 1966b; Hill and Porter, 1971) but not others (Heddle *et al.*, 1975). Purified β-lysin (Donaldson *et al.*, 1964) which contributed to serum killing of *E. coli* (Donaldson *et al.*, 1974) was shown to contain several components (Carroll and Martinez, 1979). Much remains to be learned about these substances; some confusion in earlier work resulted from extrapolation between different host species and bacterial test strains.

Fibronectin in its soluble form is another *non-specific humoral factor (reviewed by Mosher, 1980) which may have important antibacterial activity. It is reported to opsonize (Saba and Jaffe, 1980) and to interact with complement components (Harris *et al.*, 1981; Isliker *et al.*, 1982) and has also been shown to bind to bacteria, for example to *Staphylococcus aureus* (Doran and Raynor, 1981) causing clumping (Espersen and Clemmensen, 1981) distinct from that mediated by fibrinogen. A fibronectin receptor has now been isolated from *S. aureus* (Espersen and Clemmensen, 1982).

An acute phase protein which has long interested bacteriologists is C-reactive protein (CRP), originally demonstrated by its ability to precipitate the pneumococcal cell wall C-polysaccharide. Recently a protective role for CRP against *Streptococcus pneumoniae* infection in mice (Mold *et al.*, 1981) and the enhancement of inflammation (Ahlstedt, 1980) and activation of complement by CRP (Edwards *et al.*, 1982a) have been demonstrated, suggesting that this protein may function as a non-specific humoral antibacterial substance.

III. BACTERIAL ENVELOPE COMPONENTS

A. Cell wall

The basic cell wall backbone is the peptidoglycan network which is a "unimolecular" bag-shaped macromolecule surrounding the entire bacterium. It is a monolayer and a relatively minor constituent in most Gram-negative bacterial cell walls, but a more substantial three-dimensional structure which may be covalently linked to teichoic acid, polysaccharide or protein in Gram-positives. Peptidoglycan consists of polysaccharide chains of alternating N-acetylglucosamine and N-acetylmuramic acid, cross linked through pentapeptide chains containing D- and L-alanine, glutamic acid and usually lysine, ornithine or diaminopimelic acid (Rogers et al., 1980; Ghuysen et al., 1968; Tipper and Wright, 1979). These reviews describe our very detailed knowledge of the biochemistry of peptidoglycan and associated macromolecules such as teichoic acids, but we know surprisingly little about their function and role in infection. Exposed peptidoglycan would presumably be liable to attack by lysozyme, and teichoic acids are said to protect against this (Wilson and Miles, 1975). O-acetylation of peptidoglycan also gives some protection against lysozyme activity (Rosenthal et al., 1982). Stewart-Tull (1980) has reviewed immunological aspects and the potent inflammatory properties of peptidoglycan constituents. Peterson et al. (1978) showed that peptidoglycan is the prime target for opsonization of staphylococci, probably through the activation of complement. Winkelstein and Tomasz (1977) reported the activation of the alternative pathway by pneumococcal cell walls, and Greenblatt et al. (1978) showed that streptococcal peptidoglycan was very active in this respect, provided it was not broken down to small fragments by lysozyme or ultrasonification. Among Gram-negatives, release of peptidoglycan fragments has been described by Rosenthal (1979), and complement consumption by gonococcal peptidoglycan was subsequently demonstrated by Petersen and Rosenthal (1982) who also reviewed the interaction of peptidoglycan with the complement system. The importance of lysozyme in the physical lysis of Gram-negative bacteria, which may occur after bacterial death, has been shown (see above), and lysozyme itself may also enhance killing. Clearly it may be disadvantageous to the organism in infection to have peptidoglycan exposed on the surface, although Hill (1968) reported that a peptidoglycan–protein complex from skin-virulent staphylococci suppressed aspects of the inflammatory response, which may be important in some staphylococcal infections (Easmon, 1981).

Other wall components which may interact with humoral defences are the C polysaccharide of pneumococci, reactive with C-reactive protein (see above), and the M proteins of streptococci. The latter inhibit phagocytosis (Lancefield, 1962) again probably by masking reactive components such as peptidoglycan by the formation of an external layer somewhat analogous to a capsule (Swanson et al., 1969). The protein A of S. aureus strains (Grov et al., 1964), present in cell walls of most strains and able to combine specifically with the Fc portion of IgG (Forsgren and Sjoquist, 1966) has been shown to interfere with phagocytosis of staphylococci (Dossett et al., 1969) probably by complexing extracellularly with both IgG and complement which it is able to activate (Peterson *et al.*, 1977; Quie *et al.*, 1981).

Considerable further work is needed to define the role in virulence of interactions between cell wall components and host defence mechanisms in Gram-positive bacteria, a field which has perhaps been eclipsed by the rapid developments in studies of the Gram-negative outer membrane.

B. Outer membrane

Constituents of the outer membrane of Gram-negative bacteria have long excited the interest of medical microbiologists, and former concentration on lipopolysaccharide (LPS) in relation to its endotoxic, antigenic and chemical properties has been succeeded by an explosion of interest in the proteins of the outer membrane. Until quite recently the outer membrane was regarded as an integral part of the cell wall (e.g. Mandelstam and McQuillen, 1973). However, definition of its function as a barrier against access by potentially harmful substances to the subsceptible cell wall layers and cytoplasmic membrane by Nikaido (1973), Nakae and Nikaido (1975) and others (reviewed by Wright and Tipper, 1979) led to acceptance of the outer membrane as a functionally separate entity. In most Gram-negative bacterial pathogens vesicles of outer membrane may bud off and be released to exert the harmful effects characteristic of endotoxin (which in this case is behaving more as an exotoxin). This occurs particularly with pathogenic *Neisseria* species (Devoe and Gilchrist, 1973).

Structurally the outer membrane is a bilayer, with predominantly phospholipid in the inner leaflet and lipopolysaccharide in the outer leaflet (Smit *et al.*, 1975). Into this are incorporated lipoprotein which may be covalently linked to peptidoglycan (in *E. coli* the "Braun" lipoprotein is partially bound and partially free (Braun, 1975)) and outer membrane proteins including porins which traverse the outer membrane forming hydrophilic diffusion channels (Smit *et al.*, 1975; Di Rienzo *et al.*, 1978; Osborn and Wu, 1980; Wright and Tipper, 1979).

The biochemistry of LPS of the enterobacteria has been very thoroughly explored (Luderitz *et al.*, 1968; Galanos *et al.*, 1977; Wright and Tipper, 1979). The structure of the molecule has three main regions: lipid A, responsible for most of the toxin activities (Galanos *et al.*, 1977) is linked to 2-keto-3-deoxy-octonate which is part of the core polysaccharide also containing heptose, glucose and galactose. The core is in turn linked to a polysaccharide side chain which carries immunodominant O-antigenic determinants in many wild-type strains of enteric bacteria. Despite extremely detailed knowledge of the chemistry of these antigens, understanding of their exact role in survival of bacteria in infection is often rudimentary. Like peptidoglycan, and to a greater extent, LPS is very active as an inflammatory mediator and toxin (Kadis *et al.*, 1971; Kass and Wolff, 1973). As an antigen it reacts either with ubiquitous natural antibody or with specific antibody following prior infection or immunization, to fix complement by the classical pathway potentially leading to bactericidal or opsonic activity. LPS will also activate complement by either the classical (Morrison and Kline, 1977; Cooper and Morrison, 1978) or alternative pathway (Galanos *et al.*, 1977) in the absence of antibody. Exposure of LPS on the surface of bacteria might therefore be detrimental to their survival in the face of host defences. However, wild-type strains isolated from patients generally have large amounts of "smooth" LPS (i.e. with complete polysaccharide side chains), while "rough" LPS mutants lacking side chains and including those with defective synthesis of the LPS core—"deep rough" mutants of the Ra→Re series (Luderitz *et al.*, 1971)—are invariably less virulent. Smooth LPS clearly has a protective role against host defences, presumably because the side chain projects outwards from the bacterial surface to mask the core and lipid A region which is the toxic and reactive part, most liable to stimulate the non-specific host defences.

Conclusive evidence for the molecular basis of anti-phagocytic activity or resistance of bacteria to humoral bactericidins associated with possession of smooth LPS has been found difficult to obtain (Roantree, 1971). A successful approach to this problem has been the use of genetic analysis of LPS biosynthesis (Stocker and Makela, 1971; Makela and Stocker, 1981), leading to production of *Salmonella* mutants differing only in the fine structure of LPS side chains (Makela *et al.*, 1973) and shown to differ in mouse virulence (Valtonen *et al.*, 1975; Valtonen, 1977). Subsequent work has shown that differences may lie in the differential ability of different polysaccharide side chain structures to fix complement, independently of antibody, thus becoming opsonized (Liang-Takasaki, *et al.*, 1982). This suggests a critical role for fixation of complement as opsonin in host defence, which must occur at or near the exposed surface if phagocytosis mediated by C3b receptors on phagocytes is to occur. Similar considerations apply in the case of bacterial capsules (see below). Further evidence for intrinsic variability in susceptibility to host defences dependent on physicochemical properties of LPS has come from studies of surface properties (Stendahl *et al.*, 1979) which showed that smooth hydrophilic LPS side chains conferred resistance to phagocytosis, and that strains carrying rough hydrophobic LPS were more susceptible than smooth strains unless acidic polysaccharide capsules were present. McCabe *et al.* (1978) reported a preponderance of certain "O" types among strains of *E. coli* resistant to serum bactericidins, again suggesting that certain chemical structures of these side chains are intrinsically less liable to interact with humoral bactericidins.

Difficulties remain in the interpretation of the role of the outer membrane in resistance or susceptibility to serum bactericidins. If it is accepted that the outer membrane is a prime target for attack by complement in susceptible strains (Swanson and Goldschneider, 1969; Olling, 1977), then the LPS of resistant smooth strains must protect the outer membrane from attack or render it insusceptible. This protection must be twofold: first to shield the inner regions (lipid A, core polysaccharide) of LPS, known to activate complement (Galanos *et al.*, 1977); and second to be intrinsically non-reactive with either complement or natural antibody. The latter consideration applies because although some smooth strains may be totally resistant to serum killing even in the presence of specific antibody to the smooth side-chain (Reynolds and Pruul, 1971), anti-O antibody may also in some cases be bactericidal to smooth strains (Muschel, 1965). Thus the argument that smooth LPS confers resistance because complement is activated too far from susceptible locations in the cell wall for the lethal effects to be exerted (Rowley, 1971) cannot be universally applied. It also follows that the antigenic structure of a protective, smooth LPS side chain should preferably be relatively unusual in comparison with antigenic determinants exposed on commensal or other ubiquitous bacteria responsible for induction of natural antibody.

An outer membrane component apparently related to LPS through some shared biosynthetic pathways is the enterobacterial common antigen (Makela and Mayer, 1976). This is present as a hapten on the surface of nearly all enterobacteria, but is only able to stimulate antibody formation in a few strains such as *E. coli* type O14 strains. The hapten may have some toxic and virulence-related properties.

Many of the proteins found in the outer membrane are exposed on the surface and may be significant in infection. At the time when the attention of those studying outer membrane constituents was focused on lipopolysaccharide biochemistry and chemistry, efforts were often made to eliminate protein from their preparations and interest in the proteins was minimal (Luderitz *et al.*, 1968). Only very recently (Goldman *et al.*, 1981) this "contaminant" protein has been shown to comprise several of the outer membrane proteins described below. Development of methods for separation and purification of the intact outer membrane (Miura and Mizushima, 1968; Schnaitman, 1970; Osborn *et al.*, 1972) allowed investigation of its protein content, although the hydrophobic nature of these proteins made them difficult to analyse by conventional methods. While many proteins were present in minor amounts, a small number (1–4) comprised the greater amount of the total outer membrane protein

(Rosenbusch, 1974; Schnaitman, 1970, 1974). In the last decade much has been learnt of these major outer membrane proteins. Some are porins, able to form transmembrane diffusion channels for small hydrophobic molecules (Tokunaga et al., 1979). Others are "heat-modifiable" in their behaviour after solubilization by sodium dodecyl sulphate, i.e. the apparent molecular weight on polyacrylamide gel electrophoresis is greater after solubilization by boiling than, for example, at 37°C. These proteins, similar to the OmpA protein of E. coli, occur widely among Gram-negative bacteria (Beher et al., 1980b).

Most of the outer membrane proteins are antigenic (Dankert and Hofstra, 1978) and stimulate formation of antibodies especially to the portion exposed on the outer surface of the membrane. Their occurrence is highly variable, especially among pathogenic bacteria, and this variation is often interlinked with other changes in the outer membrane, for example lipopolysaccharide structure (Galanos et al., 1977; Beher et al., 1980a), which may cause difficulties for the biologist attempting to correlate changes in LPS or proteins with changes in virulence attributes. Variability in molecular weight and antigenicity of outer membrane proteins has also been widely reported in pathogenic bacteria (e.g. Johnston et al., 1976; Jann and Jann, 1980; Zollinger and Mandrell, 1980; Tsai et al., 1981) and this capacity for variation may have a role in pathogenicity. Only in the case of *Neisseria gonorrhoeae* has this been demonstrated in any detail. Expression of heat-modifiable outer membrane proteins was shown to be associated with gonococcal colony opacity (Swanson, 1978), which also correlated with enhanced expression of virulence-associated properties.

Components of the outer membrane have been strongly implicated in the resistance of gonococci to humoral bactericidins. Gonococci isolated from infections confined to mucosal surfaces are frequently serum-susceptible, whereas isolates from cases of disseminated infection tend to be resistant (Schoolnik et al., 1976). Resistance to serum killing may be subject to rapid change of phenotype to susceptibility, demonstrable on subculture of clinical isolates (Ward et al., 1970), and the "susceptible" strains isolated from mucosal infections might have shown resistance if tested on isolation without subculture. Organisms removed from chambers implanted subcutaneously in guinea-pigs also show resistance which may be phenotypically reversible on subculture (Penn et al., 1976; Rittenberg et al., 1977), and phenotypic change back to resistance may occur in the presence of serum or other host components *in vitro* (Watt et al., 1972; Goldner et al., 1979; McCutchan et al., 1976). Importantly, substances in human sera and genital secretions may also induce phenotypic resistance (Martin et al., 1982a, b). The determinants of this type of resistance are unknown. In contrast, outer membrane constituents have been implicated in "constitutive" resistance of the type observed for isolates from disseminated infection and expressed on growth in artificial media. While Hildebrandt *et al.* (1978) demonstrated co-transformation of serum resistance and an altered major outer membrane protein into susceptible strains, and it was also shown that LPS was not altered in such transformants (unpublished observations cited by Buchanan and Pearce, 1979), Guymon *et al.* (1978) and Cannon *et al.* (1981) showed that a gene conferring serum resistance (*sac-1*) was distinct from that controlling major outer membrane protein (*nmp2*) and that LPS structure was also affected following transformation to serum resistance. Lipopolysaccharide mutants of *N. gonorrhoeae* selected by pyocin resistance also showed enhanced serum sensitivity, correlated with lack of heptose, glucose, galactose and *N*-acetyl glucosamine from the core oligosaccharide (Guymon *et al.*, 1982). It appears likely that serum resistance in the gonococcus requires multiple genes (Shafter *et al.*, 1982), but outer membrane constituents appear to be critical.

An additional factor in serum resistance of *N. gonorrhoeae* appears to be the binding of non-lytic, "blocking" antibodies to outer membrane components (McCutchan *et al.*, 1978). These antibodies, present in normal human serum, are IgG. A similar phenomenon has been reported in the blocking of bactericidal activity towards *Salmonella enteritidis* of normal bovine serum by rabbit specific IgG (Normann *et al.*, 1973). Blocking of serum killing of *Neisseria meningitidis* by IgA has also been reported (Griffis and Bertram, 1977).

Outer membrane proteins can confer resistance to serum killing of *E. coli* (Taylor and Parton, 1977). Carriage of drug resistance plasmids (Reynard and Beck, 1976; Taylor and Hughes, 1978) or Col V plasmids (Binns *et al.*, 1979) conferred enhanced serum resistance to laboratory strains of *E. coli*. The resistance genes have been identified by DNA cloning techniques, and those from R factors coded for the *traT* outer membrane protein (Moll *et al.*, 1980; Binns *et al.*, 1982). The product of the serum resistance gene *iss* from the plasmid ColV, I-K94 (Binns *et al.*, 1979) has not yet been identified. Both *tra T* and *iss* gene products (which were not identical) allowed consumption of terminal complement components, but appeared to inhibit the lytic action of the complete complement complex (Binns *et al.*, 1982). It should be emphasized that in some of this work the relatively enhanced resistance of genetically manipulated rough laboratory strains of *E. coli* was being studied, and how far this relates to the complete resistance of smooth, virulent strains is not always clear. Resistance is probably multifactorial, so that the ability of plasmids or plasmid-determined proteins to enhance resistance may depend also on their interactions with smooth LPS (Taylor and Hughes, 1978). The influence of both LPS and an outer membrane protein on serum resistance was also reported in an interesting recent study by Munn *et al.* (1982) of the resistance of the fish pathogen *Aeromonas salmonicida* to killing by fish serum.

Recently intra-strain variation in the antigenicity of heat-modifiable outer membrane proteins of gonococci was reported (McBride *et al.*, 1981; Diaz and Heckels, 1982; Swanson, 1982), suggesting the intriguing possibility that gonococcal survival in the host, especially in the face of an immune response, may be enhanced by alteration of the outer membrane antigens to those most favourable for the organism. This might be considered a limited analogy to the capacity for antigenic shift in the surface glycoprotein of trypanosomes (Cross, 1975), which allows them to persist in the face of an immune response. If confirmed, this would be the first example of such behaviour in a procaryote for which the molecular basis has been determined. Older work on the *Borrelia* of relapsing fever (Felsenfeld, 1975) deserves further investigation of its molecular basis.

C. Capsules

Capsules have caused some semantic difficulties for students of pathogenicity. They may be defined functionally by their ability to mask cell wall structures, for example from combination with antibody as shown by lack of agglutination by O- (i.e. LPS-) specific antibody unless the K (capsular) antigens are destroyed by boiling the cells (Orskov *et al.*, 1977). They may also be defined morphologically by light or electron microscopy as a distinct layer external to the cell wall or outer membrane (e.g. Melly *et al.*, 1979). Ideally, though, they should be defined both functionally and morphologically and by their biochemical composition before being accepted as true capsules. Capsules are probably the longest known and most investigated biologically of the bacterial virulence factors. Early work correlating pneumococcal virulence with encapsulation, and S→R (smooth→rough, not to be confused with LPS designations) colony variation associated with loss of capsular polysaccharide and of virulence (Ward and Enders, 1933; Wood and Smith, 1949; MacCleod and Krauss, 1950), is a classic example (reviewed by Wilson and Miles, 1975).

Pneumococci require capsules in order to resist phagocytosis in normal individuals. In group A streptococci, the hyaluronic acid capsule is a virulence factor through its impairment of phagocytosis (Kass and Seastone, 1944; Foley and Wood, 1959). It has also been shown recently that sialic acid in the capsules of group B streptococci inhibits activation of the alternative complement pathway (Edwards *et al.*, 1982b). Encapsulated staphylococci are more virulent than others (Melly *et al.*, 1974) due to their antiphagocytic capsular material (Wilkinson *et al.*, 1979). Encapsulated *Haemophilus influenzae* type b are more virulent than other capsular types, apparently due to their resistance to the bactericidal action of complement (Corrall *et al.*, 1982; Sutton *et al.*, 1982; Yogev and Moxon, 1982). Despite the apparent ability of capsules of *H. influenzae* to protect bacteria from host killing, it is interesting to note that several proteins including some from the outer membrane are exposed for combination with antibody on or beneath the cell surface (Hansen *et al.*, 1981). This may relate to the comments of Wilkinson *et al.* (1979) mentioned below. Among the many known types of *E. coli*, those associated with certain diseases are encapsulated, for example in urinary tract infection (Kaijser *et al.*, 1977), and virulence has been linked with encapsulation which conferred resistance to both bactericidal activity and phagocytosis (Glynn and Howard, 1970; Howard and Glynn, 1971). It appeared that quantity and distribution of K antigen, as well as its quality, were important in resistance to complement action. These correlations have not proved to be universally applicable (Taylor and Parton, 1977). Robbins *et al.* (1980) pointed out that there was an association between the presence of a sialic acid or the structurally related 2-keto-3-deoxy-octonate (KDO) in capsular polysaccharides and the ability to cause invasive disease, for example meningococcal meningitis, or *E. coli* meningitis or urinary tract infection. Sialic acid in these polysaccharides may enhance virulence by aiding the binding of the $\beta1H$ inhibitory factor of the alternative complement pathway to surface-bound C3b (see above), thus reducing activation of complement and its bactericidal and opsonic consequences.

In *Salmonella typhi*, the Vi capsular polysaccharide confers virulence (Felix and Pitt, 1934) and Nagington (1956) showed that excess Vi antigen, even in the presence of anti-Vi antibody, inhibits bactericidal action. Virulent strains of *N. meningitidis* are encapsulated, and antibody to the group A and C polysaccharides confers protection which is correlated with serum bactericidal activity, suggesting a role for capsules in protection of the bacterium against bactericidal effects (Goldschneider *et al.*, 1969). The bactericidal activity of antibody against capsular polysaccharides is difficult to explain in the light of resistance of some bacteria in the presence of specific antibody, for example against smooth LPS (see above). It might be expected that a capsule would activate complement, in the presence of specific antibody, too far from targets of complement lethality to do any harm, as postulated by Rowley (1971) for smooth LPS. A possible mechanism for lethal action of anti-capsular antibody and complement might be the presence of capsular polysaccharide in the process of synthesis or export on the cytoplasmic membrane: if antibody and complement were able to penetrate the capsular layer and there was also some outer membrane damage, access to such sites might occur and lethal damage to the cytoplasmic membrane might result.

The role of capsules in protection of Gram-positive bacteria against bactericidins other than complement and antibody has received little attention, although Keppie *et al.* (1963) showed that the polyglutamic acid capsule of *Bacillus anthracis* inhibited the bactericidal effect of serum on susceptible strains.

Capsules have also been observed on gonococci (Richardson and Sadoff, 1977; James and Swanson, 1977), and some correlation made with virulence (Hendley *et al.*, 1977) but the biochemical nature and mechanism of action of the material responsible is not clear, emphasizing that morphological evidence alone for a capsule is sometimes not sufficient to identify a capsule in the sense described above.

The mode of action of capsules which have been examined thoroughly as virulence factors is very often to inhibit phagocytosis. Horwitz and Silverstein (1980) considered this role of capsules of *E. coli*, and concluded that *E. coli* are not ingested or killed effectively by phagocytes unless complement is fixed to their surface; in the absence of antibody, the capsule blocks complement fixation to the bacterial surface, probably by masking surface components, such as lipopolysaccharide, capable of fixing complement; and the capsule imposes a requirement for specific antibody for complement fixation. These conclusions are compatible with many of the observations of the interaction of encapsulated bacteria with host defence systems (e.g. those described above; Van Dijk *et al.*, 1979a, b; Bortolussi *et al.*, 1979). Often it appears that complement is more essential as an opsonin than as a bactericidal agent, and so successful capsular materials must not fix complement in the absence of antibody, and must form a thick enough layer to prevent contact between any complement which penetrates and is activated by internal layers, and the complement receptors on the phagocyte surface. This is the explanation put forward by Wilkinson *et al.* (1979) for the apparent paradox that some encapsulated strains can be shown to react with antibody or fix complement, and yet to resist phagocytosis.

A special category of capsules, the filamentous proteins K88 and K99 of *E. coli,* are considered in the next section.

D. Filamentous surface structures

These include fimbriae or pili, and flagella, neither of which is thought to be much involved in bacterial defence against humoral factors although they are antigenic and will be considered briefly here.

Among the fimbriae, the most significant role in pathogenicity appears to be as ligands for adhesion of bacteria to host surfaces, which is considered elsewhere in this symposium. The fibrillar proteins K88 and K99 mediate adhesion of *E. coli* to piglet and calf intestinal epithelia respectively (Jones and Rutter, 1972; Smith and Linggood, 1972). Specific antibody interferes with this adhesion but is not known to have any bactericidal or opsonic effect: the infections caused are in any case confined to the gut where such antibacterial mechanisms are unlikely to be effective. Other bacteria which bear fimbriae associated with virulence include *N. gonorrhoeae* (Jephcott et al., 1981; Swanson et al., 1971), *N. meningitidis* (Devoe and Gilchrist, 1975), and certain *E. coli* types pathogenic for man, such as those causing urinary tract infection (Klemm et al., 1982) and some diarrhoea strains (Evans et al., 1978). Although some evidence has been put forward for association of fimbriation of gonococci with resistance to phagocytosis (Punsalang and Sawyer, 1973), this may result from association of fimbriation with other virulence factors, and the direct role of fimbriation in virulence is more likely to be as an adhesion factor.

Flagella of Gram-negative bacteria have been recognized as antigens for many decades, but antiflagellar antibodies are not opsonins (Felix and Olitzki, 1926; Bhatnagar, 1935) nor do they enhance complement-mediated killing (Muschel et al., 1958). Kaijser and Olling (1973) showed that anti-flagellar antibodies do not protect against pyelonephritis. These observations suggest that flagella are unlikely to confer virulence by protecting against humoral bactericidal mechanisms or opsonins. Flagella are, however, associated with virulence in some motile bacteria: non-motile mutants of *Vibrio cholerae* are less virulent (Guentzel and Berry, 1975), but the exact role of flagella in enhancement of infection has not been defined: motility may enable the organisms to reach maximally effective sites for the development of disease, possibly by the chemotactic penetration of mucus towards epithelial cells (Allweiss et al., 1977; Freter et al., 1981).

IV. CONCLUSIONS

This survey has shown that host factors, like bacterial virulence factors, are usually multiple in the challenge of host defences by a bacterium, and the outcome of that challenge may be affected by changes in one or more of a number of systems. There is often no single answer to the questions "what is the host defence mechanism operative against this bacterium?" or "what is the virulence factor of this bacterium?", unlike the definitive answers which can be sought and have often been found to questions of chemical structure of envelope components. Thus there remains much work to be done by the biologists to complete our knowledge of the relation of structure to function.

The most interesting current development seems to be the ever-increasing range of possible interactions of bacterial envelope components with the complement system, and the central role played by complement in most of the humoral interactions discussed here. Although the opsonizing action of complement appears to be generally more important than its bactericidal action against pathogens, it must be remembered that many non-virulent bacteria which happen to enter the body through wounds or abrasions will be susceptible to complement killing, which in contributing to the total host defence system is undoubtedly important.

ACKNOWLEDGEMENT

Thanks are due to Professor H. Smith and Dr I. Allan for critical reading of the manuscript and helpful comments.

REFERENCES

Adinolfi, M., Glynn, A. A., Lindsay, M. and Milne, C. M. (1966a). *Immunology* **10**, 517–526.
Adinolfi, M., Mollison, P. L., Polley, M. J. and Rose, J. M. (1966b). *J. Exp. Med.* **123**, 951–967.
Ahlstedt, S. (1980). *Intern. Arch. Allergy & Appl. Immunol.* **62**, 341–345.
Allweiss, B. J., Dostal, K. C., Edwards, T. and Freter, R. (1977). *Nature* **266**, 448–450.
Alper, C. A., Abramson, N., Johnston, R. B., Jandl, J. H. and Rosen, F. S. (1970). *N. Engl. J. Med.* **282**, 349–354.
Baker, C. J., Edwards, M. S., Webb, B. J. and Kasper, D. L. (1982). *J. Clin. Invest.* **69**, 394–404.
Beher, M., Pugsley, A. and Schnaitman, C. (1980a). *J. Bacteriol.* **143**, 403–410.
Beher, M. G., Schnaitman, C. A. and Pugsley, A. (1980b). *J. Bacteriol.* **143**, 906–913.
Betz, S. J. and Isliker, H. (1981). *J. Immunol.* **127**, 1748–1754.
Bhatnagar, S. S. (1935). *Brit. J. Exp. Path.* **16**, 375–384.
Binns, M. M., Davies, D. L. and Hardy, K. G. (1979). *Nature* **279**, 778–781.
Binns, M. M., Mayden, J. and Levine, R. P. (1082). *Infect. Immun.* **35**, 654–659.
Bladen, H. A., Gewurz, H. and Mergenhagen, S. E. (1967). *J. Exp. Med.* **125**, 767–786.
Bortolussi, R., Ferrieri, P., Bjorgsten, B. and Quie, P. G. (1979). *Infect. Immun.* **25**, 293–298.
Brandtzaeg, P. (1975). *Immunology* **29**, 559–570.

Brandtzaeg, P. and Baklien, K. (1977). *In* "Immunology of the Gut", pp. 77–108. CIBA Foundation Symposium 46, Elsevier, Amsterdam.

Braude, A. (1981). *In* "Microbial Perturbation of Host Defences" (F. O'Grady and H. Smith, eds) pp. 31–41. Academic Press, London.

Braun, V. (1975). *Biochim. Biophys. Acta* **415**, 335–337.

Brooks, G. F., Israel, K. S. and Petersen, B. H. (1976). *J. Infect. Dis.* **134**, 450–462.

Buchanan, T. M. and Pearce, W. A. (1979). *In* "Bacterial Outer Membranes: Biogenesis and Functions" (M. Inouye, ed.) pp. 475–514. Wiley, New York.

Burritt, M. F., Calvanico, N. J., Mehta, S. and Tomasi, T. B. (1977). *J. Immunol.* **118**, 723–725.

Cannon, J. G., Lee, T. J., Guymon, L. F. and Sparling, P. F. (1981). *Infect. Immun.* **32**, 547–552.

Carroll, S. F. and Martinez, R. J. (1979). *Infect. Immun.* **25**, 810–819.

Clas, F. and Loos, M. (1981). *Infect. Immun.* **31**, 1138–1144.

Cohen, I. R. and Norins, L. C. (1966). *Science* **152**, 1257–1259.

Cooper, N. R. and Morrison, D. C. (1978). *J. Immunol.* **120**, 1862–1868.

Corrall, C. J., Winkelstein, J. A. and Moxon, E. R. (1982). *Infect. Immun.* **35**, 759–763.

Coutinho, A. and Moller, G. (1975). *Adv. Immunol.* **21**, 113–236.

Cross, G. A. M. (1975). *Parasitology* **71**, 393–417.

Davis, S. D., Ianetta, A. and Wedgwood, R. J. (1972). *In* "Biological Activities of Complement" (D. G. Ingram, ed.) pp. 43–55. Karger, Basle.

Dankert, J. and Hofstra, H. (1978). *J. Gen. Microbiol.* **104**, 311–320.

Devoe, I. W. and Gilchrist, J. E. (1973). *J. Exp. Med.* **138**, 1156–1167.

Devoe, I. W. and Gilchrist, J. E. (1975). *J. Exp. Med.* **141**, 297–305.

Diaz, J. L. and Heckels, J. E. (1982). *J. Gen. Microbiol.* **128**, 585–591.

Di Rienzo, J. M., Nakamura, K. and Inouye, M. (1978). *Annual Rev. Biochem.* **47**, 481–532.

Donaldson, D. M. and Tew, J. G. (1977). *Bacteriol. Rev.* **41**, 501–513.

Donaldson, D. M., Ellsworth, B. and Matheson, A. (1964). *J. Immunol.* **92**, 896–901.

Donaldson, D. M., Roberts, R. R., Larsen, H. S. and Tew, J. G. (1974). *Infect. Immun.* **10**, 657–666.

Doran, J. E. and Raynor, R. H. (1981). *Infect. Immun.* **33**, 683–689.

Dossett, J. H., Kronvall, G., Williams, R. C. and Quie, P. G. (1969). *J. Immunol.* **103**, 1405–1410.

Dourmashkin, R. R., Hesketh, R., Humphrey, J. H., Medhurst, F. and Payne, S. N. (1972). *In* "Biological Activities of Complement" (D. G. Ingram, ed.) pp. 89–95. Karger, Basle.

Easmon, C. S. F. (1981). *In* "The Staphylococci" (A. Macdonald and G. Smith, eds) pp. 63–72. Aberdeen University Press.

Edwards, K. M., Gewurz, H., Lint, T. E. and Mold, C. (1982a). *J. Immunol* **128**, 2493–2496.

Edwards, M. S., Kasper, D. L., Jennings, H. J., Baker, C. J. and Nicholson-Weller, A. (1982b). *J. Immunol.* **128**, 1278–1283.

Espersen, F. and Clemmensen, I. (1981). *Acta Pathol. Microbiol. Scand.* **B89**, 317–321.

Espersen, F. and Clemmensen, I. (1982). *Infect. Immun.* **37**, 526–531.

Evans, D. G., Evans, D. J., Tjoa, W. S. and Dupont, H. L. (1978). *Infect. Immun.* **19**, 727–736.

Fearon, D. T. and Austen, K. T. (1980). *N. Engl. J. Med.* **303**, 259–263.

Felix, A. and Olitzki, I. (1926). *J. Immunol.* **11**, 31–80.

Felix, A. and Pitt, R. M. (1934). *Lancet* **2**, 186–191.

Felsenfeld, O. (1975). *Bacteriol. Rev.* **29**, 46–74.

Fitzgerald, T. J. (1981). *Ann. Rev. Microbiol.* **35**, 29–54.

Foley, M. J. and Wood, W. B. (1959). *J. Exp. Med.* **110**, 617–628.

Forsgren, A. and Sjoquist, J. (1966). *J. Immunol.* **97**, 822–827.

Frank, M. M. (1980). *In* "The Molecular Basis of Microbial Pathogenicity" (H. Smith, J. J. Skehel and M. J. Turner, eds) pp. 87–100. Verlag Chemie GmbH, Weinheim.

Freer, J. H. and Salton, M. R. J. (1971). *In* "Microbial Toxins". (G. Weinbaum, S. Kadis and S. J. Ajl, eds), Vol. IV (Bacterial Endotoxins) pp. 67–126. Academic Press, New York.

Freter, R., O'Brien, P. C. M. and Macsai, M. S. (1981). *Infect. Immun.* **34**, 234–240.

Galanos, C., Luderitz, O., Rietschel, E. T. and Westphal, O. (1977). *In* "International Review of Biochemistry (T. W. Goodwin, ed.), Vol. 14 (Biochemistry of Lipids II) pp. 239–335. University Park Press, Baltimore.

Gewurz, H., Snyderman, R., Mergenhagen, S. E. and Shin, H. S. (1971). *In* "Microbial Toxins" (S. Kadis, G. Weinbaum and S. J. Ajl, eds), Vol. V (Bacterial Endotoxins) pp. 127–149. Academic Press, New York.

Ghuysen, J-M., Strominger, J. L. and Tipper, D. J. (1968). *In* "Comprehensive Biochemistry" (M. Florkin and E. H. Stotz, eds), Vol. 26A, pp. 53–104. Elsevier, New York.

Gigli, I. (1977). *In* "Biological Amplification Systems in Immunology. (N. K. Day and R. A. Good, eds) pp. 295–313. Plenum, New York.

Glynn, A. A. (1969). *Immunology* **16**, 463–471.

Glynn, A. A. and Howard, C. J. (1970). *Immunology* **18**, 331–346.

Glynn, A. A. and Milne, C. N. (1967). *Immunology* **12**, 639–653.

Goldman, R. C., White, D. and Leive, L. (1981). *J. Immunol.* **127**, 1290–1294.

Goldner, M., Penn, C. W., Sanyal, S. C., Veale, D. R. and Smith, H. (1979). *J. Gen. Microbiol.* **114**, 169–177.

Goldschneider, I., Gotschlich, E. C. and Artenstein, M. S. (1969). *J. Exp. Med.* **129**, 1307–1326.

Gotze, O. and Muller-Eberhard, H. J. (1971). *J. Exp. Med.* **134**, 90s–108s.

Greenblatt, J., Boackle, R. J. and Schwab, J. H. (1978). *Infect. Immun.* **19**, 296–303.

Griffin, F. M. (1977). *In* "Biological Amplification Systems in Immunology" (N. K. Day and R. A. Good, eds) pp 85–113. Plenum, New York.

Griffis, J. M. and Bertram, M. A. (1977). *J. Infect. Dis.* **136**, 733–739.

Griffiths, E. (1971). *Eur. J. Biochem.* **23**, 69–76.

Grov, A., Myklestad, B. and Oeding, P. (1964). *Acta Pathol. Microbiol Scand.* **61**, 588–596.

Guentzel, M. N. and Berry, L. J. (1975). *Infect. Immun.* **11**, 890–897.

Guymon, L. F., Lee, T. J., Walstad, D., Schmoyer, A. and Sparling, P. F. (1978). *In* "Immunobiology of *Neisseria gonorrhoeae*" (G. F. Brooks, E. C. Gotschlich, F. E. Young, W. D. Sawyer and K. K. Holmes, eds) pp. 139–141. American Society for Microbiology, Washington D. C.

Guymon, L. F., Esser, M. and Shafer, W. M. (1982). *Infect. Immun.* **36**, 541–547.
Guze, L. B. (ed.) (1968). "Microbial Protoplasts, Spheroplasts and L-forms". Williams and Wilkins, Baltimore.
Hall, J. G. and Andrew, E. (1980). *Immunol. Today* **1**, 100–104.
Hansen, E. J., Frisch, C. F. and Johnston, K. H. (1981). *Infect. Immun.* **33**, 950–953.
Harris, C., Roth, S., Schmid, F. R. and Anderson, B. (1981). *Immunol. Commun.* **10**, 601–609.
Heddle, R. J. and Rowley, D. (1975). *Immunology* **29**, 197–208.
Hendley, J. O., Powell, K. R., Rodewald, R., Holzgrefe, H. H. and Lyles, R. (1977). *N. Eng. J. Med.* **296**, 608–611.
Heremans, J. F., Heremans, M. T. and Schultze, H. E. (1959). *Clin. Chim. Acta* **4**, 96–109.
Hildebrandt, J. F., Mayer, L. W., Wang, S. P. and Buchanan, T. M. (1978). *Infect. Immun.* **20**, 267–273.
Hill, I. R. and Porter, P. (1974). *Immunology* **26**, 1239–1250.
Hill, M. J. (1968). *J. Med. Microbiol.* **1**, 33–43.
Horwitz, M. A. and Silverstein, S. C. (1980). *J. Clin. Invest.* **65**, 82–94.
Howard, C. J. and Glynn, A. A. (1971). *Immunology* **20**, 767–777.
Humphrey, J. H. and Dourmashkin, R. R. (1970). *Adv. Immunol.* **11**, 75–115.
Isliker, H., Bing, D. H., Lahan, J. and Hynes, R. O. (1982). *Immunol. Lett.* **4**, 39–43.
Jackson, G. D., Lemaitre-Coelho, I., Vaerman, J. P., Bazin, H. and Beckers, A. (1978). *Eur. J. Immunol.* **8**, 123–126.
James, J. F. and Swanson, J. (1977). *J. Exp. Med.* **145**, 1082–1086.
Jann, B. and Jann, K. (1980). *FEMS Microbiol. Lett.* **7**, 19–22.
Jephcott, A. E., Reyn, A. and Birch-Andersen, A. (1971). *Acta Pathol. Microbiol. Scand. Sect. B*, **79**, 437–439.
Johnston, K. H., Holmes, K. K. and Gotschlich, E. C. (1976). *J. Exp. Med.* **143**, 741–758.
Jonas, W. E. and Broad, S. (1972). *Res. Vet. Sci.* **13**, 154–159.
Jones, G. W. and Rutter, J. M. (1972). *Infect. Immun.* **6**, 918–927.
Kadis, S., Weinbaum, G. and Ajl, S. J. (eds) (1971). "Microbial Toxins", Vol. V (Bacterial Endotoxins). Academic Press, New York.
Kaijser, B. and Olling, S. (1973). *J. Infect. Dis.* **128**, 41–49.
Kaijser, B., Hanson, L. A., Jodal, U., Lidin-Janson, G. and Robbins, J. B. (1977). *Lancet* **i**, 663–664.
Kass, E. H. and Seastone, C. V. (1944). *J. Exp. Med.* **79**, 319–330.
Kass, E. H. and Wolff, S. M. (eds) (1973). "Bacterial Lipopolysaccharides: Chemistry, Biology and Clinical Significance of Endotoxins." *J. Infect. Dis.*, Supplement, July.
Keppie, J., Harris-Smith, P. W. and Smith, H. (1963). *Brit. J. Exp. Pathol.* **44**, 446–453.
Klemm, P., Orskov, I. and Orskov, F. (1982). *Infect. Immun.* **36**, 462–468.
Lancefield, R. C. (1962). *J. Immunol.* **89**, 307–313.
Leddy, J. P., Frank, M. M., Gaither, T., Baum, J. and Klemperer, M. R. (1974) *J. Clin. Invest.* **53**, 544–553.
Lee, T. J., Utsinger, P. D., Snyderman, R., Yount, W. J. and Sparling, P. F. (1978). *J. Infect. Dis.* **138**, 359–368.
Leist-Welsh, P. and Bjornson, A. B. (1982). *J. Immunol.* **128**, 2643–2651.

Liang-Takasaki, C., Makela, P. H. and Leive, L. (1982). *J. Immunol.* **128,** 1229–1235.
Luderitz, O., Jann, K. and Wheat, R. (1968). *In* "Comprehensive Biochemistry" (M. Florkin and E. H. Stotz, eds) vol. 26A, pp. 105–228. Elsevier, Amsterdam.
Luderitz, O., Westphal, O., Staub, A-M and Nikaido, H. (1971). *In* "Microbial Toxins" (G. Weinbaum, S. Kadis and S. J. Ajl, eds.), Vol. IV, pp. 145–233. Academic Press, New York.
MacCleod, C. M. and Krauss, M. R. (1950). *J. Exp. Med.* **92,** 1–9.
Makela, P. H. and Mayer, H. (1976). *Bacteriol. Rev.* **40,** 591–632.
Makela, P. H. and Stocker, B. A. D. (1981). *In* "Genetics as a Tool in Microbiology" (S. W. Glover, D. A. Hopwood, eds) pp. 219–264. 31st Sympo-. sium of the Society for General Microbiology. Cambridge University Press.
Makela, P. H., Valtonen, V. V. and Valtonen, M. (1973). *J. Infect. Dis.* **128,** supplement, s81–s85.
Mandelstam, J. and McQuillen, K. (eds) (1973). "Biochemistry of Bacterial Growth", 2nd Edition. Blackwell, Oxford.
Martin, P. M. V., Patel, P. V., Parsons, N. J. and Smith, H. (1982a). *Bri. J. Vener. Dis.* (in press).
Martin, P. M. V., Patel, P. V., Parsons, N. J. and Smith, H. (1982b). *Brit. J. Vener. Dis.* (in press).
Martinez, R. and Carroll, S. F. (1980). *Infect. Immun.* **28,** 735–745.
McBride, H. M., Lambden, P. R., Heckels, J. E. and Watt, P. J. (1981). *J. Gen. Microbiol.* **126,** 69–75.
McCabe, W. R., Kaijser, B., Olling, S., Uwaydah, M. and Hanson, L A. (1978). *J. Infect. Dis.* **138,** 33–41.
McCutchan, J. A., Levine, S. and Braude, A. I. (1976). *J. Immunol.* **116,** 1652–1655.
McCutchan, J. A., Katzenstein, D., Norquist, D., Chikami, G., Wunderlich, A. and Braude, A. (1978). *J. Immunol.* **121,** 1884–1892.
McGee, Z. A., Ratner, H. B., Bryant, R. E., Rosenthal, U. S. and Koenig, M. G. (1972). *J. Infect. Dis.* **125,** 231–242.
Melching, L. and Vas, S. I. (1971). *Infect. Immun.* **3,** 107–115.
Melly, M. A., Duke, L. J., Liau, D-F. and Hash, J. H. (1974). *Infect. Immun.* **10,** 389–397.
Melly, M. A., McGee, Z., Horn, R. G., Morris, F. and Glick, A. D. (1979). *J. Infect. Dis.* **140,** 605–609.
Mergenhagen, S., Snyderman, R., Gewurz, H. and Shin, H. S. (1969). *Curr. Top. Microbiol. Immunol.* **50,** 37–77.
Michael, J. G. and Rosen, F. S. (1963). *J. Exp. Med.* **118,** 619–626.
Miura, T. and Mizushima, S. (1968). *Biochim. Biophys. Acta* **150,** 159–161.
Mold, C. S., Nakayama, S., Holzer, T. J., Gewurz, H. and DuClos, T. W. (1981). *J. Exp. Med.* **154,** 1703–1708.
Moll, A., Manning, P. A. and Timmis, K. N. (1980). *Infect. Immun.* **28,** 359–367.
Morrison, D. C. and Kline, L. F. (1977). *J. Immunol.* **118,** 362–368.
Mosher, D. F. (1980). *In* "Progress in Hemostasis and Thrombosis" (T. H. Spate, ed.) vol. 5, pp. 111–151. Grune, New York.
Munn, C. B., Ishiguro, E. E., Kay, W. W. and Trust, T. J. (1982). *Infect. Immun.* **31,** 1069–1075.
Muschel, L. H. (1965). *In* "Complement" (G. E. W. Wolstenholme and J. Knight, eds), pp. 155–169. Churchill, London.

Muschel, L. H. (1968). *In* "Microbial Protoplasts, Spheroplasts and L-forms" (L. B. Guze, ed.) pp. 19–29. Williams and Wilkins, Baltimore.

Muschel, L. H. and Fong, J. S. C. (1977). *In* "Biological Amplification Systems in Immunology" (N. K. Day and R. A. Good, eds) pp. 136–158. Plenum, New York.

Muschel, L. H. and Jackson, J. E. (1966). *J. Immunol.* **97**, 46–51.

Muschel, L. H., Chamberlin, R. H. and Osawa, E. (1958). *Proc. Soc. Exp. Biol. Med.* **97**, 376–382.

Nagington, J. (1956). *Brit. J. Exp. Pathol.* **37**, 397–405.

Nakae, T. and Nikaido, H. (1975). *J. Biol. Chem.* **250**, 7359–7365.

Nikaido, H. (1973). *In* "Bacterial Membranes and Walls" (L. Leive, ed.) pp. 131–209. Dekker, New York.

Normann, B., Schenstrom, O. and Edebo, L. (1973). *Acta Pathol. Microbiol. Scand. Section B*, **81**, 203–206.

Olling, S. (1977). *Scand. J. Infect. Dis.* Supplement.

Opferkuch, W. and Segerling, M. (1977). *In* "Biological Amplification Systems in Immunology" (N. K. Day and R. A. Good, eds) pp. 1–16. Plenum, New York.

Orlans, E., Peppard, J., Reynolds, J. and Hall, J. (1978). *J. Exp. Med.* **147**, 588–592.

Orskov, I., Orskov, F., Jann, B. and Jann, K. (1977). *Bacteriol. Rev.* **41**, 667–710.

Osborn, M. J. and Wu, H. C. P. (1980). *Ann. Rev. Microbiol.* **34**, 369–422.

Osborn, M. J., Gander, J. E., Parisi, E. and Carson, J. (1972). *J. Biol. Chem.* **247**, 3962–3972.

Penn, C. W. and Lichfield, J. (1982). *FEMS Microbiol. Lett.* **14**, 61–64.

Penn, C. W. and Rhodes, J. (1982). *Immunology* **46**, 9–16.

Penn, C. W., Sen, D., Veale, D. R., Parsons, N. J., Smith, H. and Witt, K. (1976). *J. Gen. Microbiol.* **97**, 35–43.

Perey, D. Y. E. and Milne, R. W. (1975). *Lab. Invest.* **33**, 678–686.

Petersen, B. H. and Rosenthal, R. H. (1982). *Infect. Immun.* **35**, 442–448.

Petersen, B. H., Graham, J. A. and Brooks, G. F. (1976). *J. Clin. Invest.* **57**, 283–290.

Peterson, P. K., Verhoef, J., Sabath, L. D. and Quie, P. G. (1977). *Infect. Immun.* **15**, 760–764.

Peterson, P. J., Wilkinson, B. J., Kim, Y., Schmeling, D., Douglas, S. D., Quie, P. G. and Verhoef, J. (1978). *J. Clin. Invest.* **61**, 597–609.

Porter, R. R. (1977). *Fed. Proc.* **36**, 2191–2196.

Pruul, H. and Reynolds, B. L. (1972). *Infect. Immun.* **6**, 709–717.

Punsalang, A. and Sawyer, W. D. (1973). *Infect. Immun.* **8**, 255–263.

Quie, P. G., Verhoef, J., Kim, Y. and Peterson, P. K. (1981). *In* "The Staphylococci" (A. Macdonald and G. Smith, eds) pp. 83–93. Aberdeen University Press.

Reynard, A. M. and Beck, M. E. (1976). *Infect. Immun.* **14**, 848–850.

Reynolds, B. L. and Pruul, H. (1971). *Infect. Immun.* **3**, 365–372.

Richardson, W. P. and Sadoff, J. C. (1977). *Infect. Immun.* **15**, 663–664.

Rittenberg, S. C., Penn, C. W., Parsons, N. J., Veale, D. R. and Smith, H. (1977). *J. Gen. Microbiol.* **103**, 69–75.

Roantree, R. J. (1971). *In* "Microbial Toxins" (S. Kadis, G. Weinbaum and S. J. Ajl, eds) Vol. V (Bacterial Endotoxins). Academic Press, New York.

Robbins, J. B., Schneerson, R., Egan, W. B., Vann, W. and Liu, D. T. (1980). *In*

"The Molecular Basis of Microbial Pathogenicity" (H. Smith, J. J. Skehel and M. J. Turner, eds). Verlag Chemie GmbH, Weinheim.

Rogers, H. J., Perkins, H. R. and Ward, J. B. (1980). "Microbial Cell Walls and Membranes". Chapman and Hall, London.

Rogers, H. J. and Synge, C. (1978). *Immunology* **34,** 19–28.

Rosenbusch, J. P. (1974). *J. Biol. Chem.* **249,** 8019–8029.

Rosenthal, R. (1979). *Infect. Immun.* **24,** 869–878.

Rosenthal, R. S., Blundell, J. K. and Perskins, H. R. (1982). *Infect. Immun.* **37,** 826–829.

Rowley, D. (1971). *Journal of Infect. Dis.* **123,** 317–327.

Saba, T. M. and Jaffe, E. (1980). *Amer. J. Med.* **68,** 577–594.

Schnaitman, C. A. (1970). *J. Bacteriol.* **104,** 882–889.

Schnaitman, C. A. (1974). *J. Bacteriol.* **118,** 442–453.

Schoolnik, G. K., Buchanan, T. M. and Holmes, K. K. (1976). *J. Clin. Invest.* **58,** 1163–1173.

Schoolnik, G. K., Ochs, H. D. and Buchanan, T. M. (1979). *J. Immunol.* **122,** 1771–1779.

Schultz, D. R. and Miller, K. D. (1974). *Infect. Immun.* **10,** 128–135.

Selsted, M. E. and Martinez, R. J. (1978). *Infect. Immun.* **20,** 782–791.

Shafer, W. M., Guymon, L. H. and Sparling, P. F. (1982). *Infect. Immun.* **35,** 764–769.

Shedlofsky, S. and Freter, R. (1974). *J. Infect. Dis.* **129,** 296–303.

Smit, J., Kamio, Y. and Nikaido, H. (1975). *J. Bacteriol.* **124,** 942–958.

Smith, H. W. and Linggood, M. (1972). *J. Med. Microbiol.* **5,** 243–250.

Spiegelberg, H. L. (1974). *Adv. Immunol.* **19,** 259–294.

Steele, E. J., Chaicumpa, W. and Rowley, D. (1974). *J. Infect. Dis.* **130,** 93–102.

Stendahl, O., Normann, B. and Edebo, L. (1979). *Acta Pathol. Microbiol. Scand. Section B* **87,** 85–91.

Stewart-Tull, D. E. S. (1980). *Annual Rev. Microbiol.* **34,** 311–340.

Stocker, B. A. D. and Makela, P. H. (1971). *In* "Microbial Toxins" (G. Weinbaum, S. Kadis and S. J. Ajl, eds), Vol IV, pp. 369–438. Academic Press, New York.

Sutton, A., Schneerson, R., Kendall-Morris, S. and Robbins, J. B. (1982). *Infect. Immun.* **35,** 95–104.

Swanson, J. (1978). *Infect. Immun.* **19,** 320–331.

Swanson, J. (1982). *Infect. Immun.* **37,** 359–368.

Swanson, J. and Goldschneider, I. (1969). *J. Exp. Med.* **129,** 51–80.

Swanson, J., Hsu, K. C. and Gotschlich, E. C. (1969). *J. Exp. Med.* **130,** 1063–1092.

Swanson, J., Krauss, S. and Gotschlich, E. C. (1971). *J. Exp. Med.* **134,** 886–906.

Tarr, P. J., Hosea, S. W., Brown, E. J., Schneerson, R., Sutton, A. and Frank, M. M. (1982). *J. Immunol.* **128,** 1772–1775.

Taussig, M. J. (1979). "Processes in Pathology". Blackwell, Oxford.

Taylor, P. W. (1978). *FEMS Microbiol. Lett.* **3,** 119–122.

Taylor, P. W. and Hughes, C. (1978). *Infect. Immun.* **22,** 10–17.

Taylor, P. W. and Parton, R. (1977). *J. Med. Microbiol.* **10,** 225–232.

Tipper, D. J. and Wright, A. (1979). *In* "The Bacteria" (J. R. Sokatch and L. N. Ornston, eds) vol VII, pp. 291–426. Academic Press, New York.

Tokunaga, M., Tokunaga, H. and Nakae, T. (1979). *Eur. J. Biochem.* **95,** 433–439.

Tomasi, T. B. (1976). "The Immune System of Secretions". Prentice-Hall, New Jersey.

Tomasi, T. B. and Bienenstock, J. (1968). *Adv. Immunol.* **9**, 1–96.

Tsai, C. M., Frasch, C. E. and Mocca, L. F. (1981). *J. Bacteriol.* **146**, 69–78.

Valtonen, M. V. (1977). *Infect. Immun.* **18**, 574–582.

Valtonen, M., Plosila, M., Valtonen, V. V. and Makela, P. H. (1975). *Infect. Immun.* **12**, 828–832.

Van Dijk, W. C., Verbrugh, H. A., Peters, R., VanDerTol, M. E., Peterson, P. K. and Verhoef, J. (1979a). *J. Med. Microbiol.* **12**, 123–130.

Van Dijk, W. C., Verbrugh, H. A., VanDerTol, M. E., Peters, R. and Verhoef, J. (1979b). *Infect. Immun.* **25**, 603–609.

Ward, H. K. and Enders, J. F. (1933). *J. Exp. Med.* **57**, 527–547.

Ward, M. E., Watt, P. J. and Glynn, A. A. (1970). *Nature* **227**, 382–384.

Wardlaw, A. C. (1962). *J. Exp. Med.* **115**, 1231–1249.

Watt, P. J., Glynn, A. A. and Ward, M. E. (1972). *Nature New Biol.* **236**, 186–187.

Wilkinson, B. J., Peterson, P. K. and Quie, P. G. (1979). *Infect. Immun.* **23**, 502–508.

Williams, R. C. and Gibbons, R. J. (1972). *Science* **177**, 697–699.

Wilson, G. S. and Miles, A. A. (1975). "Topley and Wilson's Principles of Bacteriology, Virology and Immunity", 6th Edition. Edward Arnold, London.

Wilson, L. A. and Spitznagel, J. J. (1968). *J. Bacteriol.* **96**, 1339–1348.

Winkelstein, J. A. and Shin, H. S. (1974). *J. Immunol.* **112**, 1635–1642.

Winkelstein, J. A. and Tomasz, A. (1977). *J. Immunol.* **118**, 451–454.

Wood, W. B. and Smith, M. R. (1949). *J. Exp. Med.* **90**, 85–95.

Wright, A. and Tipper, D. J. (1979). *In* "The Bacteria" (J. R. Sokatch and L. R. Ornston, eds) vol. VII. pp. 427–485. Academic Press, New York.

Wright, S. D. and Levine, R. P. (1981). *J. Immunol.* **127**, 1146–1151.

Yogev, R. and Moxon, E. R. (1982). *J. Clin. Invest.* **69**, 658–665.

Zollinger, W. D. and Mandrell, R. E. (1980). *Infect. Immun.* **28**, 451–458.

6 The physicochemical basis of surface interaction between bacteria and phagocytic cells

O. STENDAHL

I. INTRODUCTION

Phagocytosis is the uptake of particles by eukaryotic cells from the extracellular environment into the cytoplasm by plasma membrane-derived vesicles. Although executed by many cells, professional phagocytes, like granulocytes and macrophages, ingest foreign particles such as bacteria and particulate antigens with great efficiency. It is clear that the cellular function of phagocytosis is of prime biological importance, both in health and disease, in eliminating the host of harmful invaders and in allowing it to eliminate debris and other foreign material. Since nonspecific immune systems (phagocytosis in the absence of antibodies) appeared earlier in phylogeny than specific immune systems—the latter being found in their classical form in lower vertebrates such as the fish, but not in invertebrates—the phagocytic cells may represent a more general and ancient form of immune defence than the specific immune system in man.

A prominent feature of the surface interaction between the phagocyte and the particle being ingested is its discriminatory character. Whether a particle is accepted by the phagocyte, permitting attachment with subsequent ingestion, is determined by the surface properties of both the particle and the phagocyte. How the particle is bound to the cell and how binding subsequently directs the contractile system to engulf the particle is poorly understood in molecular terms (Elsbach, 1977).

Attempts to learn about the physical and chemical characteristics of

MEDICAL MICROBIOLOGY, 3
ISBN 0 12 228003 3

particles that do or do not incite recognition by phagocytic cells and efforts to characterize the surface moieties of phagocytes that respond to these characteristics are necessary to reveal the mechanisms of recognition. This review will focus in the recognition mechanisms between phagocytic cells and bacteria and will try to define the interacting entities in physicochemical terms.

II. THE PHAGOCYTIC PROCESS

The phagocytic process is initially a surface phenomenon that can be described in physicochemical terms (for review see Elbach, 1977; Silverstein *et al.*, 1977). However, it is important in this context to realize that when a phagocytic cell encounters a foreign particle like a bacterium, a multistep process is initiated. First the particle attaches to the cell membrane via an energy-independent process, involving either nonspecific or specific ligand–receptor interactions. If the particle is properly recognized by the cell, a triggering signal will be transduced to the effector mechanisms of the cell, rapidly eliciting several biochemical events; membrane fluidity is enhanced (Berlin and Fera, 1977), the surface potential and surface charge are altered (Gallin, 1980; Seligman and Gallin, 1980), calcium ions are mobilized (Petroski *et al.*, 1979) and the membrane-associated NADPH-oxidase is activated (Cohen, *et al.*, 1980). These events lead to changed oxidative and arachidonic acid metabolism with generation of reactive oxygen-derived metabolites (superoxide, hydrogen peroxide, hydroxyl radicals) (Root and Cohen, 1981) as well as leukotrienes and prostaglandins, formation of actomyosin microfilament network and induction of pseudopod formation (Stendahl *et al.*, 1980). The subsequent ingestion of the attached particles is not an all-or-nothing phenomenon elicited by the attachment sites of the cell-particle association. Rather, ingestion requires sequential interaction between membrane recognition sites on the phagocyte with ligands throughout the surface of the particle (Griffin *et al.*, 1975). The circumferential flow of pseudopods around the particle is governed by the calcium-dependent regulation of the actomyosin microfilament network (Stossel *et al.*, 1981). If this system is not properly activated, attachment will not lead to ingestion and subsqunt eradication of the microorganism.

   Following ingestion and phagosome formation, the lysosomal granules will rapidly fuse with the phagosome and release their contents into the vacuole, thus creating an unfavourable milieu for the microorganism. While most virulent bacteria may evade phagocytosis at the attachment-ingestion step, certain infectious agents may inhibit phagolysosomes fusion or resist intracellular killing (for review see Densen and Mandell, 1980).

III. RECOGNITION

Two main recognition mechanisms are usually considered to be operative on the phagocyte plasma membrane: one is mediated by specific receptors being defined as saturable chemical structures with high affinity for a certain ligand, and the other is mediated by more general physicochemical surface properties such as hydrophobicity and charge on the phagocyte and the prey.

At the beginning of the century (Wright and Douglas, 1903) it had already been observed that serum was able to "opsonize" virulent bacteria, thereby increasing the avidity for the phagocytes. Attempts to explain the phagocyte process and the mechanism of opsonization led at that time to theories about interfacial tension and physicochemical surface property changes (Mudd *et al.*, 1934). So, even 50 years ago, both specific and nonspecific recognition were suggested. Before discussing the physicochemical basis for bacteria–phagocyte interaction, it is necessary to review the current concepts of receptor-mediated recognition.

A. Specific recognition

Several more or less well-defined recognition sites, claimed to be specific receptors, have been shown to occur on phagocytic cells (Table 1). Both polymorphonuclear neutrophil leukocytes (PMNL) and macrophages rec-

Table 1 Different receptor sites on macrophages and PMNL with specificities for different ligands

Receptor	Characteristics		Cells
	specificity	function	
Fc (trypsin-resistant)	IgG1, IgG3	Opsonizing	Macrophage, PMNL
Fc (trypsin-sensitive)	IgG	?	Macrophage, (PMNL)[b]
C3b	C3b	Opsonizing	Macrophage, PMNL
C3b'	C3b'	Opsonizing	Macrophage, PMNL
Carbohydrates	Lectins	(Opsonizing)[a]	Macrophage, PMNL
Lectins	Carbohydrates	(Opsonizing)	Macrophage, (PMNL)
Hydrophobic interaction	General	Opsonizing	Macrophage, PMNL

[a] means that the function is unclear or weak.
[b] means that it is unclear or not determined.

ognize the Fc-moiety of IgG. Direct binding studies with aggregated immunoglobulins show that IgG_1 and IgG_3 bind with higher affinity than IgG_2 and IgG_4 (Messner and Jelinek, 1970; Henson, 1976), whereas with nonaggregated monomeric immunoglobulins only IgG_1 and IgG_3 bound to human PMNL. Macrophages have recently been shown to express two different Fc receptors (FcR); one trypsin-sensitive FcR that binds monomeric IgG, and one trypsin-resistant FcR that binds aggregated IgG or immune complexes (Heusser *et al.*, 1977; Unkeless and Eisen, 1975). Trypsin treatment of PMNL or macrophages does not inhibit phagocytosis of IgG-opsonized particles. It is thus assumed that the trypsin-resistant receptor for aggregated IgG is the FcR that mediates phagocytosis of IgG-coated particles. Whether PMNL and macrophages from different species possess the trypsin-sensitive FcR is unclear.

Recognition sites for activated forms of complement are widely distributed among mammalian cells (Nilsson, 1981). PMNL and macrophage receptors for activated forms of C3 (C3b, C3b'), termed CR1 and CR3 respectively, are functionally independent of the Fc receptors (Ross, 1980). Only a limited number of studies have utilized opsonized particles sufficiently characterized as to allow evaluation of the relative role of the CR1 and CR3 and their relationship to FcR. Several studies on macrophages have shown that whether or not the complement receptors facilitate both attachment and ingestion depends on the physiological state of the cells (Bianco *et al.*, 1975). In non-activated macrophages, the complement recognition mediates attachment but not ingestion of particles. However, in activated macrophages complement-opsonized particles are also ingested. Although both receptors are trypsin-sensitive, it is not yet clear whether activation of the cells is associated with the genesis of more receptors or whether activation establishes a previously unexpressed link with the contractile apparatus. A similar functional difference between complement receptors on activated and unactivated PMNL has also been described (Hed, 1981). It is thus evident that the expression of receptor activity can vary during differentiation, activation and as a result of inflammatory stimulation.

Several reports have shown a cooperative function between Fc and complement receptors on phagocytic cells (Mantovani *et al.*, 1972; Newman and Johnston, 1979). On a quantitative basis, the IgG molecule is extremely effective in eliciting different effector functions such as phagocytosis, metabolic activation and lysosomal enzyme release (Hed and Stendahl, 1982). However, in certain systems, increasing the number of C3b or C3b' molecules on the particles is sufficient to trigger ingestion (Henson, 1976).

Apart from binding complement or the Fc part of IgG, PMNL and macrophages recognize and bind several other ligands. Carbohydrate residues, mannose, N-acetylglucosamine, glucose and galactose, with specificities for different lectins, concanavalin A (Con A) wheat germ agglutinin (WGA) and ricinus communis agglutinin (RCA) are expressed on different phagocytic cells. Several bacterial adhesins with lectin-like properties promote attachment of certain microorganisms (Jones, 1977; Duguid and Old, 1980). Type 1 fimbriae of certain *Escherichia coli* and *Salmonella* strains exhibit mannose-sensitive binding to macrophages, Kupffer cells and PMNL (Bar-Shavit *et al.*, 1977; Leunk and Moon, 1982; Öhman *et al.*, 1982). In several ways the lectin-like interaction resembles the complement-mediated binding, in that it promotes strong attachment but is less potent in initiating ingestion. Whether the attachment leads to ingestion may depend on the underlying surface properties of the bacteria such as lipolysosaccharide and acidic capsular antigens (Horwitz and Silverstein, 1980; Öhman *et al.*, 1982). In the absence of serum, fimbriae-mediated attachment will lead to ingestion only of relatively rough-like hydrophobic bacteria, whereas smooth-like, hydrophobic ones remain attached.

In virulent *Neisseria*, fimbriae may be antiphagocytic by mediating attachment to PMNL without eliciting ingestion (Densen and Mandell, 1978). During certain infections, the infecting bacteria may also alter their ability to interact with host cells, by changing the number of fimbriae exposed (Silverblatt and Ofek, 1978; Öhman and Stendahl, unpublished observations). These findings suggest that adaptability of the bacteria to the pressures of a particular environment is a mechanism necessary for survival.

Lectin-like, trypsin-sensitive recognition sites on macrophages recognizing different carbohydrate residues (glucose mannose, N-acetylglucosamine, galactose) on glycoproteins and bacteria have been proposed (Stahl *et al.*, 1978; Freimer *et al.*, 1978). The ability of specific sugars to inhibit binding is directly related to their presence in the repeating unit or the outer core of the lipopolysaccharide (Freimer *et al.*, 1978). Whether one or several specific receptor sites on the macrophage bind these sugar residues is not clear.

Macrophages also display specific trypsin-sensitive recognition for certain particles (sheep erythrocytes, zymosan) that can activate complement via the alternate pathway (Czop *et al.*, 1978). The chemical characteristics of these structures are unrevealed, although removal of sialic acid enhances both recognition and complement activation.

The fact that several microorganisms are phagocytosed in the absence of serum factors indicates that phagocytic cells possess several mechanisms to recognize certain microbial surface structures.

B.   General physicochemical recognition

From studying phagocytic recognition of well-defined particles in the absence of antibody and complement it has become increasingly clear that also more general physicochemical properties of the prey and the phagocyte influence the outcome of the reaction; the main properties being negative surface charge and hydrophobic interaction (Edebo *et al.*, 1980; Mudd *et al.*, 1934; van Oss, 1978).

1.   *Theoretical considerations*

Thermodynamic reasoning predicts that association occurs between a bacterium (B) and a phagocytic cell (P) when the overall change of the free energy $\Delta F_{net} < 0$. For the process of engulfment:

$$F_{net} = \gamma_{PB} - \gamma_{BW},$$

where γ_{BW} is the interfacial tension between the bacteria and water (W) and γ_{PB} is the interfacial tension between the phagocyte and the bacteria. Values of γ_{PB} and γ_{BW} can be obtained by contact-angle measurements, saying that $F_{net} < 0$, when $\theta_B > \theta_P$, a situation favouring engulfment (van Oss, 1978). Thus, general physicochemical surface properties of the bacteria and the phagocyte can be defined and may determine the outcome of the interaction. However, when cell–cell interaction occurs the reaction can also be viewed as a patch-wise reaction between hydrophobic entities, which are forced into an aqueous milieu by dominating hydrophilic groups. This is an important distinction since different methods used for probing surface hydrophobicity may reflect either average or the local affinity for the probe (Magnusson, 1980).

The surface of eukaryotic cells have a negative potential that may result from ionization of various chemical groups like sialic acid carboxyl group. Increased negative charge has been shown to impair phagocytic recognition, and removal of sialic acid may increase phagocytosis. The apparent paradox that two entities, both with negative surface potential, may still attract and adhere to one another can be explained, in part, by the application of the lyophobic theories of Derjaguin and Landau (1941) and Verwey and Overbeck (1948). The so-called DLVO theory considers that the energy of interaction of two charged particles of like sign and magnitude is the sum of electrostatic energy of repulsion and the energy of attraction provided by London–van der Waals forces. The repulsive energy decreases more rapidly with distance than attractive energy. These short range attraction forces can operate with two negatively charged particles, providing the radius of curvature is small, as in microvilli and pseudopods. With respect to hydrophobic properties, decreased water content around the bacteria and displacement of water during cell–particle interaction would bring the interacting entities closer together, where the above-mentioned forces could work.

To visualize the prey–phagocyte interaction, enzyme kinetics analysis using the Lineweaver–Burke plot has been applied in certain systems. The K_m value represents the affinity for the prey, whereas V_{max} reflects the maximal rate of uptake. Applying this formula requires that the experimental design can conclusively distinguish ingestion from attachment (Liang-Takasaki et al., 1982).

IV. BACTERIA-PHAGOCYTE INTERACTION

To study general mechanisms of bacteria–phagocyte interaction, we have chosen to study Salmonella and E. coli bacteria. It has been appreciated for several years that the LPS governs the susceptibility of these bacteria to phagocytosis and intracellular killing (Medearis et al., 1968; Stendahl and Edebo, 1972; Weiss et al., 1982). Bacteria with short LPS are more susceptible to ingestion and intra-cellular killing than those with more complete polysaccharide chains. Since several bacteria with defective polysaccharide structures were phagocytosed by granulocytes in the absence of antibody and complement, more general physicochemical surface properties may influence the outcome of the interaction. To prove this we studied the surface properties of Salmonella typhimurium mutants with defined defects in their LPS structure, in relation to phagocytosis (Edebo et al., 1980).

Few methods are available to study surface charge, surface hydrophobicity and surface tension. Mudd et al. (1934) used oil/water two-phase systems and showed a relationship between hydrophobicity and phagocytosis. Using aqueous polymer two-phase systems as devised by Albertsson (1971), in which subtle changes in charge and hydrophobicity could be detected, it was possible to quantitate differences in the bacterial surface related to LPS structure (Stendahl et al., 1973b; Stendahl et al., 1977).

In two-phase systems containing dextran-T500 and polyethyleneglycol-6000 (PEG), S. typhimurium 395 MS (smooth) accumulated into the PEG-rich top phase, whereas the R mutant derived from it showed affinity for the dextran-rich bottom phase. When a uridine-galactose-4-epimerase-less mutant (MR9) was grown without galactose in the medium, the bacteria partitioned like the other R mutants, whereas growth in the presence of galactose, allowing the synthesis of the complete S-LPS, changed the partition properties to that of S bacteria (Stendahl et al., 1973a,b) which also increase the phagocytic resistance.

Since this phenotypic difference was a consequence of the synthesis of the S-specific polysaccharide side chain, the exposure of the surface polysaccharide seems to strongly influence the physicochemical properties of the bacteria. Using positively charged (trimethylamino-) and negatively charged (sulphonate-) PEG in the phase systems revealed that the R bacteria exposed negative surface charge whereas the S bacteria were virtually uncharged (Stendahl et al., 1977). When PEG esterified with fatty acids (palmitoyl-) were included in the phase system, the partition of the bacteria were governed by hydrophobic interaction between the fatty acid moiety and the particle surface. The partition of S bacteria was not influenced by the hydrophobic polymer, whereas the partition of R mutants changed towards the hydrophobic top phase (Magnusson et al., 1977).

For further analysis of liability to hydrophobic binding of bacteria, we employed hydrophobic interaction chromatography (HIC). When the Salmonella mutants were chromatographed on phenyl- or octyl-sepharose, the rough mutants bound to the column, confirming exposure of hydrophobic sites (Stjernström et al., 1977), whereas the S bacteria eluted in the void volume. To measure the overall interfacial tension of bacterial monolayers, contact-angle measurements have been employed. Analysis of S. typhimurium mutants fits well with the hydrophobicity and liability to phagocytosis of the R mutants and hydrophilicity and resistance to phagocytosis of the S bacteria (Cunningham et al., 1975).

Recently, we have shown that also among wild-type clinical isolates of Salmonella strains, there is a correlation between hydrophobicity and interaction with PMNL. Certain serotypes (C1 and E4) of these Salmonella strains were more liable to hydrophobic interaction and phagocytosis (Jiang et al., unpublished observations).

The following pattern emerges with respect to the interaction of S. typhimurium bacteria and phagocytic cells: on smooth bacteria the long repeating polysaccharide side chain gives the surface hydrophilic, uncharged characteristics which will impair phagocytic recognition; with shorter polysaccharide chains, the bacteria becomes less hydrophilic and expose hydrophobic and negatively charged sites, both of which will enhance interaction with phagocytes. However, qualitative differences in the polysaccharide structures may also influence the bacteria–phagocyte interaction directly or through its effect on complement activation (Smith, 1977; Liang-Takasaki et al., 1982; Jiang et al., 1983) (Table 2).

Compared to the LPS-dominated surface of Salmonella, E. coli bacteria show a more complex surface structure with LPS, acidic capsular polysaccharides and adhesion-promoting factors such as pili and colonizing factors (Duguid and Old, 1981). It is evident that quantitative and qualitative differences in the LPS, like in *Salmonella*, influence phagocytic resistance (Medearis *et al.*, 1968; Stendahl *et al.*, 1979). The negatively charged capsular (K) antigen constituting the outermost layer of the bacteria may impair phagocytic interactions (Howard and Glynn, 1971; Rottini *et al.*, 1975). However, when evaluating the effect of K antigens on phagocytosis, the role of the underlying LPS must be accounted for. On bacteria with smooth-type, hydrophilic LPS, the increased negative charge provided by K antigens will not significantly influence phagocytosis in a serum-free system. In contrast, when K antigens increase the negative charge of bacteria with rough-type, hydrophobic LPS, phagocytosis may be impeded (Stendahl *et al.*, 1979) (Table 2).

As discussed earlier, *Salmonella* and *E. coli* expose specific adhesins, such as fimbriae with specific recognition sites on the phagocytes. Several investigators observed that mannose-specific recognition will enhance phagocytosis in PMNL and macrophages (Rottini *et al.*, 1979; Bar-Shavit *et al.*, 1977; Mangan and Snyder, 1979). Since the physicochemical surface properties of *E. coli* and *Salmonella* may differ extensively, the role of the fimbriae may vary accordingly. Certain virulent *E. coli* strains isolated from patients with acute pyelonephritis attach strongly to PMNL in a mannose-sensitive way, but are not ingested, since they also expose smooth-like LPS and acidic K antigen (Öhman *et al.*, 1982). However, when rough-like hydrophobic bacteria adhere to PMNL via mannose-sensitive fimbriae, they will be readily ingested. Importantly, both types of bacteria will elicit a metabolic response with release of reactive oxidative metabolites. The adhesive surface properties of these bacteria may thus not only be relevant as virulence attributes in the interplay with non-professional phagocytes such as epithelial cells (Ofek *et al.*, 1977) in governing the outcome of mucosal-associated infections, but also as elicitors of inflammation in their interaction with granulocytes and macrophages. When evaluating hydrophobic pili or other adhesins as ligands mediating phagocytosis, it is thus vital to consider the other surface properties governing the bacterial-phagocyte interface such as charge and hydrophobicity and use methods where attachment and ingestion can be properly evaluated (Hed, 1981). The described interaction between certain well-characterized *E. coli* strains and phagocytes represents a good model for studying the cooperative effect of "specific" and "non-specific" interaction.

A. Physicochemical effects of opsonization

It is well known that IgG antibodies increase phagocytosis and subsequent killing by PMNL and macrophages. This effect is mediated as discussed

Table 2 Biochemical and physicochemical surface properties of *Salmonella typhimurium* and *Escherichia coli* in relation to phagocytosis

Bacteria	Surface structure	Physicochemical effect			Phagocytic interaction	
		hydrophilicity	hydrophobicity	negative charge	attachment	ingestion
Salmonella	S-LPS	++	0	0	—	—
	R-LPS	0	++	+	++	+
E. coli	S-LPS	++	0	0	—	—
	R-LPS	0	++	+	+	+
	K-antigen	+	0	++	—	—
	pili (type 1)	0	++	n.d.	++	+/—

0 = lack of indicated effect.
+/— = weak or varying effect.
+ = strong effect.
++ = very strong effect.
— = inhibitory effect.
n.d. = not detected.

before at least in part by specific ligand-receptor interactions. It has become evident that binding of IgG antibodies to the surface of certain bacteria also alter their general surface properties in several respects. When smooth *S. typhimurium* bacteria were opsonized with IgG antibodies, their surface properties changed in a way that mimicked an S → R mutation (Stendahl *et al.*, 1974; Stjernström *et al.*, 1977). The affinity for the hydrophobic octyl-sepharose gel was increased and their two-phase partition changed. Similarly, the contact angle was increased (Cunningham *et al.*, 1975). It is thus evident that when IgG antibodies bind to hydrophilic bacteria, their liability to hydrophobic interaction increases. The same number of IgG molecules (2–4000 molecules/bacterium) were required to enhance hydrophobic interaction and phagocytosis. Both the physico-chemical and phagocytosis-promoting effects of IgG were enhanced by complement (Stendahl *et al.*, 1974; Stjernström *et al.*, 1977).

To focus on the lipophilic property of the Fc part of IgG, we employed an artificial liposomal membrane model. This phospholipid bilayer, presumably lacking specific receptors, was very effectively perturbed by *Salmonella* bacteria opsonized with IgG, but not by non-opsonized smooth-type bacteria (Tagesson *et al.*, 1977). We thus visualize that when opsonizing IgG antibodies bind to the smooth *S. typhimurium* bacteria, the hydrophilic polysaccharide is covered and hydrophobic sies are exposed via the Fc part of the molecule. Thermodynamic calculations by van Oss (1978) of the interfacial free energy needed for engulfment seem to fit with the experimental data. Whereas IgG opsonization and S → R mutation favour phagocytosis, the binding of the carbohydrate-rich secretory IgA (SIgA) antibodies, present on mucosal membranes, to rough *S. typhimurium* bacteria produces the opposite effect; hydrophobic interaction and negative surface charge were reduced, thus rendering the bacteria less liable to interact with phagocytic cells (Magnusson *et al.*, 1978). In fact, in a mutual interplay, SIgA can mask the effect of the more hydrophobic IgG and vice versa (Magnusson and Stjernström, 1982) (Table 3).

Table 3 Similarities in the biochemical, physicochemical and adhesive properties between smooth and rough *Salmonella* bacteria and SIgA and IgG antibodies

	Salmonella		Antibodies	
	smooth	rough	SIgG	IgG
Hydrophobic interaction	—	+	—	+
Association to phagocytic cells	—	+	—	+
Carbohydrate exposure	+	—	+	—

B. Alterations of the phagocyte surface in relation to phagocytosis

To combat bacteria, the host does not only alter the surface of the invader, but also the phagocytic cells as a response to inflammation. During differentiation and activation, several physicochemical membrane changes occur that are relevant to phagocytosis. During maturation the negative surface charge decreases, with a subsequent increase in phagocytosis (Lichtman and Weed, 1972). Reduction of sialic acid by neuraminidase treatment may also enhance phagocytosis (Weiss *et al.*, 1966). Furthermore, during cultivation of macrophages the complement-recognition sites are selectively reduced (Rabinovitch and DeStefano, 1973). Also during activation and phagocytosis several membrane changes occur. Lysosomal granulae secretion during interaction with chemotactic factors, immune complexes and bacteria reduce the negative surface charge (Gallin, 1980), increase hydrophobic interaction (Dahlgren and Stendahl, 1982) and adhesiveness (Gallin, 1980). Recycling of membrane and chemical modifications rather than *de novo* synthesis are responsible for these changes.

Similar results were obtained in another model. Studying the surface properties of a myeloid leukaemic cell line (HL60) during differentiation, it was observed that hydrophobic surface properties increased. Concurrently phagocytosis of IgG- and C3b-opsonized particles increased, as did the chemotactic response (Stendahl *et al.*, 1982). Although several cell properties relevant to phagocytosis such as specific receptors and contractile proteins may be modulated during the course of differentiation, the collected evidence strongly suggests that increased hydrophobic interaction will enhance phagocytosis of certain preys.

By exposing granulocytes and other cells with lysosomal vesicles it is possible to alter the plasma membrane properties (Inbar and Shinitzky, 1974; Dahlgren *et al.*, 1977). The negative surface charge, tendency to hydrophobic interaction and membrane fluidity were reduced, with a concomitant reduced capacity to phagocytose non-opsonized and IgG-opsonized *S. typhimurium* bacteria. It is thus possible that modulation of the phospholipid bilayer influences the fate of the particle–phagocyte interaction. Dianzini *et al.* (1976) have also shown that increase in plasma membrane cholesterol is accompanied by a significant reduction in the phagocytic uptake of latex particles by macrophages.

During phagocytosis the recognition sites are segregated and selectively removed from the plasma membrane (Berlin *et al.*, 1975). Recent work has shown that glycoproteins of phagocytic vacuole membranes are recycled to the plasma membrane (Muller *et al.*, 1980) and that a membrane and receptor reservoir can be made available to the surface (Petty *et al.*, 1981).

It is thus evident that the membrane of the phagocytic cell can modulate its specific and non-specific recognition sites in order to meet the requirements during inflammation.

V. CONCLUSION

Several recognition mechanisms in the host–bacteria interaction are governed by the physicochemical surface properties of the interacting entities. Although our understanding of the molecular events at the microbial envelope that govern the fate of microorganisms exposed to phagocytes is incomplete, certain characteristics are established. Liability to hydrophobic interaction favours phagocyte recognition and will increase the susceptibility of certain bacteria to phagocytosis, whereas hydrophilicity will enhance resistance of most microbes. Negative surface charge will, depending on the topography of the bacterial envelope and the cell involved, either enhance or impair phagocytic recognition. Where specific carbohydrate-binding sites are integrated components of the bacterial surface or of the phagocyte membrane, these ligands may cooperate with more general physicochemical properties in promoting attachment, subsequent ingestion and release of inflammatory mediators. Opsonizing IgG antibodies and complement will enhance both specific ligand-receptor interaction as well as rendering the bacterial surface more liable to hydrophobic interaction. On the other hand, increasing the hydrophilic properties of bacteria with SIgA or polysaccharides will decrease the bacterial interaction with phagocytic as well as with other host cells. This antiphagocytic effect of SIgA could function as an aseptic protective mechanism at the mucosal surfaces. Progress in the surface characterization of microorganisms and of the phagocyte membrane and how they can be modulated may provide new insights into phagocyte–microbe interactions and host-defence in general.

ACKNOWLEDGEMENTS

This work has been supported by grants from The Swedish Medical Research Council (2168 and 5968) and from Östergötlands Läns Landsting.

REFERENCES

Albertsson, P. Å. (1971). "Partition of Cell Particles and Macromolecules", 2nd Ed. Almqvist & Wiksell, Uppsala.

Bar-Shavit, Z., Ofek, I., Goldman, R., Mirelman, D. and Sharon, N. (1977). *Biochem. Biophys. Res. Commun.* **78,** 455–459.

Berlin, R. D. and Fera, J. P. (1977). *Proc. Nat. Acad. Sci. (USA)* **74,** 1072–1076.

Berlin, R. D., Oliver, M. J., Ukena, T. E. and Yin, H. E. (1975). *New Engl. J. Med.* **292,** 515–521.

Bianco, S., Griffin, F. M. and Silverstein, S. M. (1975). *J. Exp. Med.* **141,** 1278–1290.

Cohen, H. J., Chovaniec, M. E. and Davies, W. A. (1980). *Blood* **55,** 355–363.

Cunningham, R. K., Söderström, T. O., Gillman, C. F. and van Oss, C. J. (1975). *Immunol. Commun.* **4,** 429–442.

Czop, J. K., Fearon, D. T. and Austen, K. F. (1978). *Proc. Nat. Acad. Sci.* **75,** 3831–3834.

Dahlgren, C. and Stendahl, O. (1982). *Inflammation* (in press).

Dahlgren, C., Kihlström, E., Magnusson, K.-E., Stendahl, O. and Tagesson, C. (1977). *Exp. Cell Res.* **108,** 175–184.

Densen, P. and Mandell, G. L. (1978). *J. Clin. Invest.* **62,** 1161–1171.

Densen, P. and Mandell, G. L. (1980). *Rev. Infect. Dis.* **2,** 817–838.

Derjaguin, B. V. and Landau, L. (1941). *Acta Physiochem. USSR* **14,** 633–662.

Dianzini, M. U., Torrielli, M. V., Canuto, R. A., Carcea, R. and Feo, F. (1976). *J. Pathol.* **118,** 193–199.

Duguid, J. P. and Old, D. C. (1980). Adhesive properties of enterobacteriaceae. *In* "Bacterial Adherence" (E. H. Beachey, ed.) Receptors and Recognition, Ser. B, Vol. 6, pp. 187–217. Chapman and Hall, London, New York.

Edebo, L, Kihlström, E., Magnusson, K.-E. and Stendahl, O. (1980). *In* "Cell Adhesion and Motility" (A S. G. Curtis and J. D Pitts, eds) pp. 65–101. Cambridge University Press.

Elsbach, P. (1977). *In* "The Synthesis, Assembly and Turnover of Cell Surface Components" (G. Poste and G. Nicolson, eds) pp. 363–402. Elsevier/North Holland Biomedical Press, Amsterdam.

Freimer, N. B., Ögmundsdottir, H. M., Blackwell, C. C., Sutherland, I. W., Graham, L. and Weir, D. M. (1978). *Acta Pathol. Microbiol. Scand. Sect. B.* **86,** 53–57.

Gallin, J. I. (1980). *J. Clin. Invest.* **65,** 298–306.

Griffin, F. M., Griffin, J. A., Leider, J. E. and Silverstein, S. C. (1975). *J. Exp. Med.* **142,** 1263–1274.

Hed, J. (1981). *Monogr. Allerg.* **17,** 92–111.

Hed, J. and Stendahl, O. (1982). *Immunology* **45,** 727–736.

Henson, P. M. (1976). *Immun. Commun.* **5,** 757–772.

Heusser, C. H., Anderson, C. L. and Grey, H. M. (1977). *J. Exp. Med.* **145,** 1316–1327.

Horwitz, M. A. and Silverstein, S. C. (1980). *J. Clin. Invest.* **65,** 82–94.

Howard, C. J. and Glynn, A. A. (1971). *Immunology* **20,** 767–777.

Inbar, M. and Schinitzky, M. (1974). *Proc. Nat. Acad. Sci. USA,* **71,** 2128–2130.

Jiang, Hui Xiu, Magnusson, K.-E., Stendahl, O. and Edebo, L. (1983). *J. Gen. Microbiol.* (in press).

Jones, G. W. (1977) The attachment of bacteria to the surface of animal cells. *In* "Receptors and Recognition, Microbial Interaction" (Reissig, ed.), Series B, Vol. 3, pp. 139–184. Chapman and Hall, London.

Leunk, R. D. and Moon, R. J. (1982). *Infect. Immun.* **36,** 1168–1174.

Liang-Takasaki, C. J., Mäkelä, H. P. and Leive, L. (1982). *J. Immunol.* **128,** 1229–1235.

Lichtman, M. L. and Weed, R. I. (1972). *Blood* **39**, 301–316.
Magnusson, K.-E. (1980). *Scand. J. Infect. Dis.* suppl., **24**, 131–134.
Magnusson, K.-E. and Stjernström, I. (1982). *Immunology* **45**, 239–748.
Magnusson, K.-E., Stendahl, O., Tagesson, C., Edebo, L and Johansson, G. (1977). *Acta Pathol. Microbiol. Scand.* **85**, 212–218.
Magnusson, K.-E., Stendahl, O., Stjernström, I. and Edebo, L. (1979). *Immunology* **36**, 439–497.
Mangan, D. F. and Snyder, I. S (1979). *Infect. Immun.* **26**, 520–527.
Mantovani, M., Rabinovitch, M. and Nussenzweig, V. (1972). *J. Exp. Med.* **135**, 780–792.
Medearis, D. N., Camitta, B. M. and Heath, E. C. (1968). *J. Exp. Med.* **128**, 399–404.
Messner, R. P. and Jelinek, J. (1970). *J. Clin. Invest.* **49**, 2165–2171.
Mudd, S., McCutcheon, M. and Lucké, B. (1934). *Physiol. Review* **14**, 210–275.
Muller, W. A., Steinman, R. M. and Cohn, Z. A. (1980). *J. Cell Biol.* **86**, 304–314.
Newman, S. L. and Johnston, R. B. Jr. (1979). *J. Immunol.* **135**, 1839–1845.
Nilsson, U. R. (1981). *Monographs in Allergy* **17**, 70–91.
Ofek, I., Mirelman, D. and Sharon, N. (1977). *Nature* **265**, 623–625.
Öhman, L., Hed, J. and Stendahl, O. (1982). *J. Infect. Dis.* **146**, 751–757.
Petroski, R. J., Naccache, P. H., Becker, E. L. and Sha'afi, R. I. (1979). *Amer. J. Physiol.* **237**, C39.
Petty, H. R., Hafeman, D. G. and McConnell, H. M. (1981). *J. Cell Biol.* **89**, 223–232.
Rabinovitch, M. and DeStefano, M. J. (1973). *J. Immunol.* **110**, 695–701.
Root, R. K. and Cohen, M. S. (1981). *Rev. Infect. Dis.* **3**, 565–598.
Ross, G. D. (1980). *J. Immun. Meth.* **37**, 197–204.
Rottini, G., Dri, P., Soranzo, M. R. and Patriarca, P. (1975). *Infect. Immun.* **11**, 417–423.
Rottini, G., Ciah, F., Soranzo, M. R., Alberigo, R. and Patriarca, P. (1979). *FEBS Letters* **105**, 307–317.
Seligmann, B. E. and Gallin, J. I. (1980). *J. Clin. Invest.* **66**, 493–503.
Silverblatt, F. J. and Ofek, I. (1978). *J. Infect. Dis.* **38**, 664–667.
Silverstein, S. C., Steinman, R. M. and Cohn, Z. A. (1977). *Ann. Rev. Biochem.* **46**, 669–722.
Smith, H. (1977). *Bacteriol. Rev.* **41**, 485–500.
Stahl, P. D., Rodman, J. S., Miller, M. J. and Schlesinger, P. H. (1978). *Proc. Nat. Acad. Sci.* **75**, 1399–1403.
Stendahl, O. and Edebo, L. (1972). *Acta Pathol. Microbiol. Scand. Sect. B* **80**, 481–488.
Stendahl, O., Magnusson, K.-E., Tagesson, C., Cunningham, R. and Edebo, L. (1973a). *Infect. Immun.* **7**, 573–577.
Stendahl, O., Tagesson, C., and Edebo, M. (1973b). *Infect. Immun.* **8**, 36–41.
Stendahl, O., Tagesson, C. and Edebo, L. (1974). *Infect. Immun.* **10**, 316–319.
Stendahl, O., Edebo, L., Tagesson, C., Magnusson, K.-E. and Hjertén, S. (1977). *Acta Pathol. Microbiol. Scand. Sect. B* **85**, 334–340.
Stendahl, O., Normann, B. and Edebo, L. (1979). *Acta Pathol. Microbiol. Scand. Sect. B* **87**, 85–91.
Stendahl, O., Hartwig, J. H., Brotchi, E. A. and Stossel, T. P. (1980). *J. Cell Biol.* **84**, 215–224.
Stendahl, O., Dahlgren, C. and Hed, J. (1982). *J. Cell Physiol.* **112**, 217–221.

Stjernström, I., Magnusson, K.-E., Stendahl, O. and Tagesson, C. (1977). *Infect. Immun.* **18,** 261–265.

Stossel, T. P., Hartwig, J. H. and Yin, H. L. (1981). *Cell Surface Rev.* (in press).

Tagesson, C., Magnusson, K.-E. and Stendahl, O. (1977). *J. Immunol.* **119,** 609–613.

Thornburg, R. W., Day, J. F., Baynes, J. W. and Thorpe, S. R. (1980). *J. Biol. Chem.* **225,** 6820–6826.

Unkeless, J. C. and Eisen, H. N. (1975). *J. Exp. Med.* **142,** 1520–1533.

van Oss, C. J. (1978). *Ann. Rev. Microbiol.* **32,** 19–39.

Verwey, E. J. W. and Overbeck, J. T. G. (1978). "Theory of the Stability of Lyophobic Colloids." Elsevier, Amsterdam.

Weiss, L., Mayhew, E. and Ulrich, K. (1966). *Lab. Invest.* **15,** 1304–1309.

Weiss, J., Victor, M., Stendahl, O. and Elsbach, P. (1982). *J. Clin. Invest.* **69,** 959–970.

Wright, A. E. and Douglas, S. R. (1903). *Proc. Roy. Soc. B. Biol. Sci.* **72,** 357–372.

7 Availability of iron and survival of bacteria in infection

ELWYN GRIFFITHS

I. INTRODUCTION

The basic requirement for a rational approach to the management and treatment of patients with infections, and to the development and use of vaccines, is a clear understanding of the way pathogenic organisms produce infection and, consequently, pathological changes in the tissues of the natural host. The factors involved in an infection are, clearly, numerous and complex, and may vary with the infecting organism. However, one common and essential factor in all infections is the ability of the invading pathogen to multiply in the host. This property is now known to be greatly influenced by the availability of iron. Animals injected with various forms of iron are much more susceptible to infection with a variety of bacterial pathogens than are the untreated controls (Table 1); iron compounds also abolish the antibacterial effects of body fluids *in vitro* (Bullen *et al.*, 1978; Weinberg, 1978; Griffiths, 1981). For example, iron can abolish the bactericidal action of serum on *Pasteurella septica* and abolish the passive

Table 1 Examples of bacteria whose virulence in experimental infections is enhanced by injecting iron compounds

Aeromonas hydrophilia	Miles *et al.* (1979)	*N. meningitidis*	Calver *et al.* (1976)
Clostridium welchii	Bullen *et al.* (1967)	*Pasteurella septica*	Bullen *et al.* (1968b)
C. oedematis	Miles *et al.* (1979)	*Pseudomonas aeruginosa*	Forsberg and Bullen (1972)
Corynebacterium renale	Henderson *et al.* (1978)	*Salmonella typhimurium*	Kaye *et al.* (1965)
Escherichia coli	Bullen *et al.* (1968a)	*Staphylococcus aureus*	Gladstone and Walton (1971)
Klebsiella pneumoniae	Miles *et al.* (1979)	*Vibrio cholerae*	Ford and Hayhoe (1970)
Listeria monocytogenes	Sword (1966)	*V. vulnificus*	Wright *et al.* (1981)
Neisseria gonorrhoeae	Payne and Finkelstein (1975)	*Yersinia pestis*	Jackson and Burrows (1956)

MEDICAL MICROBIOLOGY, 3
ISBN 0 12 228003 3

protection afforded by *P. septica* antiserum *in vivo* (Bullen *et al.*, 1968b; Griffiths, 1975). In addition to abolishing the passive protection of antiserum, iron affects the susceptibility of normal animals to infection by reducing the lethal dose of bacteria. Thus, the lethal dose of *Escherichia coli* for normal guinea-pigs is about 10^8 cells, but in guinea-pigs treated with ferric ammonium citrate this dose can be reduced to about 10^3 cells (Bullen *et al.*, 1968a). Only iron has been found to act in this way and the investigation of the phenomenon has led not only to an explanation of the changes in resistance which sometimes accompany clinical alterations in the iron status of the host, but has also increased our understanding of the mechanisms involved in microbial pathogenicity.

II. AVAILABILITY OF IRON *IN VIVO*

Although there is plenty of iron present in the body fluids of vertebrates, the amount of free iron, which might be readily available to bacteria, is extremely small. Body iron is held primarily intracellularly, as ferritin, haemosiderin or haem, and that which is extracellular in serum or other body fluids is attached to the high affinity iron-binding glycoproteins transferrin and lactoferrin (Table 2; Bezkorovainy and Zschocke, 1974; Bullen *et al.*, 1978; Aisen, 1980; Morgan, 1980, 1981). Transferrin is found mainly in serum and lymph and lactoferrin in secretions and milk, where it occurs in relatively high concentrations (Masson and Heremans, 1966; Masson *et al.*, 1966a,b; Mason and Taylor, 1978). Lactoferrin is also found in the secretory granules of polymorphonuclear leukocytes (Masson *et al.*, 1969; Bullen, 1981). A related protein, ovotransferrin, occurs in avian egg white (Schade and Caroline, 1944; Alderton *et al.*, 1946; Bezkorovainy and Zschocke, 1974). These proteins have molecular weights of about 80 000

Table 2 Distribution of iron-binding proteins

Lactoferrin	Saliva
	Tears
	Nasal secretion
	Bronchial secretion
	Intestinal fluid
	Seminal fluid
	Cervical mucus
	Colostrum
	Milk (human)
	Polymorphonuclear leukocytes
Transferrin	Serum
Ovotransferrin	Avian egg white

and each is capable of reversibly binding two ferric ions with the simultaneous incorporation of two bicarbonate ions (Bezkorovainy and Zschocke, 1974; Bezkorovainy, 1980; Morgan, 1981). Since they are normally only partially saturated with Fe^{3+} and have an association constant of approximately 10^{36}, the amount of free iron in equilibrium with the iron-binding proteins is about 10^{-18} M, which is far too low for normal bacterial growth (Bullen et al., 1978; Bullen, 1981). In addition, during infection the host reduces the total amount of iron bound to serum transferrin (Cartwright et al., 1946). This decrease, called the hypoferraemia of infection, in which there is a movement of iron from serum to the iron stores, can be reproduced by injecting small amounts of bacterial endotoxin (Baker and Wilson, 1965). Endotoxin acts by stimulating the release from polymorphonuclear leukocytes of a factor which appears identical to leukocytic pyrogen (Merriman et al., 1977). Leukocyte pyrogen induces fever, leukocytosis and the release of the contents of specific granules from polymorphs (Leffell and Spitznagel, 1974; Klempner et al., 1978). Van Snick et al. (1974) have shown that it is the lactoferrin released from polymorphs that is responsible for lowering serum iron. Lactoferrin removes iron from transferrin and the Fe^{3+}-lactoferrin is taken up by macrophages and removed rapidly from the circulation by the reticuloendothelial system. Furthermore, it has been shown that lactoferrin accumulates at the site of inflammation and appears to be involved in regulating granulopoiesis (Broxmeyer et al., 1978). Unlike transferrin, whose iron-binding affinity is diminished below pH 6, lactoferrin retains its iron-binding properties in the more acidic conditions which often prevail at sites of inflammation (McClelland and van Furth, 1976; Aisen, 1980; Morgan, 1980; Ainscough et al., 1980).

III. ACQUISITION OF IRON BY PATHOGENIC BACTERIA

In spite of the virtual absence of freely available iron in normal body fluids, and of the hypoferraemia of infection, many pathogenic organisms can multiply successfully in blood, mucosal secretions and other body fluids. Since all known bacterial pathogens need iron to multiply, and thus to establish an infection, they must possess mechanisms for assimilating protein bound iron or for acquiring it from liberated haem. One possibility is that iron is removed from the iron-binding proteins by a direct interaction between receptors on the bacterial cell surface and the Fe^{3+}-protein complex in a manner analogous to the reaction occurring between transferrin and the reticulocyte (Witt and Woodworth, 1978; Morgan, 1981). Proteolytic cleavage of transferrin, which would disrupt the iron-binding site and release Fe^{3+}, is another possibility. So far there is no direct evidence that either system operates in bacteria, although it has been suggested that the removal of iron from transferrin by *Neisseria meningitidis* may occur via a cell-bound iron transport system (Archibald and DeVoe, 1979; Simonson *et al.*, 1982). It is known, however, that many microorganisms combat the biological unavailability of iron in aerobic environments, where iron exists exclusively in the ferric state, and as such forms insoluble ferric hydroxide at neutral pH (Bullen *et al.*, 1978; Raymond and Carrano, 1979), by producing low molecular weight iron-chelating compounds known as siderophores (Lankford, 1973; Raymond and Carrano, 1979; Neilands, 1981). Siderophores are also produced by several pathogenic organisms and these chelators can remove iron from iron-binding proteins.

The best studied of the high affinity iron-sequestering systems is that in the bacteria of the genera *Salmonella*, *Escherichia* and *Klebsiella* which secrete the iron-chelator enterochelin (Fig. 1), also known as enterobactin,

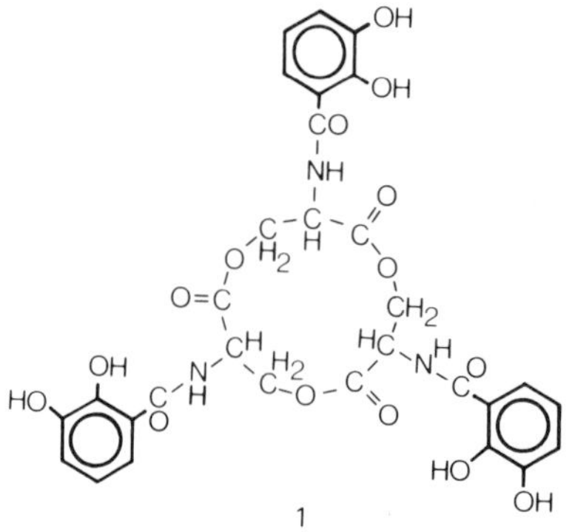

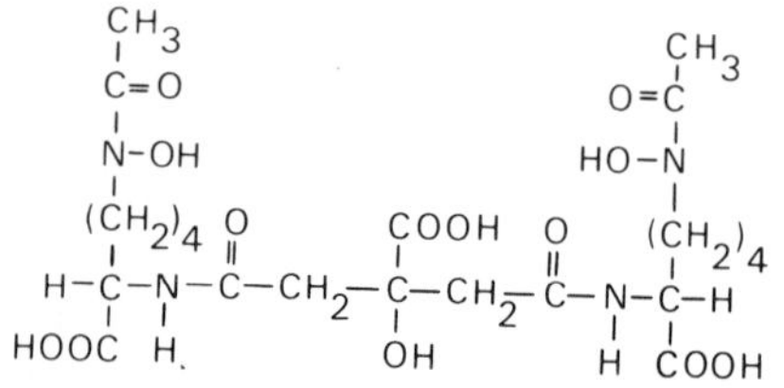

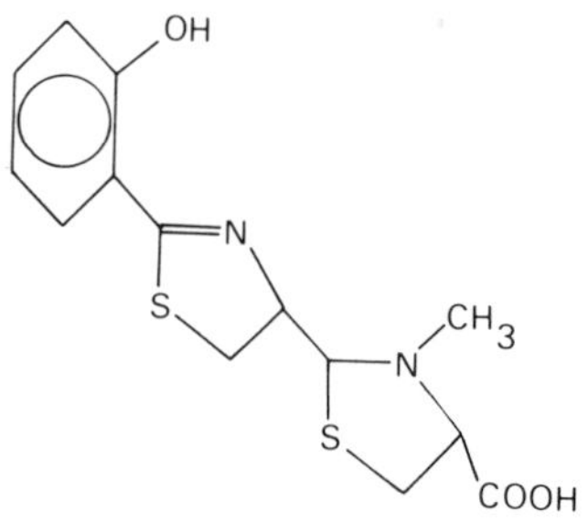

Fig. 1 Structural formulae of three bacterial siderophores 1. enterochelin; 2. aerobactin; 3. pyochelin.

a cyclic trimer of 2,3-dihydroxy-*N*-benzoyl-L-serine (Rosenberg and Young, 1974; Rogers *et al.*, 1977). This compound is produced only under iron-restricted conditions and it efficiently removes iron from iron-binding proteins, promoting bacterial growth at extremely low concentrations (0·01 μM) (Rogers, 1973; Miles and Khimji, 1975; Rogers *et al.*, 1977; Carrano and Raymond, 1979). Enterochelin is known to be produced *in vivo* during fatal infections with *E. coli* (Griffiths and Humphreys, 1980) and the loss by mutation of the ability to synthesize this chelator greatly reduces the virulence of *Salmonella typhimurium* for mice and inhibits its ability to grow in human serum (Yancey *et al.*, 1979). Although enterochelin-mediated iron uptake is the primary indigenous system used by these organisms for accumulating iron in media containing very low levels of available iron, they also have the remarkable capability for obtaining iron via a variety of hydroxamate type siderophores, such as ferrichrome and ferrioxime B, which are produced by other microorganisms (Leong and Neilands, 1976; Raymond and Carrano, 1979; Konisky, 1979; Schneider *et al.*, 1981). It is not known if such systems normally operate *in vivo*, but exogenously supplied desferrioxime B certainly enhances both *Klebsiella* (Khimji and Miles, 1978) and *Salmonella* (Jones *et al.*, 1977) infections. The enterobacteriaceae themselves synthesize neither desferrioxime nor ferrichrome, but several enteric species do synthesize another hydroxamate iron chelator called aerobactin, a dihydroxamate derivative of citric acid (Fig. 1; Gibson and Magrath, 1969; Arceneaux *et al.*, 1973; Payne, 1980). Recently, it was reported that the plasmid-specified siderophore secreted by invasive *E. coli* is also aerobactin (Braun, 1981; Warner *et al.*, 1981). This plasmid-mediated iron-sequestering system is found in strains of *E. coli* which harbour certain Col V plasmids and which are associated with bacteraemia in humans and domestic animals (Smith, 1974; Smith and Huggins, 1976; Davies *et al.*, 1981). Another plasmid-mediated iron-sequestering system has been described in the fish pathogen *Vibrio anguillarum* (Crosa, 1980), but the nature of the chelator is not yet known; only bacteria which carry this plasmid, and which can therefore assimilate protein bound iron, are pathogenic.

The secretion of aerobactin is thought to play an important part in the virulence of the invasive *E. coli* strains (Williams, 1979; Stuart *et al.*, 1980; Williams and Warner, 1980; Warner *et al.*, 1981), but how this siderophore confers a selective advantage on organisms which are already capable of synthesizing enterochelin is not clear. At pH 7·4, the normal physiological pH, enterochelin is thermodynamically and kinetically the most effective siderophore yet characterized (Harris *et al.*, 1979a,b; Carrano and Raymond, 1979). Stuart *et al.* (1980) have proposed that Col V-plasmid specified aerobactin is bound to the cell wall and is, therefore, functionally different and more efficient than the secreted enterochelin in acquiring iron from iron-binding proteins. However, this conclusion contrasts with the known relative effectiveness of the two compounds as iron chelators and the cell-free mode of action suggested for aerobactin by genetic data (Williams and Warner, 1980; Warner *et al.*, 1981). Aerobactin is, in fact, secreted into the culture media both of the Col V-plasmid bearing *E. coli* strains and of other aerobactin producing organisms, which in addition make enterochelin (Gibson and Magrath, 1969; Payne, 1980; Braun, 1981; Warner *et al.*, 1981; van Tiel-Menkveld *et al.*, 1982). There is also a receptor for aerobactin in the outer membrane of these organisms (Grewal *et al.*, 1982). One important difference between the mode of action of enterochelin and the hydroxamate siderophores, such as aerobactin, is the fact that the latter can be re-used. Enterochelin is used only once for transporting iron into the cell; Fe^{3+}-enterochelin is hydrolysed by an esterase in order to release the iron and is so converted into 2,3-dihydroxybenzoylserine which is then discarded (Rosenberg and Young, 1974; Konisky, 1979). It is, therefore, an energetically expensive way of assimilating iron (Raymond and Carrano, 1979). In contrast, iron can be removed from the hydroxamates by simple reduction of Fe^{3+} to Fe^{2+} and without destruction of the chelator (Harris *et al.*, 1979b; Hartmann and Braun, 1980; Schneider *et al.*, 1981). Harris *et al.* (1979b) consider that the high affinity low capacity, and energetically expensive, iron transport system using enterochelin would operate under conditions of extreme iron stress, and the low affinity high capacity system, using aerobactin, under conditions of mild iron stress. In contrast, others conclude that enterochelin is produced under conditions of mild iron limitation and that aerobactin production is maximal under iron deficient conditions (van Tiel-Menkveld *et al.*, 1982). However, results seem to show that both chelators are produced simultaneously, although aerobactin is synthesized mainly in the late logarithmic and stationary phases of growth (Gibson and Magrath, 1969; Stuart *et al.*, 1980; van Tiel-Menkveld *et al.*, 1982). The relevance of these findings, obtained with bacteria in iron-deficient media, in which the quantity of iron is limiting and the organisms iron-starved, to the situation *in vivo* during infection, in which it is the availability of iron that is limiting, is debatable. A clear distinction should be made between the quantity of iron present in a medium and its availability to bacteria. Although there is plenty of iron present in body fluids, it is not readily available because of the iron-binding proteins. This is quite a different situation from that found in media made iron deficient by chemical means. The responses of iron-starved bacteria may be quite different from those of iron-restricted organisms.

Iron -sequestering systems based on siderophores and similar to those of the enteric bacteria, have been found in other pathogens although, in general, much less is known about them or their role *in vivo* during infection. *Vibrio cholerae*, for example, produces a phenolate iron chelator (Payne and Finkelstein, 1978a; Sigel and Payne, 1982) and *Pseudomonas aeruginosa* iron chelators of both phenolate and the hydroxamate types (Liu and Shokrani, 1978; Cox and Graham, 1979; Cox, 1980). The cholera chelator has not yet been characterized but the structure of the siderophore from *Pseudomonas*, called pyochelin, has recently been reported (Fig. 1; Cox *et al*, 1981). Pyochelin, which promotes experimental *Pseudomonas* infection in mice (Cox, 1982), appears to be derived from one molecule of salicyclic acid and two molecules of cysteine and is quite unlike any previously described siderophore. Although *Pseudomonas* does not synthesize enterochelin, it can utilize this chelator as well as pyochelin (Liu and Shokrani, 1978). In addition, *Pseudomonas* can, like certain strains of *E. coli* (Frost and Rosenberg, 1973; Reiter *et al*., 1975; Griffiths and Humphreys, 1977; Hussein *et al*., 1981), utilize ferric citrate as a source of iron, even though citrate is not excreted by these organisms (Cox, 1980). Ferric citrate also functions as an iron source for *Neisseria meningitidis* and *Neisseria gonorrhoeae* (Archibald and DeVoe, 1980; Michelson and Sparling, 1981; Yancey and Finkelstein, 1981a) and for *Mycobacterium smegmatis* and *Mycobacterium bovis* BCG *in vitro* (Messenger and Ratledge, 1982). However, it remains to be seen if iron chelated to traces of citrate *in vivo* can serve as a source of iron for any of these organisms.

The assimilation of iron by mycobacteria has been shown to involve two iron chelators, mycobactin and exochelin, but their exact roles in the pathogenesis of mycobacterial infections remains to be established (Kochan, 1973; Stephenson and Ratledge, 1979). Again, whilst there is no doubt that pathogenic *Neisseria* species can remove iron from iron-binding proteins, the means by which this is accomplished also remains obscure and there is conflicting evidence regarding the role of cell-free or surface associated siderophores (Norrod and Williams, 1978; Payne and Finkelstein, 1978b; Archibald and DeVoe, 1979; Yancey and Finkelstein, 1981a,b; Holbein, 1981; Michelson and Sparling, 1981; Michelson *et al*., 1982; Simonson *et al*., 1982). Recently, Yancey and Finkelstein (1981b) reported finding small amounts of hydroxamate-type iron chelators in culture supernatants of *N. gonorrhoeae* and *N. meningiditis* although a large part of the siderophore remained associated with the cell. Others have failed to find siderophores and have suggested that iron is acquired by these organisms via a mechanism involving an interaction between the iron-binding protein and the bacterial cell surface (Archibald and DeVoe, 1979; Simonson *et al*., 1982).

In addition to obtaining iron from the iron-binding proteins, there are indications that some pathogenic bacteria may also, under certain conditions, obtain sufficient iron *in vivo* from cell-free haem. Organisms which can utilize the iron in haem, or in haemoglobin, include *N. gonorrhoeae, N. meningiditis, E. coli, Clostridium welchii, Yersinia pestis, P. septica* and *Ps. aeruginosa* (Bullen *et al.*, 1968a,b; Rogers *et al.*, 1970; Bullen *et al.*, 1974a; Perry and Brubaker, 1979; Michelson and Sparling, 1981; Yancey and Finkelstein, 1981a). Normally, there is only a trace of free haem in serum, and this is bound to haemopexin or serum albumin (Morgan, 1980). Although there might be enough haem present to promote the growth of some bacteria, such as *Y. pestis* (Perry and Brubaker, 1979; Bullen, 1981), it may be necessary to liberate haemoglobin from erythrocytes, through haemolysis, in order to promote the growth of other pathogens. Recent work suggests that the Hly plasmid, which determines the production of α-haemolysin in *E. coli*, probably acts in this way and functions as a virulence factor by enabling the haemolytic Hly positive *E. coli* to obtain iron for growth from the lysed erythrocytes of infected animals (Welch *et al.*, 1981; Linggood and Ingram, 1982). Such a mechanism would, of course, only be important for growth of the bacteria in blood and the possession of the Hly plasmid should have no effect on growth on mucosal surfaces, such as in the gut, as indeed appears to be the case (Smith and Linggood, 1971). It is also interesting to note that the concentration of haptoglobin, a naturally occurring haemoglobin-binding protein, increases dramatically in the plasma of patients with both acute and chronic infections (Owen *et al.*, 1964; Chiancone *et al.*, 1968).

IV. ADAPTATION TO GROWTH *IN VIVO*

Pathogenic organisms which depend on the iron associated with iron-binding proteins for multiplication clearly have to adapt to a severely iron-restricted environment and produce systems for assimilating protein bound iron. This involves not only the synthesis of enzymes for making the siderophores but also the production of outer-membrane protein receptors and enzymes which are involved in the uptake and release of iron from the chelators. *E. coli* and *S. typhimurium* produce several new outer-membrane proteins, with apparent molecular weights in the range 74 000–83 000 when grown under iron restricted conditions *in vitro* (Braun *et al.*, 1976; Bennett and Rothfield, 1976; McIntosh and Earhart, 1977; Ichihara and Mizushima, 1977; Konisky, 1979; Reeves, 1979; Klebba *et al.*, 1982).

In *E. coli* these proteins are usually designated according to their apparent molecular weights, 83 000, 81 000, 78 000 and 74 000 proteins. The 81 000 protein (FepA protein) is the receptor for Fe^{3+}-enterochelin and is the product of the *fep* gene (Hollifield and Neilands, 1978; Konisky, 1979), mapping in the *ent fep fes* gene cluster at approximately 13 min. This gene cluster controls enterochelin biosynthesis, enterochelin uptake and enterochelin hydrolysis (Rosenberg and Young, 1974; Bachmann and Low, 1980). The 78 000 protein (Ton A protein) is the receptor for ferrichrome and the product of the *ton* A gene (Konisky, 1979). The functions of the 83 000 protein and of the 74 000 protein (Cir protein), which is the product of the *cir* gene (Hancock *et al.*, 1977; Konisky, 1979), are currently unknown. In addition, another outer-membrane protein, with an apparent molecular weight of about 81 000 (FecA protein) is produced by *E. coli* growing in iron restricted media containing 1 mM citrate (Hancock *et al.*, 1976; Konisky, 1979; Wagegg and Braun, 1981). This protein is thought to be part of the citrate-dependent iron transport system (Hussein *et al.*, 1981; Wagegg and Braun, 1981). Recently, yet another outer-membrane protein specified by a Col V plasmid, and involved in aerobactin-mediated iron transport by Col V strains of *E. coli* has been reported (Grewal *et al.*, 1982); this iron-regulated plasmid-specified protein has an apparent molecular weight of 74 000 and is only revealed in *cir* mutants which lack the 74 000 Cir protein. In *S. typhimurium* three outer-membrane proteins are expressed when iron is limiting (Bennett and Rothfield, 1976; Ernst *et al.*, 1978). These have apparent molecular weights of 82 000, 79 000 and 77 000 and have been designated OM1, OM2 and OM3.

Although most work on the iron-regulated outer-membrane proteins has been carried out with laboratory strains of *E. coli*, it has recently been shown that pathogenic *E. coli* produce the same new outer-membrane proteins when grown *in vitro* in the presence of iron-binding proteins (Griffiths *et al.*, 1983). There was, however, considerable variation in the relative abundance of the 83 000, 81 000, 78 000 and 74 000 proteins expressed in different strains. The same iron-regulated outer-membrane proteins were also present in the outer-membrane of the pathogenic strain *E. coli* O111 recovered directly from the peritoneal cavities of lethally infected guinea-pigs (Griffiths *et al.*, 1983), clearly showing that these proteins can indeed be expressed by organisms growing *in vivo* during infection (Fig. 2). It is interesting to note that the pathogenic strains of *E. coli* produced considerably more of the iron-regulated outer membrane proteins than did *E. coli* K12, a laboratory strain, when grown under the same conditions. For example, the iron-regulated outer-membrane proteins of *E. coli* O111 growing *in vitro* in broth containing ovotransferrin, or *in vivo* during infection, were present in amounts equal to, or even slightly greater than the so-called "major" outer-membrane proteins with apparent molecular weights in the range 30 000–42 000 (Overbeeke and Lugtenberg, 1980).

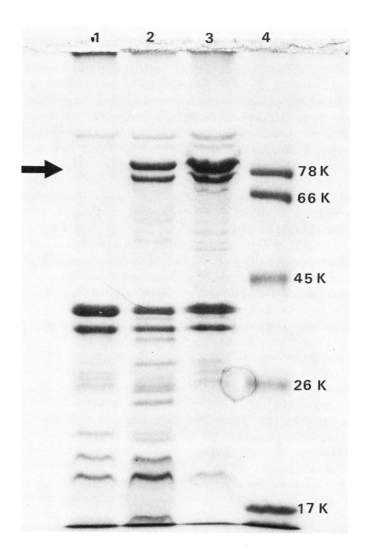

Fig. 2 Polyacrylamide gel electrophoresis of the outer membrane proteins from *Escherichia coli* O111 grown in 1. trypticase soy broth; 2. trypticase soy broth containing ovotransferrin; 3. in the peritoneal cavities of lethally infected guinea-pigs. Lane 4 carried molecular weight markers, the sizes of which are indicated. The positions of the iron regulated outer-membrane proteins are shown by the arrow (Griffiths *et al.*, 1983).

Other pathogenic bacteria have also been shown to produce new outer-membrane proteins when growing under iron restricted conditions *in vitro*. However, our knowledge of these new proteins and of their relationship to the assimilation of iron, and to growth *in vivo*, is still rather limited. *V. cholerae* has been shown to produce at least six new proteins in its outer membrane during iron starvation (Sigel and Payne, 1982). Five of these proteins have apparent molecular weights in the range 62 000–77 000 and it has been suggested that one or more may be part of the uptake system for iron-siderophores. Three new proteins, with molecular weights of 76 000, 86 000 and 92 000, have been seen in the outer membranes of iron starved *N. gonorrhoeae* (Norqvist *et al.*, 1978) and iron related changes have been noted in the outer membrane protein composition of *N. meningitidis* (Brener *et al.*, 1981). Analysis of the outer-membrane proteins synthesized by plasmid-containing *V. anguillarum* strains has shown that two proteins are induced under iron-limited conditions, a 78 000 protein and an 86 000 protein, the latter being specifically associated with the presence of the plasmid, the presence of which correlates with virulence (Crosa, 1980; Crosa and Hodges, 1981; Buckley *et al.*, 1981). The 86 000 protein is induced by iron restriction only in those cells which contain the virulence plasmid. On losing the plasmid *V. anguillarum* loses its virulence for fish and also its ability to grow under conditions of iron limitation imposed by iron-binding proteins (Crosa, 1980).

Although a considerable amount of information is available about some of the siderophores and about their outer-membrane receptors, especially those of *E. coli*, little is known about the way these high affinity iron-sequestering systems are regulated, except, of course, to say that their synthesis is repressed when iron is freely available in the medium (Konisky, 1979). In *E. coli*, the biosynthesis of enterochelin, and of some of the outer-membrane protein receptors, appears to be co-ordinately regulated by the intra-cellular content of iron even though the genes are not all included in the same transcriptional unit (McIntosh and Earhart, 1977; Bachmann and Low, 1980; Klebba *et al.*, 1982). The 83 000, 81 000, and 74 000 proteins are regulated together but the synthesis of the 78 000 protein is controlled separately (Plastow *et al.*, 1981; Klebba *et al.*, 1982). However, the recent production of constitutive mutants of *E. coli* K12 in which the 83 000, 81 000, 78 000, 74 000 and FecA proteins are all expressed in an iron-rich medium seems to suggest that there is a regulatory mechanism functioning which covers all iron-uptake systems and which is superimposed on the regulation of the individual systems (Hantke, 1981). These constitutive mutants have been called *fur* mutants, for Fe^{3+} uptake regulation, and were originally discovered in *S. typhimurium* (Ernst *et al.*, 1978). The *fur* mutants of *S. typhimurium* express OM1, OM2 and OM3 proteins constitutively irrespective of the iron concentration in the medium. The induction of the FecA protein, which is probably the receptor for Fe-citrate, is very interesting since it depends not only on low levels of iron, but in addition, on relatively high concentrations of citrate (Hussein *et al.*, 1981). Only exogenous ferric citrate induces the FecA protein. In fact the intracellular citrate and iron concentrations are about 10–100 times higher than those outside the cell (Hussein *et al.*, 1981). This exogenous induction of the citrate-dependent iron transport system resembles the induction of the transport system for glucose-6-phosphate in *E. coli* (Dietz, 1976); glucose-6-phosphate generated intracellularly does not lead to the synthesis of the transport system.

Quite apart from the more obvious phenotypic changes discussed above, other more fundamental changes take place when bacteria adapt to grow under the iron-restricted conditions imposed by iron-binding proteins. Of particular interest are the changes which occur in transfer RNA (tRNA) molecules. In *E. coli*, as in other prokaryotes, tRNA genes are transcribed as polynucleotide precursor molecules. These molecules then undergo a maturation process involving both a reduction in the size of the transcribed polynucleotide chain by a cleavage reaction and the modification of certain nucleosides (Smith, 1976). Iron is specifically involved in the synthesis of the hypermodified nucleoside 2-methylthio-N^6-($\triangle^2$-isopentenyl)-adenosine (ms^{2}i^{6}A) which occurs next to the 3' end of the anticodon of tRNA molecules recognizing codons with a 5'-terminal uridine (UXY codons) (Rosenberg and Gefter, 1969; Hall, 1971). Under conditions of iron deficiency, altered species of tRNAs appear which elute earlier on chromatography than the usual tRNAs (Wettstein and Stent, 1968; Rosenberg and Gefter, 1969; Juarez *et al.*, 1975). Similar chromatographic changes occur in the tRNAs of pathogenic *E. coli* growing *in vitro* in body fluids, or in defined media, containing iron-binding proteins (Griffiths, 1972; Griffiths and Humphreys, 1978). These chromatographically altered tRNA species lack the methylthio (ms^2) moiety of ms^{2}i^{6}A (Griffiths and Humphreys, 1978; Buck and Griffiths, 1982); the change in structure is shown in Fig. 3 for phenylalanine tRNA (tRNA^{phe}). Transfer RNA alterations have also been found in *S. typhimurium, Klebsiella pneumoniae* and *Ps. aeruginosa* when grown *in vitro* in the presence of ovotransferrin (McLennan *et al.*, 1981; Whittle and Griffiths, unpublished data). The *E. coli* tRNAs which are altered during iron restriction include tRNA^{phe}, tRNA^{trp}, tRNA^{tyr} and two minor tRNA^{ser} species, and recent work suggests a regulatory role for these changes (Griffiths and Humphreys, 1978; Buck and Griffiths, 1981, 1982; Buck and Griffiths, unpublished data). Variations in the extent of modification of the adenosine located next to the anticodon influence codon–anticodon interactions and lead to

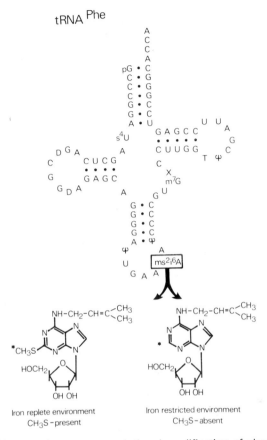

Fig. 3 Effect of iron on the post-transcriptional modification of phenylalanine tRNA from *Escherichia coli* (Griffiths, 1981).

changes in the translational efficiency of the tRNA. The loss of the ms^2 group reduces the translational efficiency of the tRNA molecule and this, in turn, effects an increase in the expression of certain operons through a mechanism called attenuation (Yanofsky and Soll, 1977; Zurawski *et al.*, 1978; Eisenberg *et al.*, 1979; Buck and Griffiths, 1982). Attenuation is also regulated by the level of charged tRNA; this control depends upon the availability of the amino acid (Yanofsky, 1981). It is thought that such regulatory features in the phenylalanine and tryptophan operons and possibly other operons in the aromatic amino acid biosynthetic pathway, may be involved with adapting *E. coli* for growth in iron restricted environments (Buck and Griffiths, 1982). Since enterochelin is synthesized from chorismic acid by way of a branch of the aromatic amino acid biosynthetic pathway (Rosenberg and Young, 1974), derepression of the enterochelin system will require adjustment to the whole aromatic pathway to ensure production of the amino acids and other aromatic compounds, if required. In addition, iron is itself essential for the biosynthesis of all aromatic compounds in *E. coli*; it is a component of 3-deoxy-D-arabino-heptulosonate-7-phosphate synthase, the first enzyme in the common pathway (McCandliss and Herrmann, 1978). The ability to control the expression of various operons in this pathway through the level of charging of tRNA and by the degree of modification of tRNA, in turn dependent upon iron levels, may well provide the cell with useful regulatory flexibility. Methylthiolation of tRNA also influences aromatic amino acid transport in *E. coli* (Buck and Griffiths, 1981), although the way in which the under-modified tRNAs function to increase the uptake of phenylalanine, tryptophan and tyrosine is not clear. The ability of the bacterial cell to scavenge the environment for these amino acids rather than synthesize them may, however, be a helpful feature of cellular economy when enterochelin synthesis is necessary for continued growth in an iron restricted environment. It remains to be seen, of course, if there are further metabolic effects stemming from the tRNA alterations. However, in any work on infection it is essential to show, as far as is possible, that biochemical mechanisms studied *in vitro* really do apply to conditions in the animal body during infection. It is significant, therefore, that the same iron-related tRNA changes have been shown to occur in *E. coli* recovered directly from the peritoneal cavities of lethally infected animals (Fig. 4; Griffiths *et al.*, 1978). This finding strengthens the notion that these phenotypic changes are important for bacterial growth *in vivo* and provides an insight into some of the more subtle changes that occur in the organisms.

V.   EFFECTS OF FREELY AVAILABLE IRON

The metabolic changes discussed above, the synthesis and secretion of siderophores, the production of new outer membrane proteins and the changes in the tRNAs can be considered to be features of cellular economy during the stress of iron restriction. Generally, bacteria under these conditions multiply more slowly than the iron-replete organisms. *E. coli*, for example, has a doubling time of about 35 min when growing in the presence of iron-binding proteins *in vitro*, but this is reduced by 10 min when iron is freely available in the medium (Griffiths and Humphreys, 1978). Similarly, iron-replete *Ps. aeruginosa* grows with a doubling time of

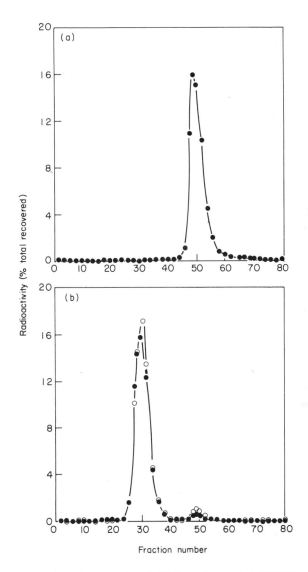

Fig. 4 Chromatography of tryptophanyl-tRNA on benzoylated-DEAE cellulose. (a) ^{3}H-tryptophanyl-tRNA extracted from iron-replete *Escherichia coli* O111. (b) Co-chromatography of (○) ^{14}C-tryptophanyl-tRNA isolated from *E. coli* O111 grown in the guinea-pig peritoneum, (●) ^{3}H-tryptophanyl-tRNA from *E. coli* O111 grown in broth containing ovotransferrin. (a) was chromatographed separately on the same column (Griffiths *et al.*, 1978).

about 30 min but in the presence of transferrin or lactoferrin this time is increased to 72 min (Bullen *et al.*, 1974b). These relatively small differences in doubling times can make a big difference to the size of a bacterial population over a matter of hours and this may be a crucial factor in deciding the outcome of an infection. Supplying free iron in one form or another will bypass the effects of the iron-binding proteins on the bacteria and will abolish the need for a pathogen to go into what might be called the iron-stressed state. The bacteria will grow faster and will be phenotypically different from the iron-restricted organisms; no siderophores will be produced, the tRNAs will be unchanged and no new proteins would be expected in the outer membranes. The increased rate of growth may be sufficient to tip the balance in favour of an invading pathogen, the host defences then being unable to contain the more rapidly multiplying bacterial population and thus to control the infection. This is well illustrated by experimental peritoneal infections in rabbits using *Ps. aeruginosa* and in guinea-pigs using *E. coli* (Bullen *et al.*, 1968a, 1974b). In both cases, sublethal doses of bacteria grew for a few hours and then declined, the infection being contained by the polymorphonuclear leukocyte response; in animals injected with ferric ammonium citrate or haematin, however, the same sublethal dose multiplied rapidly and killed the animals even though the cellular response was the same as before. The enhancement of bacterial infections in normal animals by iron compounds thus appears to be due to iron acting as a nutrient although there is evidence which suggests that iron may also interfere with the activity of some antibacterial systems in immune animals (Kochan *et al.*, 1978). It has been suggested that a distinction should be made between the role of iron compounds in providing an essential growth factor and their ability to abolish the bactericidal action of certain sera (Griffiths, 1975). The mechanism by which iron inhibits the bactericidal action of immune sera is unknown. Polymorphs also contain lactoferrin and this seems to be required for the functioning of their bactericidal system (Masson *et al.*, 1969; Bullen and Wallis, 1977; Bullen and Armstrong, 1979). However, they are relatively impermeable to iron salts and their bactericidal activity is not affected by freely available iron (Gladstone and Walton, 1970; Bullen and Wallis, 1977).

Since an increased availability of iron exerts such a marked effect on experimental bacterial infections in animals (Table 1), and can abolish the need for a pathogen to adapt to the normally iron-restricted environment of the host, it might be expected that similar alterations in the availability of iron might lead to reduced resistance to infection in man. In general, increasing the availability of iron does predispose man to infection. The life-threatening combination of *E. coli* and haemoglobin in the peritoneal cavity is a well-documented case (Davis and Yull, 1964; Bornside *et al.*, 1968; Bornside and Cohn, 1968; Bullen *et al.*, 1978). This combination may arise from any form of trauma, such as strangulation of a loop of gut (Davis and Yull, 1964), and experimental work has shown that it is the iron in haemoglobin that is responsible for stimulating bacterial growth (Bornside *et al.*, 1968; Bullen *et al.*, 1968a; Lee *et al.*, 1979). Recently it has been shown that the administration of haptoglobin, a protein which binds free haemoglobin in plasma, protects against experimental infections promoted by haemoglobin (Eaton *et al.*, 1982). Such work has suggested a possible use for haptoglobin in the treatment of potentially fatal haemoglobin induced bacterial infection. Individuals with other haemolytic conditions such as sickle cell anaemia (Barrett-Conner, 1971), bartonellosis (Cuadra, 1956) and malaria (Kaye *et al.*, 1967) also show increased susceptibility to bacterial infections. Of course, other contributory factors may be operating in some of these diseases, such as the suppression of the immune system in malaria, but there is no doubt that freely available haem plays an important part in lowering resistance. Haemochromatosis, with its chronic iron overload, is an example of a condition in which the serum transferrin is often, but not always, fully saturated with Fe^{3+} (Powell and Halliday, 1980). However, this disease is not noted for problems with infections (Anonymous, 1974; Bullen *et al.*, 1974a, 1978) although infections with *Vibrio vulnificus*, resulting in septicaemia with high mortality, have recently been reported (Blake *et al.*, 1979; Wright *et al.*, 1981). A particularly striking example of the adverse effect of injected iron has been described by Barry and Reeve (1977) and by Farmer (1976). They found that the intramuscular administration of iron-dextran to newborn Polynesian infants greatly increased the incidence of neonatal sepsis and meningitis due mainly to *E. coli*. When this practice was stopped then the high rate of infection also ceased. Subsequent studies showed that the sera of infants given intramuscular iron-dextran had markedly reduced antibacterial activity against *E. coli* compared with pre-treatment and control sera (Becroft *et al.*, 1977). Since incidents such as these are rare, it is likely that the deleterious effect of injected iron is seen only in high risk populations subject to considerable environmental contamination much in the same way that the protective effects of breast-feeding against infections can best be demonstrated in the lower socio-economic population of the underdeveloped countries (Chandra, 1977). The adverse effect of iron therapy on infection has also been found during treatment of children with kwashiorkor; these individuals have very low levels of serum transferrin (McFarlane *et al.*, 1970; Masawe and Rwabwago-Atenyi, 1973) and many of those given iron as part of the initial treatment died immediately afterwards. It is suggested that some of the deaths in the treated children were due to overwhelming infection induced by the availability of iron which in turn was due to the inability of the low amounts of transferrin present to bind the iron supplied (McFarlane *et al.*, 1970, 1972). In the light of their work, McFarlane *et al.* (1972) recommend that iron therapy should be delayed until transferrin levels have increased satisfactorily following refeeding.

Of course, the enhancement of infection occurs not only with excess iron but also during severe iron deficiency (Sussman, 1974; Chandra, 1977). This is an entirely separate aspect of the effects of iron on infections and is probably due to the decline in cell-mediated immunity that occurs in severe iron-deficiency anaemia (Joynson *et al.*, 1972; MacDougall *et al.*, 1975). Polymorphs show a reduction in bactericidal activity during iron deficiency, due to a reduction in iron-dependent myeloperoxidase activity and this can be corrected by giving iron (Klebanoff, 1970; Arbeter *et al.*, 1971; Chandra, 1973).

VI. PHENOTYPIC CHANGES, VACCINES AND ANTIBACTERIAL AGENTS

Whilst iron clearly modulates the interactions between host and pathogen, freely available iron generally predisposing man and animals to infection, the key to its importance lies in the fact that it is not normally readily available to invading organisms. As we have seen, many organisms adapt to this severely iron-restricted environment by synthesizing and secreting competitive iron chelators that can remove iron from iron-binding proteins and transport it back to the bacterial cell. The host's ability to interrupt or to interfere with this process can, therefore, be considered as a defensive mechanism. One such mechanism is the inhibition of siderophore production by elevated temperatures. It has been proposed that this is one of the mechanisms behind the adaptive or beneficial role of fever (Garibaldi, 1972; Grieger and Kluger, 1978; Kluger and Rothenburg, 1979; Buck *et al.*, 1979). Limiting the availability of iron by reducing a pathogen's ability to synthesize iron chelators, or by increasing the rate of their destruction in tissue fluids, by higher temperatures, would clearly restrict an organism's ability to multiply well in the presence of iron-binding proteins. Other defensive processes depend upon the immune system. Recent work has shown that normal human serum contains antibodies specific for enterochelin which, when acting in concert with transferrin, limit the growth of *E. coli* (Moore *et al.*, 1980; Moore and Earhart, 1981). The evidence suggests that antibody blocks enterochelin mediated Fe^{3+} uptake but not the uptake of Fe^{3+} from ferrichrome or citrate. Since enterochelin is an aromatic molecule it may well adhere to protein and act as a hapten for generating antibodies. An alternative immune mechanism has been described by Fitzgerald and Rogers (1980) who studied serotype specific horse serum antibodies and secretory IgA in human milk. These antibodies, which act in conjunction with transferrin or lactoferrin to give bacteriostasis, appear to interfere with enterochelin synthesis or secretion. They recognize colitose which is the terminal sugar of the O-specific side chain of the lipopolysaccharide of the *E. coli* used (*E. coli* O111), and block the production of enterochelin, thus depriving the bacteria of essential iron (Bullen *et al.*, 1978). Although the mechanisms involved in blocking enterochelin production are unknown it is thought that the bacteriostatic action of IgA and lactoferrin plays an important part in breast milk's protective action against neonatal enteritis caused by *E. coli* (Bullen *et al.*, 1972; Bullen, 1976, 1981).

Since surface components play such an important part in host–bacteria interactions, the alterations induced in the bacterial cell envelope by iron-binding proteins are clearly of interest, especially since it has now been shown that the new outer membrane proteins do appear in *E. coli* growing *in vivo* during infection (see above). Although it remains to be seen if *E. coli* colonizing body sites other than the peritoneal cavity also express these proteins, the possibility that the receptors for ferric chelates are important protective antigens is worth exploring. It has already been shown that some of the iron regulated outer-membrane proteins are exposed on the surface of the pathogenic strain *E. coli* O111 and can interact with large protein molecules in solution (Griffiths *et al.*, 1983). Such antigens would, of course, only appear during growth and multiplication of the bacteria *in vivo* or *in vitro* in iron-restricted media. Whole cell vaccines made from the iron-replete organisms would lack these proteins and might therefore be incomplete as regards antigenic determinants.

The better understanding of the environment encountered by bacteria growing *in vivo* during infection and of the way they adapt to such conditions, has also led to ideas concerning the development of new antibacterial agents. Since enterochelin is produced *in vivo* during infection and is indeed an essential growth factor for some organisms, it was reasoned that it might be possible to use complexes of enterochelin with ions other than Fe^{3+} as antimetabolites to Fe^{3+}-enterochelin (Rogers *et al.*, 1980). Enterochelin forms complexes with a number of Group III and transition metal ions but only the complexes of scandium (Sc^{3+}) and indium (In^{3+}) have shown any significant antibacterial activity. The Sc^{3+} and In^{3+} complexes each exerted a bacteriostatic effect on *K. pneumoniae* (Rogers *et al.*, 1980) and on a number of pathogenic serotypes of *E. coli*, including those carrying either the K1 antigen or the Col V plasmid (Rogers *et al.*, in press); inhibition only occurred in an iron-restricted environment. The Sc^{3+}-complex also exerted a significant therapeutic effect on *K. pneu-*

moniae and *E. coli* infections in mice. Although it is clearly too early to say how successful such compounds might be for therapeutic purposes in man, an investigation of the mechanisms involved in their antibacterial action might suggest further possibilities for the synthesis of new compounds. Preliminary work indicates that the Sc^{3+} complex acts as a competitive inhibitor of the Fe^{3+}-enterochelin, although other changes beyond an interruption of the iron supply might also be taking place in *E. coli*.

VII. CONCLUDING REMARKS

As the limitations of vaccination and antibiotic therapy become apparent for some infectious diseases, it is clear that a better understanding of the mechanisms of microbial pathogenicity is needed for the development of more effective control measures. Understanding the various processes involved in an infection in detail, at the molecular level, is essential and it is the only way that meaningful progress can now be made. One important development has been the realization that the genetic determinants for certain virulence characteristics, such as haemolysins, toxins and adhesive factors, can be carried by plasmids (Cabello and Timmis, 1979). The presence of a plasmid is not, however, always required for virulence nor is it the only factor involved. As we have seen in this paper, the ability of an organism to adapt to and multiply in the iron restricted environment of the host also plays a decisive role, although this process itself may sometimes depend upon the presence of a plasmid (Williams, 1979; Crosa, 1980). Much of our understanding of what may be happening as pathogenic bacteria adapt to and grow in the iron-restricted environment of the host has come from studies with *E. coli*. This is because the organism forms such an ideal experimental model; we already know a great deal about its biochemistry and its genetics and it is, also, the causative agent of important infections in man and animals. The work with *E. coli* has established the principle that pathogenic bacteria can undergo considerable phenotypic changes both in their metabolism and in the composition of their outer membrane when growing *in vivo* during infection. It is hoped that this information will now serve as a guideline for the often more difficult investigation of other pathogenic bacteria.

REFERENCES

Ainscough, E. W., Brodie, A. M., Plowman, J. E., Bloor, S. J., Loehr, J. S. and Loehr, T. M. (1980). *Biochemistry* **19**, 4072–4079.
Aisen, P. (1980). *In* "Iron in Biochemistry and Medicine" (A. Jacobs and M. Worwood, eds), Vol. 2, pp. 87–129. Academic Press, New York and London.

Alderton, G., Ward, W. H. and Fevold, H. L. (1946). *Arch. Biochem. Biophys.* **11**, 9–13.

Anonymous (1974). *Lancet* **2**, 325–326.

Arbeter, A., Echeverri, L., Franco, D., Munson, D., Velez H. and Vitale, J. J. (1971). *Fed. Proc.* **30**, 1421–1428.

Arceneaux, J. E. L., Davies, W. B., Downer, D. N., Haydon, A. H. and Byers, B. R. (1973). *J. Bacteriol.* **115**, 919–927.

Archibald, F. S. and DeVoe, I. W. (1979). *FEMS Microbiol. Letts.* **6**, 159–162.

Archibald, F. S. and DeVoe, I. W. (1980). *Infect. Immun.* **27**, 322–334.

Bachmann, B. J. and Low, K. B., (1980). *Microbiol. Revs.* **44**, 1–56.

Baker, P. J. and Wilson, J. B. (1965). *J. Bacteriol.* **90**, 903–910.

Barrett-Connor, E. (1971). *Medicine* **50**, 97–112.

Barry, D. M. J. and Reeve, A. W. (1977). *Pediatrics* **60**, 908–912.

Becroft, D. M. O., Dix, M. R. and Farmer, K. (1977). *Arch. Dis. Child.* **52**, 778–781.

Bennett, R. L. and Rothfield, L. I. (1976). *J. Bacteriol.* **127**, 498–504.

Bezkorovainy, A. (1980). "Biochemistry of Non-heme Iron". Plenum Press, New York.

Bezkorovainy, A. and Zschocke, R. H. (1974). *Arzneim. Forsch.* **24**, 476–485.

Blake, P. A., Merson, M. H., Weaver, R. E., Hollis, D. G. and Heublein, P. C. (1979). *N. Engl. J. Med.* **300**, 1–5.

Bornside, G. H. and Cohn, I. (1968). *Amer. Surg.* **34**, 63–67.

Bornside, G. H., Bouis Jr. P. J. and Cohn Jr. I. (1968). *J. Bacteriol.* **95**, 1567–1571.

Braun, V. (1981). *FEMS Microbiol. Lett.* **11**, 225–228.

Braun, V., Hancock, R. E. W., Hantke, K. and Hartmann, A. (1976). *J. Supramol. Struct.* **5**, 37–58.

Brener, D., DeVoe, I. W. and Holbein, B. E. (1981). *Infect. Immun.* **33**, 59–66.

Broxmeyer, H. E., Smithyman, A., Eger, R. R., Meyers, P. A. and De Sousa, M. (1978). *J. Exp. Med.* **148**, 1052–1067.

Buck, M. and Griffiths, E. (1981). *Nucleic Acids Res.* **9**, 401–414.

Buck, M. and Griffiths, E. (1982). *Nucleic Acids Res.* **10**, 2609–2624.

Buck, M., Humphreys, J. and Griffiths, E. (1979). *Soc. Gen. Microbiol. Quart.* **7**, 9–10.

Buckley, J. T., Howard, S. P. and Trust, T. J. (1981). *FEMS Microbiol. Letts.* **11**, 41–46.

Bullen, J. J. (1976). *Ciba Found. Symp.* **42**, 149–169.

Bullen, J. J. (1981). *Rev. Infect. Dis.* **3**, 1127–1138.

Bullen, J. J. and Armstrong, J. A. (1979). *Immunology* **36**, 781–791.

Bullen, J. J. and Wallis, S. N. (1977). *FEMS Microbiol. Letts.* **1**, 117–120.

Bullen, J. J., Cushnie, G. H. and Rogers, H. J. (1967). *Immunology* **12**, 302–312.

Bullen, J. J., Leigh, L. C. and Rogers, H. J. (1968a). *Immunology*, **15**, 581–588.

Bullen, J. J., Wilson, A. B., Cushnie, G. H. and Rogers, H. J. (1968b). *Immunology* **14**, 889–898.

Bullen, J. J., Rogers, H. J. and Leigh, L. (1972). *Brit. Med. J.* **1**, 69–75.

Bullen, J. J., Rogers, H. J. and Griffiths, E. (1974a). "Microbial Iron Metabolism" (J. B. Neilands, ed.) pp. 517–551. Academic Press, New York and London.

Bullen, J. J., Ward, C. G. and Wallis, S. N. (1974b). *Infect. Immun.* **10**, 443–450.

Bullen, J. J., Rogers, H. J. and Griffiths, E. (1978). *Curr. Top. Microbiol. Immunol.* **80**, 1–35.

Cabello, F. and Timmis, K. N. (1979). *In* "Plasmids of Medical, Environmental

and Commercial Importance" (K. N. Timmis and A. Pühler, eds) pp. 55–69. Elsevier-North Holland, New York.
Calver, G. A., Kenny, C. P. and Lavergne, G. (1976). *Can. J. Microbiol.* **22**, 832–838.
Carrano, C. J. and Raymond, K. N. (1979). *J. Amer. Chem. Soc.* **101**, 5401–5404.
Cartwright, G. E., Lauritsen, A., Humphreys, S., Jones, P. J., Merrill, I. M. and Wintrobe, M. M. (1946). *J. Clin. Invest.* **25**, 81–86.
Chandra, R. K. (1973). *Arch. Dis. Child.* **48**, 864–866.
Chandra, R. K. (1977). *Ciba Found. Symp.* **51**, 249–262.
Chandra, R. K. (1978). *Nutr. Rev.* **36**, 265–272.
Chiancone, E., Alfsen, A., Ioppolo, C., Vecchini, P., Finazzi Agro, A., Wyman, J. and Antonini, E. (1968). *J. Mol. Biol.* **34**, 347–356.
Cox, C. D. (1980). *J. Bacteriol.* **142**, 581–587.
Cox, C. D. (1982). *Infect. Immun.* **36**, 17–23.
Cox, C. D. and Graham, R. (1979). *J. Bacteriol.* **137**, 357–364.
Cox, C. D., Rinehart Jr., K. L., Moore, M. L. and Cook, Jr. J. C. (1981). *Proc. Natl. Acad. Sci. (US)* **78**, 4256–4260.
Crosa, J. H. (1980). *Nature* **284**, 566–568.
Crosa, J. H and Hodges, L. L. (1981). *Infect. Immun.* **31**, 223–227.
Cuadra, M. (1956). *Tex. Rep. Biol. Med.* **14**, 97–113.
Davies, D. L., Falkiner, F. R. and Hardy, K. G. (1981). *Infect. Immun.* **31**, 574–579.
Davis, J. H. and Yull, A. B. (1964). *J. Trauma* **4**, 84–90.
Dietz, Jr., G. W. (1976). *Adv. Enzymol.* **44**, 237–259.
Eaton, J. W., Brandt, P., Mahoney, J. R. and Lee, Jr., J. T. (1982). *Science* **215**, 691–693.
Eisenberg, S. P., Yarus, M. and Soll, L. (1979). *J. Mol. Biol.* **135**, 111–126.
Ernst, J. F., Bennett, R. L. and Rothfield, L. I. (1978). *J. Bacteriol.* **135**, 928–934.
Farmer, K. (1976). *N.Z. Med. J.* **84**, 286–287.
Fitzgerald, S. P. and Rogers, H. J. (1980). *Infect. Immun.* **27**, 302–308.
Ford, A. and Hayhoe, J. P. V. (1976). *J. Biol. Stand.* **4**, 353–366.
Forsberg, C. M. and Bullen, J. J. (1972). *J. Clin. Pathol.* **25**, 65–68.
Frost, G. E. and Rosenberg, H. (1973). *Biochim. Biophys. Acta* **330**, 90–101.
Garibaldi, J. A. (1972). *J. Bacteriol.* **110**, 262–265.
Gibson, F. and Magrath, D. I. (1969). *Biochim. Biophys. Acta* **192**, 175–184.
Gladstone, G. P. and Walton, E. (1971). *Brit. J. Exp. Pathol.* **52**, 452–464.
Grewal, K. K., Warner, P. J. and Williams, P. H. (1982). *FEBS Lett.* **140**, 27–30.
Grieger, T. A. and Kluger, M. J. (1978). *J. Physiol.* **279**, 187–196.
Griffiths, E. (1972). *FEBS Lett.* **25**, 159–164.
Griffiths, E. (1975). *J. Gen. Microbiol.* **88**, 345–354.
Griffiths, E. (1981). *In* "Nutritional Factors: modulating Effects on Metabolic processes" (R. F. Beers and E. G. Bassett, eds) pp. 463–476. Raven Press, New York.
Griffiths, E. and Humphreys, J. (1977). *Infect. Immun.* **15**, 396–401.
Griffiths, E. and Humphreys, J. (1978). *Eur. J. Biochem.* **82**, 503–513.
Griffiths, E. and Humphreys, J. (1980). *Infect. Immun.* **28**, 286–289.
Griffiths, E., Humphreys, J., Leach, A. and Scanlon, L. (1978). *Infect. Immun.* **22**, 312–317.
Griffiths, E., Stevenson, P. and Joyce, P. (1983). *FEMS Microbiol. Lett.* **16**, 95–99.

Hall, R. H. (1971) "The Modified Nucleosides in Nucleic Acids." Columbia University Press.

Hancock, R. E. W., Hantke, K. and Braun, V. (1976). *J. Bacteriol.* **127**, 1370–1375.

Hancock, R. E. W., Hantke, K. and Braun, V. (1977). *Arch. Microbiol.* **114**, 231–239.

Hantke, K. (1981). *Mol. Gen. Genet.* **182**, 288–292.

Harris, W. R., Carrano, C. J., Cooper, S. R., Sofen, S. R., Avdeef, A. E., McArdle, J. V. and Raymond, K. N. (1979a). *J. Amer. Chem. Soc.* **101**, 6097–6104.

Harris, W. R., Carrano, C. J. and Raymond, K. N. (1979b). *J. Amer. Chem. Soc.* **101**, 2722–2727.

Hartmann, A. and Braun, V. (1980). *J. Bacteriol.* **143**, 246–255.

Henderson, L. C., Kadis, S. and Chapman, Jr. W. L. (1978). *Infect. Immun.* **21**, 540–545.

Holbein, B. E. (1981). *Infect. Immun.* **34**, 120–125.

Hollifield, Jr. W. C. and Neilands, J. B. (1978). *Biochemistry* **17**, 1922–1928.

Hussein, S., Hantke, K. and Braun, V. (1981). *Eur. J. Biochem.* **117**, 431–437.

Ichihara, S. and Mizushima, S. (1977). *J. Biochem (Tokyo)* **81**, 749–756.

Jackson, S. and Burrows, T. W. (1956). *Brit. J. Exp. Pathol.* **37**, 577–583.

Jones, R. L., Peterson, C. M., Grady, R. W., Kumbaraci, T. and Cerami, A. (1977). *Nature* **267**, 63–64.

Joynson, D. H. M., Jacobs, A., Walker, D. M. and Dolby, A. E. (1972). *Lancet* **2**, 1058–1059.

Juarez, H., Skjold, A. C. and Hedgcoth, C. (1975). *J. Bacteriol.* **121**, 44–54.

Kaye, D., Merselis, Jr. J. G. and Hook, E. W. (1965). *Proc. Soc. Exp. Biol. Med.* **120**, 810–813.

Kaye, D., Gill, F. A. and Hook, E. W. (1967). *Amer. J. Med. Sci.* **254**, 205–215.

Khimji, P. L. and Miles, A. A. (1978). *Brit. J. Exp. Path.* **59**, 137–147.

Klebanoff, S. J. (1970). *Science* **169**, 1095–1097.

Klebba, P. E., McIntosh, M. A. and Neilands J. B. (1982). *J. Bacteriol.* **149**, 880–888.

Klempner, M. S., Dinarello, C. A. and Gallin, J. I. (1978). *J. Clin. Investig.* **61**, 1330–1336.

Kluger, M. J. and Rothenburg, B. A. (1979). *Science* **203**, 374–376.

Kochan, I. (1973). *Curr. Top. Microbiol. Immunol.* **60**, 1–30.

Kochan, I., Wasynczuk, J. and McCabe M. A. (1978). *Infect. Immun.* **22**, 560–567.

Konisky, J. (1979). *In* "Bacterial Outer Membranes' Biogenesis and Functions" (M. Inouye, ed.) pp. 319–359. John Wiley and Sons, New York.

Lankford, C. E. (1973). *CRC Crit. Rev. Microbiol.* **2**, 273–331.

Lee, Jr. J. T., Ahrenhoz, D. H., Nelson, R. D. and Simmons, R. L. (1979). *Surgery* **86**, 41–48.

Leffell, M. S. and Spitznagel, J. K. (1974). *Infect. Immun.* **10**, 1241–1249.

Leong, J. and Neilands, J. B. (1976). *J. Bacteriol.* **126**, 823–830.

Linggood, M. A. and Ingram, P. L. (1982). *J. Med. Microbiol.* **15**, 23–30.

Liu, P. V. and Shokrani, F. (1978). *Infect. Immun.* **22**, 878–890.

MacDougall, L. G., Anderson, R., McNab, G. M. and Katz, J. (1975). *J. Pediatr.* **86**, 833–843.

Masawe, A. E. J. and Rwabwogo-Atenyi, J. (1973). *Arch. Dis. Child.* **48**, 927–931.

Mason, D. Y. and Taylor, C. R. (1978). *J. Clin. Pathol.* **31**, 316–327.

Masson, P. L. and Heremans, J. F. (1966). *Protides Biol. Fluids. Proc. Collq.* **14**, 115–124.

Masson, P. L., Heremans, J. F. and Dive, C. (1966a). *Clin. Chim. Acta* **14**, 735–739.

Masson, P. L., Heremans, J. F., Pignot, J. J. and Wauters, G. (1966b). *Thorax* **21**, 538–544.

Masson, P. L., Heremans, J. F. and Schonne, E. (1969). *J. Exp. Med.* **130**, 643–658.

McCandliss, R. J. and Herrmann, K. M. (1978). *Proc. Natl. Acad. Sci.* (US) **75**, 4810–4813.

McClelland, D. B. L. and van Furth, R. (1976). *Clin. Exp. Immunol.* **25**, 442–448.

McFarlane, H., Reddy, S., Adcock, K. J., Adeshina, H., Cook, A. R. and Akene, J. (1970). *Brit. Med. J.* **4**, 268–270.

McFarlane, H., Okubadejo, M. and Reddy, S. (1972). *Amer. J. Clin. Pathol.* **57**, 587–591.

McIntosh, M. A. and Earhart, C. F. (1977). *J. Bacteriol.* **131**, 331–339.

McLennan, B. D., Buck, M., Humphreys, J. and Griffiths, E. (1981). *Nucleic Acids Res.* **9**, 2629–2640.

Merriman, C. R., Pulliam, L. A. and Kampschmidt, R. F. (1977). *Proc. Soc. Exp. Biol. Med.* **154**, 224–227.

Messenger, A. J. M. and Ratledge, C. (1982). *J. Bacteriol.* **149**, 131–135.

Michelson, P. A. and Sparling, F. P. (1981). *Infect. Immun.* **33**, 555–564.

Michelson, P. A., Blackman, E. and Sparling, F. P. (1982). *Infect. Immun.* **35**, 915–920.

Miles, A. A. and Khimji, P. L. (1975). *J. Med. Microbiol* **8**, 477–490.

Miles, A. A., Khimji, P. L. and Maskell, J. (1979). *J. Med. Microbiol.* **12**, 17–28.

Moore, D. G. and Earhart, C. F. (1981). *Infect. Immun.* **31**, 631–635.

Moore, D. G., Yancey, R. J., Lankford, C. E. and Earhart, C. F. (1980). *Infect. Immun.* **27**, 418–423.

Morgan, E. H. (1980). *In* "Iron in Biochemistry and Medicine" (A. Jacobs and M. Worwood, eds), Vol. II, pp. 641–687. Academic Press, New York and London.

Morgan, E. H. (1981). *Mol. Aspects Med.* **4**, 1–123.

Neilands, J. B. (1981). *Ann. Rev. Biochem.* **50**, 715–731.

Norqvist, A., Davies, J., Norlander, L. and Normark S. (1978). *FEMS Microbiol. Lett.* **4**, 71–75.

Norrod, P. and Williams, R. P. (1978). *Curr. Microbiol.* **1**, 281–284.

Overbeeke, N. and Lugtenberg, B. (1980). *J. Gen. Microbiol.* **121**, 373–380.

Owen, J. A., Smith, R., Padanyi, R. and Martin, J. (1964). *Clin. Sci.* **26**, 1–6.

Payne, S. M. (1980). *J. Bacteriol.* **143**, 1420–1424.

Payne, S. M. and Finkelstein, R. A. (1975). *Infect. Immun.* **12**, 1313–1318.

Payne, S. M. and Finkelstein, R. A. (1978a). *Infect. Immun.* **30**, 310–311.

Payne, S. M. and Finkelstein, R. A. (1978b). *J. Clin. Invest.* **61**, 1428–1440.

Perry, R. D. and Brubaker, R. R. (1979). *J. Bacteriol.* **137**, 1290–1298.

Plastow, G. S., Pratt, J. M. and Holland, I. B. (1981). *FEBS Letts.* **131**, 262–264.

Powell, L. W. and Halliday, J. W. (1980). *In* "Iron in Biochemistry and Medicine" (A. Jacobs and W. Worwood, eds), Vol. II, pp. 461–498. Academic Press, New York and London.

Raymond, K. N. and Carrano, C. J. (1979). *Accounts Chem. Res.* **12**, 183–190.

Reeves, P. (1979). *In* "Bacterial Outer Membranes: Biogenesis and Functions" (M. Inouye, ed.) pp. 255–291. John Wiley & Sons, New York.

Reiter, B., Brock, J. H. and Steel, E. D. (1975). *Immunology.* **28,** 83–95.

Rogers, H. J. (1973). *Infect. Immun.* **7,** 445–456.

Rogers, H. J., Bullen, J. J. and Cushnie, G. H. (1970). *Immunology* **19,** 521–538.

Rogers, H. J., Synge, C., Kimber, B. and Bayley, P. M. (1977). *Biochim. Biophys. Acta* **497,** 548–557.

Rogers, H. J., Synge, C. and Woods, V. E. (1980). *Antimicrob. Ag. Chemother.* **18,** 63–68.

Rosenberg, A. H. and Gefter, M. L. (1969). *J. Mol. Biol.* **46,** 581–584.

Rosenberg, H. and Young, I. G. (1974). *In* "Microbial Iron Metabolism" (J. B. Neilands, ed.) pp. 67–82. Academic Press, New York and London.

Schade, A. L. and Caroline L. (1944). *Science* **100,** 14–15.

Schneider, R., Hartmann, A. and Braun, V. (1981). *FEMS Microbiol. Lett.* **11,** 115–119.

Sigel, S. P. and Payne, S. M (1982). *J. Bacteriol.* **150,** 148–155.

Simonson, C., Brener, D. and DeVoe, I. W. (1982). *Infect. Immun.* **36,** 107–113.

Smith, H. W. (1974). *J. Gen. Microbiol.* **83,** 95–111.

Smith, H. W. and Huggins, M. B. (1976). *J. Gen. Microbiol.* **92,** 335–350.

Smith, H. W. and Linggood, M. A. (1971). *J. Med. Microbiol.* **4,** 467–485.

Smith, J. D. (1976). *Prog. Nucleic Acid Res. Mol. Biol.* **16,** 25–73.

Stephenson, M. C. and Ratledge, C. (1979). *J. Gen. Microbiol.* **110,** 193–202.

Stuart, S. J., Greenwood, K. T. and Luke, R. K. J. (1980). *J. Bacteriol.* **143,** 35–42.

Sussman, M. (1974). *In* "Iron in Biochemistry and Medicine" (A. Jacobs and W. Worwood, eds) pp. 649–679. Academic Press, New York and London.

Sword, C. P. (1966). *J. Bacteriol.* **92,** 536–542.

Van Snick, J. L., Masson, P. L. and Heremans, J. F. (1974). *J. Exp. Med.* **140,** 1068–1084.

van Tiel-Menkveld, G. J., Mentjox-Vervuurt, J. M., Oudega, B. and De Graaf, F. K. (1982). *J. Bacteriol.* **150,** 490–497.

Wagegg, W. and Braun, V. (1981). *J. Bacteriol.* **145,** 156–163.

Warner, P. J., Williams, P. H., Bindereif, A. and Neilands, J. B. (1981). *Infect. Immun.* **33,** 540–545.

Weinberg, E. D. (1978). *Microbiol. Rev.* **42,** 45–66.

Welch, R. A., Dellinger, E. P., Minshew, B. and Falkow, S. (1981). *Nature* **294,** 665–667.

Wettstein, F. O. and Stent, G. S. (1968). *J. Mol. Biol.* **38,** 25–40.

Williams, P. H. (1979). *Infect. Immun.* **26,** 925–932.

Williams, P. H. and Warner, P. J. (1980). *Infect. Immun.* **29,** 411–416.

Witt, D. P. and Woodworth, R. C. (1978). *Biochemistry* **17,** 3913–3917.

Wright, A. C., Simpson, L. M. and Oliver, J. D. (1981). *Infect. Immun.* **34,** 503–507.

Yancey, R. J. and Finkelstein, R. A. (1981a). *Infect. Immun.* **32,** 592–599.

Yancey, R. J. and Finkelstein, R. A. (1981b). *Infect. Immun.* **32,** 600–608.

Yancey, R. J., Breeding, S. A. L. and Lankford, C. E. (1979). *Infect. Immun.* **24,** 174–180.

Yanofsky, C. (1981). *Nature* **289,** 751–758.

Yanofsky, C. and Soll, L. (1977). *J. Mol. Biol.* **113,** 663–677.

Zurawski, G., Elseviers, D., Stauffer, G. V. and Yanofsky, C. (1978). *Proc. Natl. Acad. Sci.* (*US*) **75,** 5988–5992.

8 Exploitation of the bacterial envelope: rational design of antibacterial agents

PETER S. RINGROSE

I. INTRODUCTION

The bacterial cell envelope provides one of the most selective targets in chemotherapy (Gale *et al.*, 1981). Most components of the envelope are structurally unique to bacteria and are vital for survival *in vivo*. In contrast to multicellular organisms, unicellular bacteria are limited in their ability to control the environment in which they exist. Clearly the envelope must not only provide physical protection against often hostile conditions but it also has to control the cell's internal environment by regulating the flow of nutrients and ions (Saier, 1979). As a result of this need to respond to changing cultural conditions, bacteria have developed an envelope which is both structurally "plastic" in terms of its overall composition (Brown, preface) as well as functionally "highly tuned", particularly in terms of its ability to scavenge low levels of essential nutrients and ions (Koch, 1971; Kadner, 1978).

It is essentially these adaptive features which will be discussed as molecular devices for exploiting the envelope. The very same pores, binding proteins and permeases necessary for survival under nutrient- or ion-limiting conditions are often the ones that are used for facilitating the uptake of antibiotics or antibiotic-carrier systems. Likewise, the pathways for peptidoglycan and lipopolysaccharide biosynthesis are usually the most vulnerable to attack when the cell is trying to survive under extreme conditions.

Two strategies for drug design will therefore be discussed. First, the exploitation of bacterial transport systems by antibiotics as a means of

MEDICAL MICROBIOLOGY, 3
ISBN 0 12 228003 3

facilitating cell entry and second, the selective inhibition of enzymes involved in the biosynthesis of important envelope components. Other envelope-related approaches for drug design, such as attempting to influence pathogenicity mechanisms by interfering with adhesion, phago-cytic killing, serum resistance, haemolysin production and iron-utilization are discussed elsewhere (Vosbeck and Mett, Chapter 2; Chabanon, 1981; Penn, Chapter 5; Griffiths, Chapter 7; Braun and Hantke, 1981).

II. EXPLOITATION OF TRANSPORT SYSTEMS

Although some lipophilic antibiotics manage to arrive at their target sites by simply diffusing through membranes, an increasing number of hydro-philic antibiotic molecules have been shown to penetrate bacteria by means of a carrier- or pore-mediated process (see Franklin, 1973, 1974; Fischer and Braun, 1981; Chopra and Ball, 1982). Many of the permeases, pores and high affinity binding proteins implicated in antibiotic uptake, however, have been shown to be primarily produced by the bacterium in response to potentially hostile environments as a result of limiting levels of nutrients, ions and vitamins (Kadner, 1978; Leonard *et al.*, 1981; Alper and Ames, 1978).

The detailed mechanisms by which naturally occurring antibiotic mole-cules exploit already existing bacterial transport systems has been exten-sively reviewed elsewhere (Chopra and Ball, 1982). This topic will, therefore, only be briefly commented upon here. After giving an overview of the various transport systems in the envelope that are exploited by different antibiotic types, three mechanistically different examples will be discussed in greater detail in section III, in the context of their overall action as peptidoglycan biosynthesis inhibitors. The examples will be (i) the natural and synthetic amino acid mimetics, D-cycloserine and α-fluoro-D-alanine, which exploit the D-alanine permease, (ii) the natural and synthetic dipeptides bacilysin and alafosfalin, which exploit both dipeptide and oligopeptide permeases, and (iii) the epoxy- and hydroxamate-phosphonates fosfomycin and fosmidomycin which exploit both glycerol-phosphate and hexose-phosphate permeases. The transport systems of the bacterial inner and outer membranes that are implicated in facilitating the uptake of antibiotic molecules are listed in Tables 1 and 2.

A. Inner membrane

The permeases involved in the uptake of amino acids and peptides are usually constitutive, although nutrient levels in the medium and in the

Table 1 Antibiotic exploitation of inner membrane transport systems.

TRANSPORT SYSTEM	ANTIBIOTIC
amino acid	D-cycloserine
dipeptide	bacilysin alafosfalin
tripeptide	phosphinothricyl-Ala-Ala
glycero 3-phosphate	fosfomycin fosmidomycin
sugar	nojirimycin streptozotocin
nucleoside	showdomycin
polyamine	aminoglycoside
C_4 dicarboxylate	tetracycline

Table 2 Antibiotic exploitation of outer membrane transport systems.

TRANSPORT SYSTEM	ANTIBIOTIC	PHAGE
Fe-ferrichrome/FhuA	Col M albomycin	$T_1 T_5$ $\emptyset_{80}$
Fe-enterochelin/FepA	Col B_1D	
Fe-aerobactin	Col V Clo DF_{13}	
vitamin B_{12}/BtuB	Col $E_1 E_2 E_3$	BF_{23}
maltose/LamB		lambda
nucleosides/Tsx	Col K showdomycin	T_6
porin/OmpF	β-lactams	T_2 TuIa

cytoplasm will influence permease activity for both influx and efflux (Payne, 1980b; Oxender *et al.*, 1980). In terms of exploitation, however, the broad peptide transport systems offer more potential since they are far less discriminatory in their substrate specificities than the many different highly selective amino acid permeases (Payne, 1980a; Anraku, 1978). The only amino acid mimetics of any real therapeutic interest have been those exploiting the D-alanine permease, i.e. D-cycloserine and α-fluoro-D-alanine (Neuhaus and Hammes, 1981) (see section III.C.1). However, there are many examples of natural antimetabolites which use the L-amino acid permeases (Fig. 1) (Scannel and Pruess, 1974).

The many structurally diverse examples of di- and tripeptide antibiotics give support to the possibilities of using this transport system for

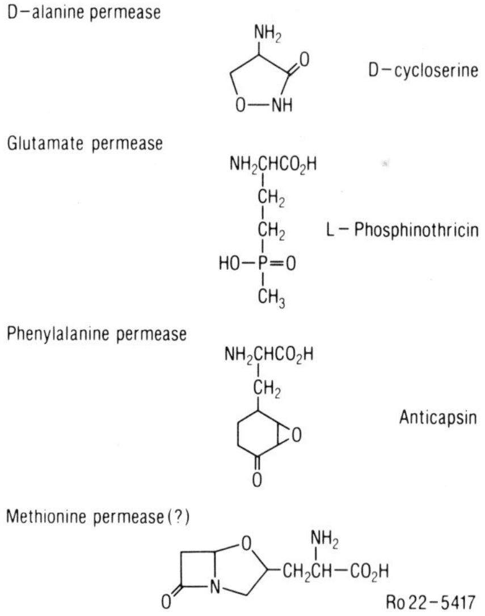

D–alanine permease

NH$_2$

D–cycloserine

O—NH

Glutamate permease

NH$_2$CHCO$_2$H
|
CH$_2$
|
CH$_2$ L – Phosphinothricin
|
HO—P=O
|
CH$_3$

Phenylalanine permease

NH$_2$CHCO$_2$H
|
CH$_2$

Anticapsin

O

Methionine permease (?)

NH$_2$
|
—CH$_2$CH—CO$_2$H

Ro 22–5417

Fig. 1 Antibiotics using amino acid permeases.

facilitating the uptake of "designed mimetics" (Ringrose, 1980) (Fig. 2). Most antibacterial peptides of this type, however, utilize another interesting mechanistic feature during their uptake, i.e., warhead-delivery (see section III.C.2). The intracellularly active principle is not usually the peptide itself but an amino acid mimetic metabolite, which is released only after being "smuggled" into the cells disguised as a peptide (see Ames *et al.*, 1973; Fickel and Gilvarg, 1973; Matthews and Payne, 1975; Gilvarg, 1981). This is necessary since the amino acid warhead is normally very poorly transported by itself. The warhead moiety can be at either the *N* or *C* terminus of the peptide and the "carrier" amino acid(s) can be almost any L-α-amino acid, although those with hydrophobic residues are usually preferred (Atherton *et al.*, 1979a,b, 1980; Ringrose, 1980).

The overall structural features of the peptide mimetic must always conform with the specificities of the peptide permeases (Payne, 1980a). Such requirements are, however, sometimes difficult to reconcile with the need for the peptide to be stable against human tissue peptidases. Antibacterial peptides that use peptide permeases and yet remain intact inside the cells are also known but are therapeutically uninteresting (Ringrose, 1980).

The carbohydrate transport systems, in contrast to those for amino acids and peptides, are mostly inducible and subject to catabolite repression (Dills *et al.*, 1980). Fosfomycin and fosmidomycin (Fig. 3) exploit the

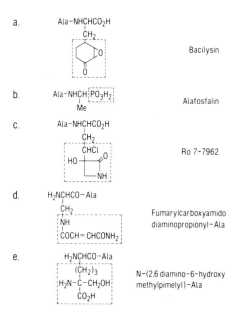

Fig. 2 Antibiotics using the dipeptide permease (dipeptides with L-Ala as carrier).

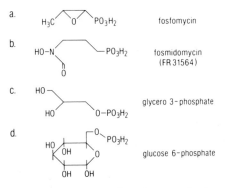

Fig. 3 Antibiotics using the glycero 3-phosphate and glucose-6-phosphate permeases.

constitutive permease for glycerol phosphate and in certain organisms also the inducible hexose phosphate transport system (Kahan *et al.*, 1974; see section III.B.5). Unlike the antibacterial peptides, these two compounds do not require metabolism in order to interact with their intracellular target sites. Nojirimycin and streptozotocin exploit the glucose and *N*-acetyl-glucosamine permeases (Ammer *et al.*, 1979; Lengeler, 1979), which are part of the group-translocation phosphotransferase system (Hays, 1978). Both sugar analogues therefore appear in the cytoplasm as the phosphates and are only active in this form (Ammer *et al.*, 1979; Lengeler, 1979, 1980). The nucleoside analogue, showdomycin (Fig. 4), however, is only phosphorylated after being taken up via one of the nucleoside permeases, nupC (Komatsu and Tanaka, 1972; Munch-Peterson *et al.*, 1979).

There has been much discussion concerning the uptake of the last two antibiotics listed in Table 1 (see Hancock, 1981a b; Chopra and Howe, 1978). It has been thought for sometime that both aminoglycosides and

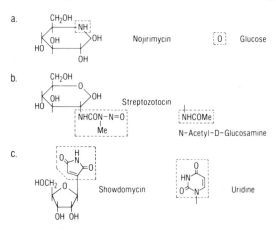

Fig. 4 Antibiotics using sugar and nucleoside permeases.

tetracyclines are taken up by cells, at least in part, by an energy-driven carrier-mediated process. The exact nature of the carrier or permease is, however, a matter of some controversy but it has been suggested that aminoglycosides exploit an inducible permease normally used for polyamine uptake (Höltje, 1978, 1979b), whilst the tetracyclines use a C_4-(dicarboxylate transport) system (Plakunov, 1973; Lo, 1979).

B. Outer membrane

The existence of specific receptor proteins on the outer surface of Gram-negative bacteria for colicins and bacteriophages has been known for some time (see Braun *et al.*, 1976). However, the discovery that most of these proteins are normally used under limiting conditions for the uptake of ions, vitamins and certain nutrients came in 1973, when Di Masi *et al.*, showed that the E group of colicins used the receptor normally used for vitamin B_{12} transport (BtuB). Subsequently, it was demonstrated that colicins of the B group used the siderophore transport systems (Table 2) (Braun and Hantke, 1981a; Konisky, 1979) and that colicin K used the nucleoside Tsx protein (Hantke, 1976; Krieger-Brauer and Braun, 1980).

Although the colicins are high molecular weight proteins they are still antibiotics and would appear to act as macromolecular warhead delivery

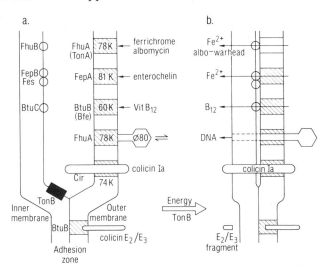

Fig. 5 Scheme for ton B-dependent systems and their exploitation by sideromycins, colicins and phage. (Adapted from Konisky, 1979 and produced with permission of the author and the publisher, John Wiley & Sons, New York.)

systems. During the translocation process across the inner and outer cell membranes, a C-terminal portion of the colicin molecule is cleaved off and subsequently interacts with the target site directly (Watson and Sherratt, 1979). In the case of colicins E_2 and E_3 the warheads have specific enzymic activity, i.e. DNase and a highly selective RNase respectively (Konisky and Tokuda, 1979). Colicin E_1 like colicins K and I form ion-channels in the inner membrane (De Graaf, 1979). Another intriguing fact is that during receptor recognition of the N-terminal sequence, a small protective immunity protein is "peeled away" from the colicin thus "unsheathing" the lethal molecule and "arming the warhead". The colicins are generally long thin molecules and are able to span the two membranes during uptake either at natural adhesion points (e.g. the E-colicins) or at tonB-induced regions of adhesion (e.g. B-group colicins) (Fig. 5) (Konisky, 1978; Kadner et al., 1979). The "new" generation of peptide warhead delivery systems (e.g. alafosfalin) may, therefore, be regarded as mechanistically "mini-versions" of the colicins.

The important involvement of the iron-transport systems in determining pathogenicity and their responsiveness to Fe-limiting conditions has been discussed by Griffiths (Chapter 7). In addition to its exploitation by colicins, the ferrichrome system (FhuA) is also exploited by the sidero-mycin antibiotic, albomycin (Knüsel and Zimmermann, 1975) (see Fig. 6).

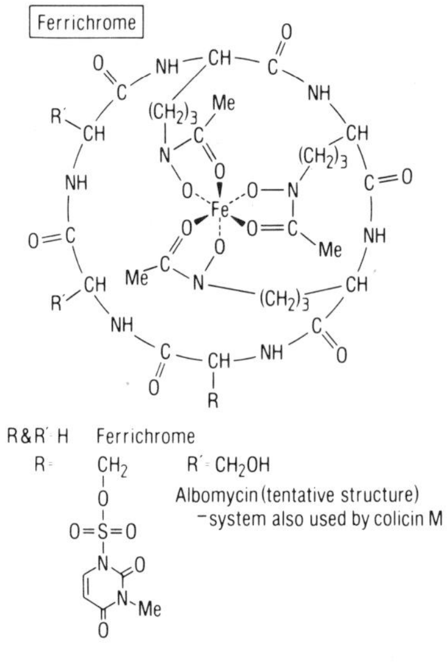

Fig. 6 Outer membrane Fe-transport systems—albomycin.

Although the detailed structure of this antibiotic is still uncertain (Maehr, 1971; and personal communication), it is clear that part of the molecule resembles the natural substrate, ferrichrome, and thus acts as a carrier for a warhead moiety, which is subsequently released and accumulated intracellularly (Hartmann *et al.*, 1979). There have been some attempts to attach other warheads to similar carrier systems but with only limited success (Zähner *et al.*, 1977).

It is also possible that the nucleoside antibiotic showdomycin may use the Tsx protein in preference to the less-selective porin channels. The important role of the porins in the initial uptake stages of most hydrophilic antibiotics has been discussed by Lambert (Chapter 1) and will not be further discussed here, except to say that during any "rational" synthesis of new antibacterial agents, the specificities of the porins, in particular OmpF for *Escherichia coli*, must be taken into account with regard to overall charge characteristics, molecular size and hydrophilicity (Nikaido and Rosenberg, 1981; Nikaido, 1981).

C. Design features

When considering the general picture of permease-mediated or binding protein-mediated antibiotic uptake, it is clearly advantageous for a drug to use multiple transport systems (re resistance development) which are either constitutive or are maximally induced under the environmental conditions experienced *in vivo*. The carrier-warhead principle would also seem to be a general feature which is not restricted to peptides and could have applications in facilitating the uptake of other molecular types. The initial stage in the uptake of most agents active against Gram-negative organisms, is, however, transport through the negatively-charged voltage-gated porin channels. The molecular specificity and species differences of these pores, when properly understood, should considerably facilitate design concepts. In conclusion, it would seem unlikely that both animal and bacterial cells should have developed transport systems and membrane receptors for agents (viruses, toxins) whose sole purpose is ultimately to destroy the cell. Design of antibiotics and other chemotherapeutic agents (e.g. antiviral drugs), based on ideas of receptor-exploitation could in the future prove beneficial.

III. SELECTIVE TARGET SITES IN THE ENVELOPE

The bacterial envelope is unique as a target in chemotherapy, in particular the biosynthesis and subsequent polymerization of cell wall peptidoglycan and the assembly of the Gram-negative outer membrane lipopolysac-charide. The biochemical events involved in these biosynthetic pathways are largely understood (Gale *et al.*, 1981) and provide many opportunities for attempts at the rational design of new or improved antibacterial agents.

A. Lipopolysaccharide biosynthesis and diazaborines

Lipopolysaccharide (LPS) is a unique feature of the Gram-negative bacterial outer-membrane and is responsible for its bilayer asymmetry and in part for the hydrophilicity and antigenicity of the envelope surface (see Nikaido and Nakae, 1979; Nikaido, 1973; Osborn, 1979; Formanek and Weidner, 1981). LPS is a complex anionic amphipathic molecule composed of three main regions. The lipid A region is usually a glucosamine-disaccharide monomer substituted with fatty acids which anchor the rest of the LPS molecule to the outer layer of the outer membrane (see Fig. 7).

The core region is made up of a KDO (2-keto-3-deoxyoctonate) acidic trisaccharide linked via a phosphate to lipid A. The three carboxyl groups of the KDO trisaccharide form a high affinity binding site for divalent cations (Schindler and Osborn, 1979). Mg^{2+} ions are necessary for

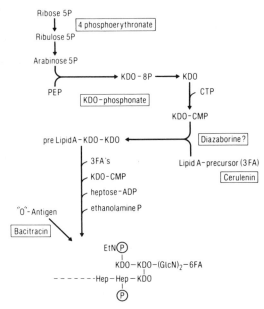

Fig. 7 Synthesis of lipid A and the core region of LPS (*Salmonella typhimurium*).

maintaining the integrity of the membrane made up by these anionic glycolipid units. The core is further extended by heptose, ethanolamine phosphate and a few assorted hexoses. The third region extends out from the core and is composed of repeating units of oligosaccharides, i.e. the O antigen chains. Rough mutants are defective in the O antigen and core regions. Re mutants of *Salmonella typhimurium* contain only the KDO trisaccharide and lipid A and are usually nonpathogenic and hypersensitive to certain antibiotics (Roantree *et al.*, 1977).

Despite the obvious attractiveness of using selective inhibitors of LPS biosynthesis, there are no examples yet of agents acting in this way that could be used in therapy. LPS-inhibitors would not necessarily be expected to be antibacterial in the traditional sense of the word but could directly influence pathogenicity *in vivo* by increasing cell surface hydrophobicity

(Dahlbäck *et al.*, 1981), and hence increasing the cell's susceptibility to phagocytosis (van Oss, 1978). Cell sensitivity to both serum killing (Taylor *et al.*, 1981) and the more hydrophobic antibiotics (Sanderson *et al.*, 1974; Tamaki and Matsuhashi, 1973) would also be increased. Defective LPS often results in patches of phospholipid not normally found on the outer surface of the outer membrane. This therefore enables easier diffusion of hydrophobic antibiotics into the cell. However, a more direct growth inhibitory effect might also be expected as a result of LPS blockade since a conditional mutation which results in a block in the synthesis of the core component sugar, KDO (at the level of KDO-8-phosphate synthetase), has been shown to be lethal (Rick and Osborn, 1977). LPS is also necessary for a properly functional outer-membrane which it has been proposed may act in certain circumstances more like a polymeric network than a fluid mosaic (Schindler *et al.*, 1980a,b).

The pathway involved in the total biosynthesis of LPS has been recently reviewed (Osborn, 1979; Lüderitz *et al.*, 1978). Of particular interest, however, are the early stages involved in the synthesis of the unusual 8-carbon sugar KDO and its subsequent addition to lipid A (see Fig. 7) (Unger, 1981). One of the earliest enzymes in the KDO pathway is D-arabinose-5-phosphate isomerase, which converts ribulose-5-phosphate to arabinose-5-phosphate. The ribulose-phosphate, however, comes from the normal pentose-phosphate pathway via the action of another aldose-ketose isomerase on ribose-5-phosphate. This enzyme has been studied by Woodruff and Wolfenden (1979), who reported on the potent inhibition shown by a transition-state analogue of the ene-diolate intermediate. 4-Phosphoerythronate has a K_i value almost 3 orders of magnitude lower than the K_m for ribose-5-phosphate. This enzyme, however, occurs in all cell types and inhibitors would therefore be expected to be non-selective. The arabinose-phosphate isomerase is, however, specific to the KDO pathway and an approach similar to that of Woodruff and Wolfenden (1979) may yield useful compounds.

KDO is formed from arabinose-5-phosphate by two enzymic steps. First arabinose-5-phosphate is combined with phosphoenol-pyruvate to give KDO-8-phosphate which is subsequently converted to KDO by a specific phosphatase (Ray, 1980; Ray and Benedict, 1980). Analogues of phosphoenol-pyruvate, such as fosfomycin (see later), have so far been ineffective as selective inhibitors of the KDO-8-phosphate synthetase. The phosphonate analogue of arabinose-5-phosphate acts as a false substrate for the synthetase, with the phosphonate analogue of KDO-8-phosphate being formed. This compound cannot act as a substrate for the subsequent phosphatase but does act as a product-inhibitor of the synthetase (Unger *et al.*, 1978).

The KDO is finally attached to the lipid A precursor molecule via the CMP-KDO intermediate by a membrane-bound CMP-KDO transferase (Osborn *et al.*, 1980). It is believed that only two KDO molecules are initially attached to the lipid A precursor which, in the case of *Salm. typhimurium*, is a phosphorylated glucosamine disaccharide containing one ester and two amide-linked residues of β-hydroxymyristate (Rick *et al.*, 1977). The precursor KDO disaccharide then receives the rest of its ester linked saturated fatty acids followed by a third KDO molecule, heptose and the rest of the core sugars plus the preformed O antigen (Walenga and Osborn, 1980a,b). Translocation of O antigen sugars requires the C_{55}-isoprenyl carrier lipid which is inhibited by bacitracin. The completed LPS molecule is believed to be translocated out to the outer membrane at the adhesion zones with the KDO-trisaccharide region possibly playing an important recognition role in this process (Osborn, 1979).

Attempts at inhibiting these terminal stages of KDO incorporation into LPS based on structural analogues of the KDO molecule have so far been largely unsuccessful (Unger, 1981). Cerulenin, a potent inhibitor of bacterial fatty acid biosynthesis, also inhibits LPS biosynthesis but does not affect the rate of conversion of preformed lipid A precursor to an under-acylated LPS product (Walenga and Osborn, 1980b).

The most encouraging class of inhibitors of the KDO pathway, however, are the diazaborines (Högenauer and Woisetschläger, 1981). Synthetic diazaborines contain one boron and two nitrogen atoms in a six-membered ring and were first described by Gronowitz *et al.* (1971) as antibacterial compounds. Their antibacterial spectrum is limited to Gram-negative organisms and subsequent biochemical investigations with the diazaborine Sa 84·474 (Fig. 8) suggested a possible site of action at the level of KDO

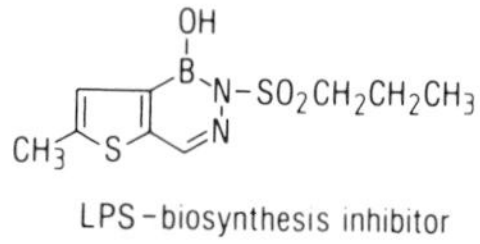

LPS-biosynthesis inhibitor

Fig. 8 Structure of diazaborine Sa 84474.

incorporation into LPS (Högenauer and Woisetschläger, 1981). The action of Sa 84·474 on LPS biosynthesis was confirmed by inhibition of labelled-galactose incorporation into the core region of a gal-epimerase *E. coli* mutant. Other cell wall inhibitors were not inhibitory. The absence of O antigen synthesis in Sa 84·474-treated *Salm. typhimurium* was also confirmed by the lack of cell binding of ferritin-labelled antibody. The diazaborines therefore represent the first hint at a possible selective-inhibition of the KDO pathway and LPS biosynthesis. Information as to the molecular mechanism of the diazaborines should help in the design of agents acting in a similar manner but without the toxicity that is presently associated with this group of molecules.

In addition to rational design, many groups have tried screening for natural LPS inhibitors, again so far without much success. Recently sideromycin was reported as originating from an LPS screen (Liu *et al.*, 1981). It is, however, unlikely that this compound primarily acts by inhibiting LPS biosynthesis. Clearly selective inhibitors of this pathway are awaited with much interest, not only as biochemical tools but also as potentially very novel therapeutic agents.

B.   Peptidoglycan biosynthesis—early stages

Peptidoglycan is the major structural component of the bacterial cell wall. This crosslinked biopolymer acts primarily to protect the delicate cytoplasmic membrane. It also provides the bacterial cell with its characteristic

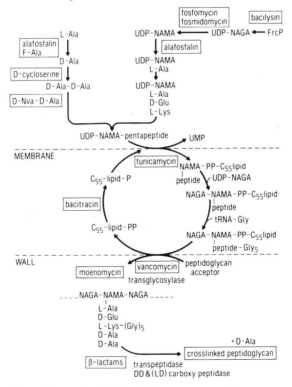

Fig. 9   Peptidoglycan biosynthesis (*Staphylococcus aureus*).

shape and also in the case of Gram-negative organisms provides an underlying matrix to which many other outer membrane proteins and periplasmic binding proteins are "anchored".

All the early stages of muramyl pentapeptide biosynthesis are located inside the cytoplasmic membrane (Fig. 9), and therefore require penetration of this membrane by potential inhibitors. The alanine pathway involving the 2 stage synthesis of D-alanyl-D-alanine from L-alanine will be discussed as the target for D-cycloserine, the haloalanines and the dipeptide mimetic alafosfalin. The other branch, i.e. synthesis of *N*-acetyl muramic acid, will be discussed as the target for bacilysin and fosfomycin.

1. *D-Cycloserine*

D-Cycloserine acts on the two enzymes (alanine-racemase and D-alanyl-D-alanine synthetase) involved in the synthesis of the peptidoglycan precursor dipeptide D-alanyl-D-alanine (Fig. 10). Early studies by Neuhaus (1968)

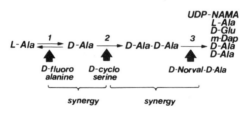

Fig. 10 Double blockade of the alanine pathway. D-F. Ala in excess will act as substrate for enzyme 2; D-Norval is converted to D-Ala-D-Norval by enzyme 2.

indicated that at low concentrations the major site of inhibition was the donor site of the synthetase. The action of D-cycloserine on the racemase enzyme, however, has led to some confusion partly owing to the fact that racemases from Gram-negative and Gram-positive organisms behave differently.

Originally it was proposed by Roze and Strominger (1966) from their studies with *Staphylococcus aureus* that D-cycloserine behaves almost like a "transition-state" analogue, in that it resembles both L- and D-alanine on the enzyme surface. In these studies L-cycloserine was ineffective and this was interpreted as being due to its having the wrong conformation. Subsequently Lambert and Neuhaus (1972) showed that racemase from *E. coli* W was inhibited by both L- and D-cycloserine. It may be that there are fundamental differences in the binding site specificities between Gram-negative and Gram-positive organisms (Neuhaus and Hammes, 1981). Similar differences were also observed with the racemase-inhibitory action of the alafosfalin warhead (see later) (Atherton *et al.*, 1979b). Originally

Lambert and Neuhaus (1972) reported that D-cycloserine was a reversible inhibitor of alanine racemase ($K_i = 6\cdot5 \times 10^{-4}$ M) but subsequent studies now clearly show that D-cycloserine is an effective suicide substrate which probably irreversibly acylates an amino group at the enzyme active site after forming a Schiff's base intermediate with the pyridoxal enzyme cofactor (Rando, 1975; Wang and Walsh, 1978; Neuhaus and Hammes, 1981). Other sites of action of D-cycloserine may also include its ability to act as an acceptor for the cell wall transpeptidase and thus inhibit the hydrolytic action of D,D-carboxypeptidase activity (Ghuysen, 1977; Neuhaus and Hammes, 1981).

D-Cycloserine is only active against whole cells by virtue of its ability to use the D-alanine/glycine transport system (Mora and Snell, 1963; Reitz *et al.*, 1967; Neuhaus, 1968; Wargel *et al.*, 1970, 1971). It is an effective inhibitor of glycine and D-alanine, but not L-alanine, accumulation in *E. coli.* Likewise glycine and D-alanine (at 10^{-5} M), but not L-alanine, antagonize the effect of D-cycloserine. However, depending on the organism and the conditions there is some overlap between the transport systems of D-cycloserine and L-alanine (Wargel *et al.*, 1970). Interestingly, *O*-carbamoyl-D-serine is a better competitive inhibitor of L-alanine uptake than D-alanine uptake (Wargel *et al.*, 1970) despite the fact that it is very poorly taken up by *E. coli.*

Recent studies with *Klebsiella* grown in chemostat cultures (Sterkenburg and Wouters, 1981) have shown that ammonia and phosphate-limited cells became more susceptible to D-cycloserine as the growth rate was increased, whereas with glucose-limited cells sensitivity was independent of growth rate. The high affinity cycloserine uptake system was present in ammonia and glucose-limited cells but not in phosphate-limited cells.

Resistance studies with cycloserine have identified basically two mechanisms of resistance (Reitz *et al.*, 1967; Wargel *et al.*, 1971). The first type involves increased synthesis of the two target enzymes, although with *O*-carbamoyl-D-serine there is only increased synthesis of the racemase. The most important resistance mechanism, however, is where the permease for D-alanine/glycine is defective or absent. Clearly when there are multiple intracellular target sites it is easier for the organism to become resistant by being defective in a single permease. In *E. coli* K12, Wargel *et al.* (1971) showed that first a high affinity permease was lost (cyc^{r1}). Subsequent step mutations resulted in the loss of the low affinity permease(s). The mutant cyc^{r1} lost 70% of its transport capacity for D-alanine and glycine and was 24-fold more resistant to D-cycloserine. A multistep mutant of *E. coli* W was 80-fold more resistant and had lost >90% of its transport capacity.

Various analogues of D-cycloserine have been synthesized in order to increase its aqueous stability and transport. The Merck enamine conjugate of cycloserine with pentanedione is essentially a prodrug (R-4[(1-methyl-3-oxo-l-butenyl)-amino]-3-isoxazolidinone, MK 642) which is slowly hydrolysed at neutral pH allowing partial circumvention of the normally high tubular resorption of the parent drug (Kollonitsch *et al.*, 1975; Jensen *et al.*, 1980). This is particularly necessary in the combination with D-fluoroalanine for treatment of urinary tract infections.

Peptides containing D-cycloserine have been tried with some limited success but only as inhibitors of isolated D,D-carboxypeptidase, e.g. Ac$_2$ Lys-D-Ala-D-cycloserine (Nieto *et al.*, 1973). Other peptides such as D-Ala-D-cycloserine (Payne and Stammer, 1968) and Ac-D-Ala-D-cycoserine (Nieto *et al.*, 1973) were inactive. Recently a naturally occurring L,L,D-tripeptide containing D-cycloserine was isolated from iron-limited *Corynebacterium*, i.e. L-α-aspartyl-L-α-*N*-hydroxyl-aspartyl-D-cycloserine (McCullough and Merkal, 1979). However, no biological activity was reported for this compound.

2. *Haloalanines*

Following the early reports of Kollonitsch *et al.* (1973), Kahan and Kropp (1975) on the antibacterial activity and alanine racemase inhibitory activity of D-3-fluoralanine, there has been considerable interest in the mechanism of action of related haloalanines, e.g. β-chloro-D- and L-alanine (Manning *et al.*, 1974; Kaczorowski *et al.*, 1975; Wang and Walsh, 1978), β,β-difluoroalanine, and β,β,β-trifluoroalanine (Silverman and Abeles, 1976; Wang and Walsh, 1981) and β-bromo-D-alanine (Soper and Manning, 1978; Manning and Soper, 1978).

As might be expected, the D-haloalanines are more selective, i.e. less toxic than their L-isomers and enter bacterial cells via the D-alanine/glycine transport system. Once inside the cell all the monohaloalanines irreversibly inhibit alanine racemase in a time-dependent manner by alkylation of a nucleophilic centre in the active enzyme (Neuhaus and Hammes, 1981). The monohaloalanines all belong to Neuhaus and Hammes (1981) category "a" racemase inhibitors in that they have good leaving groups which, after Schiff base formation with the enzyme-bound pyridoxal phosphate, form an electrophilic species capable of alkylation. This type of inhibition is characteristic of a "suicide substrate" (Walsh, 1978) but the partition ratio for the haloalanines as simple substrates (with α,β-elimination to give pyruvate) compared with their ability irreversibly to inhibit the enzyme is around 800, i.e. there are 800 molecules of pyruvate product formed for each inactivation sequence.

In an attempt to improve the partition ratio of killing efficiency, Wang and Walsh (1981) have examined D- and L-difluoralanine and D,L-trifluoroalanine. Trifluoroalanine was an extremely efficient irreversible inhibitor of alanine racemase with a partition ratio of less than 10 and like monofluoroalanine forms a stable inactivated enzyme species. The difluoralanines, however, form labile covalent enzyme derivatives with inefficient partition ratios of 5000 and 2600 for the D- and L-isomers respectively (Wang and Walsh, 1981). The K_m's for the difluoroalanines are also high and the product of catalytic HF loss is fluoropyruvate. It is not surprising therefore that the difluoralanines are ineffective as antibacterial agents. One might, however, expect that trifluoroalanine would be very active against whole cells. The fact that it is inactive is probably explained by its poor transport into the cells using the D-alanine or L-alanine carrier system. Its failure to be recognized as a transport substrate may be due to the low pKa of its amino group (pKa 5·8) thus preventing formation of a zwitterion at neutral pH (Wang and Walsh, 1981).

Other targets are also possible for the halo-D-alanines, in particular D-amino acid transaminase which is involved in producing D-glutamic acid (required in peptidoglycan biosynthesis) from D-alanine (Soper and Manning, 1978). The action of renal D-amino acid oxidase also has to be considered for any eventual therapeutic use of these mimetics. Interestingly only β-chloro-D-alanine forms chloropyruvate, however, β-bromo-D-alanine and β-fluoro-D-alanine form pyruvate. The halopyruvates react with many enzymes and are toxic (Soper and Manning, 1978; Leung and Frey, 1978; Bisswanger, 1980) thus preventing further development of the *in vivo* antibacterial activity observed for β-chloro-D-alanine (Manning *et al.*, 1974). The α-deutero- β-fluoro-D-alanine analogue however was more slowly metabolized *in vivo* and was thus selected for further studies in combination with D-cycloserine.

The effect of β-chloro-D- and L-alanines on D-alanine dependent amino acid transport in *E. coli* membrane vesicles has been reported (Kaczorowski *et al.*, 1975). Only the β-chloro-D-alanine inactivates D-alanine dehydrogenase coupled transport as well as the phosphotransferase system by forming the reactive chloropyruvate. β-Chloro-L-alanine only forms pyruvate which is subsequently metabolized and stimulates active transport.

As a result of the various findings with the haloalanines, Wang and Walsh (1978) proposed that "future antibiotic candidates targeted at alanine racemase might balance the features of being a D-amino acid isomer with a small good leaving group at the β-carbon, but one which when oxidized by an animal cell D-amino oxidase will yield a β-substituted α-keto acid of low reactivity".

A peculiar property of β-fluoro-D-alanine is its ability for "self reversal". At low concentrations the compound inhibits alanine racemase and deprives the cell of a source of D-alanine. However, at higher concentrations β-fluoro-D-alanine itself acts as an alternative source of D-alanine and is incorporated into the peptidoglycan, thus relieving the growth inhibitory effect (Kollonitsch *et al.*, 1973; Kahan and Kropp, 1975). This self reversal is prevented and potent synergy is observed when D-cycloserine (or a derivative) is used in combination with D-fluoroalanine due to double blockade of the racemase and D-Ala-D-Ala synthetase enzymes (Kahan and Kropp, 1975) (Fig. 10). However, from the transport viewpoint both inhibitors are using the same uptake systems which could give rise to competition or "transport-antagonism".

3. *Bacilysin*

Historically this dipeptide mimetic (see Fig. 11) was one of the first examples of a naturally-occurring carrier warhead peptide to be isolated

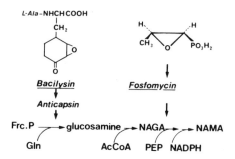

Fig. 11 Inhibition of the muramic acid pathway.

and shown to have antimicrobial activity (Abraham *et al.*, 1946). However, it was not until 1976 that its mechanism of action and uptake was properly understood (Kenig and Abraham, 1976; Kenig *et al.*, 1976). The dipeptide is produced by a strain of *Bacillus subtilis* and was first identified by its ability to lyse growing cultures of *S. aureus* (Abraham *et al.*, 1946). Bacilysin is, however, active against a wide range of Gram-positive and Gram-negative bacteria, also *Candida albicans* (Kenig and Abraham, 1976). The compound was structurally identified in 1970 (Walker and Abraham) and later shown to be identical to two other peptide antibiotics, tetaine (Kaminski and Sokolowska, 1973) and bacillin (Atsumi *et al.*, 1975).

From its structure (Fig. 11) it is seen that bacilysin is composed of an N-terminal L-alanine residue and a C-terminal epoxy-L-amino acid mimetic, known as anticapsin. Anticapsin was first isolated by the Lilly group from *Streptomyces griseoplanus* (Shah *et al.*, 1970; Neuss *et al.*, 1970) and subsequently synthesized by Richards *et al.* (1977). It is called anticapsin because of its ability to inhibit hyaluronic acid capsule formation in *Streptococcus pyogenes.* The amino acid mimetic is, however, inactive against *S. aureus.* Thus, by disguising anticapsin as a peptide in the form of bacilysin, activity is increased against a much wider range of organisms.

From the work of Kenig and Abraham (1976) and Kenig *et al.* (1976), it was clearly shown that bacilysin is transported into bacterial cells via an L,L-specific peptide permease system. Once inside the cell it is hydrolysed to release anticapsin. The inhibition of glucosamine synthesis and consequently peptidoglycan biosynthesis (Fig. 9) is therefore due entirely to the amino acid warhead and not the intact peptide. This is consistent with the earlier findings of Whitney and Fundeburk (1970) who first showed that anticapsin inhibited L-glutamine: D-fructose- 6-phosphate amino transferase (glucosamine synthase). Glucosamine is, however, important in mammalian glycoprotein biosynthesis and therefore this could give rise to toxicity problems if bacilysin were ever used therapeutically. The presence of the epoxide group probably brings about an irreversible inhibition of bacterial glucosamine synthase involving alkylation of an enzyme thiol group (see fosfomycin action). In a similar manner tetaine has been shown to inhibit mannoprotein biosynthesis in *Candida* sp. by blocking "amidotransferase" in the synthesis of glucosamine (Chmara *et al.*, 1980).

As would be expected the antimicrobial activity of bacilysin is very dependent on the composition of the growth media, being antagonized by a variety of small peptides and amino acids, also glucosamine and *N*-acetylglucosamine (Kenig and Abraham, 1976). Uptake of bacilysin in *E. coli* is primarily by the dipeptide permease (Dpp) but also in part by the oligopeptide permease (Opp) (Diddens *et al.*, 1979; Chmara *et al.*, 1981), whereas in *S. aureus* there would seem to be only one permease which transports di- and tripeptides but tetrapeptides only poorly (Perry and Abraham, 1979; Perry, 1981; Chmara *et al.*, 1981).

Bacilysin resistant mutants lose the ability to transport not only bacilysin but also related peptides such as alanyl-phenylalanine, alanyl-tyrosine and glycyl-phenylalanine as well as di- and trialanine (Perry and Abraham, 1979). Mutants have not yet been reported in which transport occurs but subsequent cleavage is absent. It is interesting to note that after the rapid intracellular cleavage of the dipeptide, efflux of anticapsin occurs in the case of bacilysin. Similarly tyrosine or phenylalanine are effluxed in the case of dipeptides containing these aromatic amino acids (Perry and Abraham, 1979).

Structural modifications of bacilysin do not seem to have been extensively pursued, probably due to the synthetic difficulties. One would imagine that alternative carrier amino acids in the *N*-terminal position could be more effective than alanine (see alafosfalin). Chmara *et al.* (1980), however, reported that the analogue L-alanyl-L-(2,3,epoxycyclohexyl-4-)-alanine is as effective as bacilysin. This suggests that the keto group in bacilysin is not necessary for activating the epoxide.

4. *Alafosfalin*

The dipeptide mimetic alafosfalin (Fig. 2) is essentially an analogue of L-alanyl-L-alanine with a phosphonic acid group instead of the usual *C*-terminal carboxyl group (Allen *et al.*, 1978). It has good overall antibacterial activity, being more active against Gram-negative species (e.g. *E. coli, Klebsiella, Serratia, Enterobacter*) than Gram-positive species (e.g. *S. aureus*) (Allen *et al.*, 1979; Maruyama *et al.*, 1979). It does, however, have good activity against *Streptococcus faecalis*, although certain oligopeptide analogues are superior against the *Streptococci* (Atherton *et al.*, 1980). It is generally bactericidal against Gram-negative organisms, it is orally absorbed and shows good activity *in vivo* (Atherton *et al.*, 1980). Like other antibacterial di- and tripeptide mimetics, its *in vitro* activity is antagonized by natural peptides in the media (Allen *et al.*, 1979). It is similar to bacilysin in that both are L,L-dipeptides with *N*-terminal alanine moieties. Both inhibit bacterial cell wall biosynthesis, although at different sites, and rely on rapid intracellular release of a warhead moiety from the peptide after being transported into the cell via the peptide permease(s). An important difference from the standpoint of therapeutic potential is that the alafosfalin warhead (AlaP) is more selective in its target site (i.e. alanine-racemase), and it is concentrated inside bacterial cells far more than is anticapsin. The phosphono-dipeptide is also much more stable in body fluids (Atherton *et al.*, 1979a,b; Allen *et al.*, 1979).

Although work on phosphonopeptides started in an attempt to synthesize mimetics of the ubiquitous bacterial cell wall peptide D-Ala-D-Ala (Gale and Smith, 1973; Smissman *et al.*, 1976; Huber *et al.*, 1975; Shiba *et al.*, 1977; Okada *et al.*, 1976; Neuhaus *et al.*, 1977), it was initially the Roche group who identified the importance of L,L-stereochemistry and hence made use of the principle of warhead delivery (Allen *et al.*, 1978). *C*-terminal derivatization of dialanine showed the phosphonates to be by far the most active, with phosphonate esters, phosphinates, sulfonates, sulfonamides, hydroxamates and tetrazoles being almost inactive despite moderate to good transport into cells (Atherton *et al.*, 1979a).

The mode of action of L-alanyl-L-1-aminoethyl-phosphonic acid (alafosfalin) involves active transport by the stereo-selective bacterial peptide permeases followed by rapid intracellular aminopeptidase cleavage to yield the L-1-aminoethyl-phosphonic acid warhead (AlaP) (Fig. 12). Probably because of the very poor ability of AlaP to penetrate cells without the aid

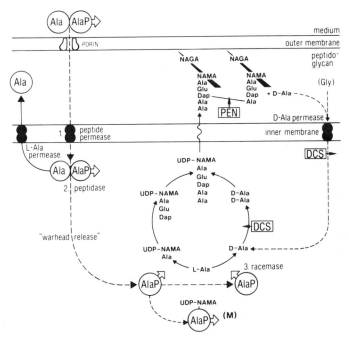

Fig. 12 Mechanism of action of alafosfalin in *Escherichia coli* (Adapted from Allen *et al.*, 1978 and produced with permission from Macmillan Journals Ltd.)

Abbrevations
AlaAlaP — Alafosfalin
DCS — D-cycloserine
PEN — penicillin
UDP-NAMA – Uridine diphospho-N-acetylmuramic acid
NAGA – N-acetylglucosamine
M – metabolite of Ala(P)

of a peptide carrier, AlaP is not able to leave the cells once it is released intracellularly from alafosfalin. As a consequence very high intracellular levels of the warhead are achieved corresponding to concentrations 100 to 1000-fold in excess of the precursor peptide in the surrounding medium (Ringrose *et al.*, 1977; Atherton *et al.*, 1979b).

The major intracellular target site of alafosfalin's warhead is alanine racemase, which it appears to inhibit reversibly in the case of Gram-negative organisms ($K_i = 30\,\mu\text{M}$ for *E. coli*) but irreversibly in the case of Gram-positive organisms (Atherton *et al.*, 1979b). A secondary target is at the level of UDP-*N*-acetylmuramyl-L-alanine synthetase (Fig. 12). AlaP is a weak competitive reversible inhibitor of this enzyme and in most

Gram-negative organisms also acts as a false substrate to give UDP-*N*-acetylmuramyl-AlaP. The weak activity at this second site, however, may be important in whole cells when one considers that intracellular levels of the warhead can achieve concentrations in the order of 40 mM (Ringrose *et al.*, 1977; Atherton *et al.*, 1979b). The lower activity of alafosfalin observed against Gram-positive organisms would seem to be due to a combination of slower transport, slower intracellular hydrolysis and higher levels of pool D- and L-alanine which compete with AlaP.

As a result of the action of alafosfalin's warhead on the early stages of muramyl-peptide biosynthesis, intracellular levels of D-alanine rapidly decrease, peptidoglycan biosynthesis ceases and cell lysis occurs within 20–40 min in sensitive organisms. Compared with other inhibitors of alanine racemase (e.g. cycloserine, haloalanines; see Neuhaus and Hammes, 1981) alafosfalin is significantly more potent in decreasing pool levels of D-alanine. This is in part due to the much more rapid initial rate of alafosfalin uptake (Ringrose and Lloyd, 1979) compared with that reported for D-cycloserine (Wargel *et al.*, 1971).

The synergy observed between alafosfalin and cycloserine (Atherton *et al.*, 1979b) may be due to double blockade at the level of the racemase and D-Ala-D-Ala synthetase. It could also be at the level of the D-Ala-permease due to D-cycloserine preventing D-alanine recycling from its liberation site in the cell wall (Fig. 12). This would be consistent with the lytic-synergy observed between alafosfalin and certain β-lactams, also between alafosfalin and glycine (Atherton *et al.*, 1979b; Atherton *et al.*, 1981).

The transport kinetics and energetics of alafosfalin (Ala-AlaP) uptake in comparison with dialanine, trialanine and Ala-Ala-AlaP have been reported by Ringrose and Lloyd (1979). In a number of respects their findings are consistent with those of Cowell (1974) who was the first to examine peptide transport kinetics and energetics in detail (see Payne, 1980b). There are, however, some important differences. Early studies of peptide transport in *E. coli* indicated the existence of two main peptide permeases, the dipeptide permease (Dpp) used exclusively by dipeptides and the oligo-peptide permease (Opp), characterized by its loss in triorinithine-resistant mutants, and used by oligopeptides as well as dipeptides (Payne, 1968). It would now seem that this view is far too simple and there exist a number of Opp's (Naider and Becker, 1975) and perhaps more than one Dpp in *E. coli* (Payne, 1980c). In other organisms, however, the picture may be different but investigations are unfortunately limited (cf. bacilysin uptake in *S. aureus*). Certain peptides may also use simple diffusion to complement permease-mediated transport (Cowell, 1974). In addition the permeases transporting dipeptides may be selectively inhibited by a peptide photoaffinity label (Staros and Knowles, 1978).

Uptake of alafosfalin is competitively inhibited by L-alanyl-L-alanine and L-alanyl-L-alanyl-L-alanine but not by tetra-alanine or Ala-Ala-AlaP and not by L,D-, D,L- or D,D-dialanine (Ringrose et al., 1977; Atherton et al., 1979a). Kinetic analysis of the nonlinear double reciprocal plot of radiolabelled alafosfalin uptake indicates the involvement of at least two non-interacting saturable permeases. In contrast the phosphono-tripeptide Ala-Ala-AlaP uses a single permease (Ringrose and Lloyd, 1979).

In triornithine-resistant mutants (TOR, Opp⁻) the transport of Ala-Ala-AlaP is completely lost, whereas the transport of alafosfalin, di- and trialanine is unaffected (Ringrose and Lloyd, 1979). Likewise in penicillin-G spheroplasts the transport of Ala-Ala-AlaP is lost but Ala-AlaP transport is retained. Interestingly both phosphonopeptides are taken up by cephalexin-induced filaments. It would therefore seem that Ala-Ala-AlaP uses only the Opp permease system described by Barak and Gilvarg (1974, 1975) and that a component of this system is a shock-sensitive periplasmic binding protein (see Payne, 1980b; Cowell, 1974).

Since alafosfalin and its corresponding tripeptide Ala-Ala-AlaP use different permeases to enter $E.$ $coli$, it is possible to demonstrate that a 1:1 combination of the two phosphono-peptides (50 μM and 50 μM) results in a 50–60% enhanced delivery of AlaP warhead compared with 100 μM of either compound alone (Ringrose and Lloyd, 1979). This result agrees with that of Diddens et al. (1976) where they found synergy by exploiting both amino acid and Opp transport systems with a combination of methionine sulfone and its tripeptide derivative.

The influence of intracellular hydrolysis on the initial rate of alafosfalin uptake was investigated using the aminopeptidase inhibitor bestatin. Although intracellular alafosfalin hydrolysis is reduced after preincubating the cells with 50 μM bestatin, the initial uptake velocity was not significantly altered (Ringrose and Lloyd, 1979). This result is consistent with that reported for peptidase-minus mutants and for peptidase-resistant peptides (Hermsdorf and Simmonds, 1980) indicating that peptide transport and accumulation are not dependent on subsequent intracellular hydrolysis. Peptidase activity, however, is directly influenced by environmental conditions (Payne, 1972).

Resistance mechanisms in $E.$ $coli$ to alafosfalin would all seem to involve changes in the permease(s) (Atherton et al., 1980) although in certain $Streptococci$ there may also be changes in the peptidase (unpublished data). Although mutation frequencies for $E.$ $coli$ of between 10^{-4} and 10^{-5} are reported for the Opp system (Barak and Gilvarg, 1974), spontaneous resistance to alafosfalin are 10^{-8} to 10^{-9} consistent with multiple-permease transport (Atherton et al., 1980). Bacilysin transport in $S.$ $aureus$ by a single permease gave rise to high frequencies of mutation (Perry and Abraham, 1979).

Since in the early studies with alafosfalin it was obvious that the peptide was acting purely as a "delivery system" for the AlaP warhead, it became necessary to optimize the peptide length and sequence for good bacterial transport, rapid cleavage in bacteria and stability in human body fluids. The warhead on the other hand was optimized against racemase inhibition. It was hoped in this way to improve transport and hence activity against "refractory" organisms such as *Pseudomonas* and *Streptococci*.

Although different organisms were found to have subtle differences in their transport specificities, it was generally found that amongst the Gram-negative organisms the more hydrophobic *N*-terminal amino acids give better transport and activity in the dipeptide series (Atherton *et al.*, 1980). Unfortunately, the more hydrophobic carrier amino acids, such as methionine, also produce peptides (Met-AlaP) that are more rapidly hydrolysed in body fluids. Peptides with aromatic amino acids are, however, poorly transported by *Pseudomonas*. Optimal activity against Gram-negative bacteria including *Pseudomonas* is found with Norvalyl-AlaP (Atherton *et al.*, 1980).

Against the *Streptococci* (e.g. *Strep. pyogenes* and *Strep. pneumoniae*), the phosphono-oligopeptides are far superior to the phosphono-dipeptides. These organisms apparently seem unable to effectively transport dipeptides. The rate of intracellular hydrolysis, i.e. warhead release, is much slower in Gram-positive organisms and this has to be taken into account with the amino acid adjacent to the AlaP moiety. An optimal tetrapeptide was identified (Sar-Nva-Nva-AlaP) whose *N*-terminal sarcosine increases stability *in vivo* (Atherton *et al.*, 1980). The size of this peptide, however, prevents oral absorption, consistent with the findings of Adibi and Morse (1977) on the absorption size limit of glycine oligopeptides in human jejunum.

Warhead optimization yielded only the GlyP analogue worthy of further investigation (Atherton *et al.*, 1982). Other substituents in the alkyl position of AlaP and other acidic groups do not, however, yield interesting compounds (Atherton *et al.*, 1979).

Other groups have also attempted further optimization of the alafosfalin lead with essentially very similar results (Okada *et al.*, 1980; Kametani *et al.* 1981, 1982). Kametani *et al.* (1981) found enhanced activity in phosphonodipeptides with the *N*-terminal amino acid being replaced by unnatural substituted phenylalanines and 5- or 6-membered hetero-aromatic ring substituted alanines. Combination of AlaP or AlaAlaP via a peptide link to nalidixic acid, however, results in the loss of antibacterial activity for both compounds (Kametani *et al.*, 1981).

5. Fosfomycin

The cell wall inhibitory antibiotic fosfomycin (L-cis-1,2-epoxypropylphosphonic acid) was first described in 1969 (Christensen et al.; Hendlin et al.) and contains what were, at that time, two unusual chemical features, an epoxide ring and a carbon–phosphorous bond (see Fig. 3). However, during the last ten years other examples of these two features have been found to be exploited in other antibiotic molecules, e.g. bacilysin and the phosphonopeptides.

Early studies with this small antibiotic molecule established that it interferes with the early stages of bacterial cell wall biosynthesis by specifically and irreversibly inhibiting the enzyme involved in attaching phosphoenolpyruvate (PEP) to UDP-N-acetyl-glucosamine (pyruvyl-transferase) to give, after reduction with NADPH, UDP-N-acetylmuramic acid, see Fig. 11 (Kahan et al., 1974). The way fosfomycin mimics phosphoenolpyruvate for this enzyme and yet does not significantly interfere with other PEP-dependent enzymes will be described later. The mechanism by which this very acidic molecule enters sensitive bacteria is, however, an equally intriguing story, that has proved to be not only exploitable therapeutically but important in determining the eventual therapeutic usefulness of the compound (see Woodruff et al., 1977).

Studies by Kahan et al. (1974) showed that the pyruvyl-transferase enzyme from several different bacterial sources is equally sensitive to fosfomycin inhibition. However, activity against whole cells ranged between 1 and 200 μM. Similarly, differences in sensitivities between enzymes isolated from sensitive strains and their resistant isolates are not observed. This clearly indicates the specific involvement of a transport process. Resistant mutants have, however, been separately isolated which possess altered pyruvyl-transferase with a decreased affinity for fosfomycin (Venkateswaren and Wu, 1972; Wu and Venkateswaren, 1974).

Further evidence (Kahan et al., 1974) indicates that there is a 15- to 50-fold intracellular accumulation of unbound intracellular fosfomycin relative to its concentration in the surrounding medium. Subsequently it was shown that one of the transport systems used by fosfomycin is that normally used by L-α-glycerophosphate (glpT). Indeed, for all bacterial strains showing sensitivity to fosfomycin there was a corresponding ability to metabolize α-glycerophosphate (Kahan et al., 1974). Likewise, with the exception of Klebsiella/Aerobacter species, all strains that acquire resistance to fosfomycin are unable to metabolize α-glycerophosphate. Conversely glpT⁻ mutants of E. coli are also fosfomycin resistant. Although there is significant intrinsic expression of α-glycerophosphate transport, isogenic mutants constitutive for the glpT function are more sensitive to fosfomycin. Further confirmatory evidence comes from competition studies, where it is shown that excess α-glycerophosphate in the medium blocks fosfomycin uptake. Phosphate ions also inhibit both fosfomycin and α-glycerophosphate uptake.

Further studies established that the permease normally responsible for the uptake of hexose phosphates (uhp) could also transport fosfomycin. The uhp system is, however, only active when cells are pre-exposed to hexose phosphates (e.g. fructose-6-phosphate or glucose-6-phosphate, less so with mannose-6-phosphate and glucose-l-phosphate) or to media containing blood (erythrocytes being a source of hexose phosphates) (Zimmermann *et al.*, 1970). The uhp system differs from the glpT system not only in its greater dependence on induction but also on its more restricted distribution, being primarily confined to the *Enterobacteriaceae* (excluding *Proteus*) and *Staphylococci*. Other organisms usually rely on extracellular or periplasmic phosphatases to hydrolyse hexose phosphates prior to transport. Kander and Winkler (1973) were also able to prove the identity of mutations in the uhp gene with fosfomycin resistance in glpT⁻ strains of *E. coli*.

Although the α-glycerophosphate transport system remains the major means of fosfomycin uptake into wild-type bacteria, the hexose phosphate transport system can play a very useful back-up role and under certain conditions can replace the glpT system. This is demonstrated particularly well by experiments with animals infected with organisms having an inducible uhp system. When glucose-6-phosphate was given s.c. or i.v. at the same time or up to 4h after fosfomycin administration (s.c.), the curative dose of fosfomycin against an *E. coli* infection is significantly reduced (Kahan *et al.*, 1974).

Fosfomycin thus represents yet another variation on the theme of an antibiotic able to exploit simultaneously more than one transport system but has the additional unusual property of showing "synergy" *in vivo* and *in vitro* with an antibacterially inactive agent by virtue of transport enhancement.

Although *in vitro* under certain conditions there is a rapid and broad development of resistance to fosfomycin with the appearance of morphologically altered colonies on agar (Tsuruoka and Yamada, 1975), these mutants are primarily transport deficient and growth defective and it is believed would probably not be a problem *in vivo* (Dulaney and Ruby, 1977). In contrast to these chromosomal mutants, transport is not affected in plasmid-containing fosfomycin resistant *E. coli* (Leon *et al.*, 1982).

In addition to the glpT and uhp transport mutations already described, other mutations have now been identified. These would appear to influence indirectly the glycerol-phosphate and hexose-phosphate transport systems of *Salmonella* via PTS-enzyme mediated regulation (Cordaro *et al.*, 1976; Saier and Moczydlowski, 1978) and cAMP-control (Alper and Ames, 1978). Similar results have also been found in *E. coli* (Tsuruoka *et al.*, 1978). Of all the many antibiotics and antimetabolites examined by Alper and Ames (1978), the uptake of fosfomycin proved to be one of the most sensitive to mutations in cAMP synthesis (cya) and in the cAMP receptor protein (crp). This clearly reflects the dependence of those antibiotics, that exploit transport systems normally used for the uptake of carbon energy sources, on the cAMP-mediated regulatory mechanisms in the cell. Under the nutrient-limiting conditions of an *in vivo* environment, therefore, intracellular cAMP levels would be expected to be high and the necessary transport systems maximally induced (Botsford, 1981; Saier *et al.*, 1982; Dills *et al.*, 1980).

Mode of action studies by Kahan *et al.* (1974) established that after transport into the cell, fosfomycin selectively inhibits the pyruvyl-transferase enzyme in the early stages of peptidoglycan biosynthesis. This step comes directly after that blocked by the bacilysin warhead (Kenig and Abraham, 1976) (see Fig. 11). The mechanism by which fosfomycin is able to mimic phosphoenol-pyruvate (PEP) at the active site of this enzyme and yet not significantly interfere with the many other enzymes that use PEP is remarkable. Inhibition of pyruvyl-transferase occurs in a time-dependent manner and is independent of the UDP-*N*-acetylglucosamine concentration. Although the initial affinity of the enzyme for fosfomycin is poor (i.e. the antibiotic is not a close structural analogue of PEP), selective irreversible inhibition is made possible by the susceptibility of the C(2)-O bond of fosfomycin to nucleophilic attack by an enzymic sulfhydryl group.

The C=C bond of PEP is believed to be analogous to the C(2)–O bond of fosfomycin and whereas an alkylated cysteine is formed on pyruvyl-transferase with both inhibitor and substrate, it is the ring opened fosfomycin adduct that remains unreactive and consequently inactivates the enzyme. The ^{14}C-labelled fosfomycin enzyme adduct has been isolated and characterized (Kahan *et al.*, 1974). The enzyme-PEP complex, however, normally reacts rapidly with UDP-*N*-acetylglucosamine to give the UDP-*N*-acetyl-glucosamine-3-enolpyruvyl ether product.

In all other cases of PEP-utilizing enzymes examined, fosfomycin has either no detectable activity or a weak competitive effect, e.g. enolase, pyruvate kinase, PEP-carboxykinase, PEP : shikimate 5-phosphate -3-enol-pyruvyl-transferase (Kahan *et al.*, 1974). Even the PEP-dependent phosphotransferase system of sugar transport is not directly inhibited by fosfomycin (Cordaro *et al.*, 1976). It also does not inhibit 3-deoxy-D-manno-2-octulosonic acid (KDO) 8-phosphate synthase which involves C–C bond formation on the C(3) of PEP (see Unger, 1981 and unpublished results).

6. Fosfomycin related compounds

Recently a novel series of phosphonic acid containing antibiotics has been isolated and characterized (Okuhara et al., 1980a,b; Iguchi et al., 1980; Kuroda et al., 1980). These natural compounds are all essentially related to FR 900098, i.e. 3-(N-acetyl-N-hydroxyamino)-propylphosphonic acid. The most active member of the series would, however, now seem to be FR 31564, i.e. 3(N-formyl-N-hydroxyamino)-propylphosphonic acid or fosmidomycin (Mine et al., 1980; Murakawa et al., 1982) (see Fig. 3). Its antibacterial activity is reported to be superior to that of fosfomycin in vitro and in vivo particularly against Pseudomonas and, like fosfomycin, its in vitro activity is enhanced when blood is added to the nutrient agar (Mine et al., 1980). It is, however, inactive against Gram-positive organisms and less active than fosfomycin against Serratia. Interestingly fosmidomycin (FR 31564) was synthesized on the basis of the FR 900098 lead before it was discovered as a natural compound (Kamiya et al., 1980; Hashimoto et al., 1980).

Present studies indicate that fosfomycin and fosmidomycin use the same transport systems (Kojo et al., 1980). Mutants resistant to fosmidomycin are usually also resistant to fosfomycin and vice versa; however, see Leon et al. (1982). In general, fosmidomycin is more effectively taken up by bacteria than fosfomycin.

In particular, Pseudomonas transports fosmidomycin ten times faster than fosfomycin. The primary transport system was further characterized to be glpT, i.e. both fosfomycin and fosmidomycin are transported by the same system. Although blood/agar stimulation of fosmidomycin uptake is consistent with induction of a hexose phosphate system, it should be noted that Pseudomonas does not possess the hexose phosphate system. The intracellular mechanism of action has not been reported in detail, but it may be related to that of fosfomycin. Synergy of fosmidomycin with β-lactam antibiotics and with trimethoprim has been reported (Yokota et al., 1981). It will be interesting, therefore, to see if these hydroxamic-phosphonates work in a manner related to the Fe-chelating hydroxamates in terms of metal ion chelation at enzyme active sites.

C. Peptidoglycan biosynthesis—Polymerization

1. β-Lactams

The biochemistry of bacterial peptidoglycan biosynthesis and the mechanism of action of the β-lactam group of antibiotics has been the subject of many recent and extensive reviews (Matsuhashi et al., 1981; Ghuysen et al., 1981; Ghuysen, 1980; Cooper, 1980; Jung et al., 1980; Mirelman, 1979;

Amanuma and Strominger, 1981; Salton and Shockman, 1981; Brown, 1981; Baddiley and Abraham, 1980). β-Lactams interfere with the terminal stages of peptidoglycan polymerization and cross-linking (Wise and Park, 1965; Tipper and Strominger, 1965) by inhibiting specific enzymes and/or functional proteins located on the outer surface of the cytoplasmic membrane (Fig. 13). The β-lactam target site is therefore outside the cytoplasmic membrane, but in the case of Gram-negative organisms it is

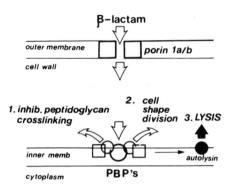

Fig. 13 Cell penetration and targets of β-lactam action.

necessary for the inhibitor molecule to penetrate the outer membrane by way of the porin channels.

The β-lactam group of antibiotics are the most widely used and probably the safest of all therapeutic agents. Their precise molecular mechanism of action is still subject to some controversy but generally they can all be regarded as site-directed acylating agents of target D,D-carboxypeptidases involved in peptidoglycan biosynthesis (Waxman *et al.*, 1980). However, the diversity of spectra, potencies and morphological effects produced by different β-lactams reflect the different specificities of their multiple membrane-bound target sites and the various degrees of difficulty different β-lactams experience in getting to the target sites, i.e. crossing the outer membrane and remaining stable to β-lactamase attack (Richmond, 1978).

As a result of the increasing body of knowledge on enzyme mechanisms at a molecular level and on inhibitor/substrate interaction at the enzyme active site, it is becoming more feasible to design useful drugs as enzyme inhibitors based on current theories of transition state analogues, suicide substrates, bi-product analogues and site-directed metal–ion chelators (Sandler, 1980; Brodbeck, 1980; Walsh, 1977; Abeles, 1980; Andrews, 1979). Much is known mechanistically about the different types of microbial and animal peptidases (Walsh, 1978a). There are essentially four main mechanistic types. The serine (trypsin) and thiol (papain) proteases involve the formation of acyl-enzyme intermediates through a "charge-relay system" (Hunkapiller *et al.*, 1976). The metallo- (carboxypeptidase A) and acid (pepsin) peptidases probably do not involve such a covalent intermediate. The ways in which all peptidases catalyse nucleophilic displacement reactions at the carbonyl of the peptide bond may, however, follow a similar sequence of events. This involves a combination of (1) electron-withdrawal at the carbonyl-O, using Zn or an amide-N at the enzyme active site; (2) nucleophilic attack on the electrophilic carbonyl-C by an active-site serine, cysteine or glutamate residue, often facilitated by a neighbouring histidine, and forming a tetrahedral sp^3 intermediate; and (3) protonation of the peptide-bond NH by histidine or tyrosine to give either the acylated enzyme intermediate, which is subsequently hydrolysed (in the case of the serine- and thiol-peptidases), or the cleaved product directly (probably in the case of the acid- and metallo-peptidases). The action of the peptidoglycan D,D-carboxypeptidases can be interpreted in terms of these current enzyme models and there are examples of serine-, thiol- and metallo-carboxypeptidases in bacteria (Ghuysen *et al.*, 1981). Based on a closer understanding of these mechanisms, it may be possible to design non-β-lactam molecules as inhibitors. Likewise the immense amount of knowledge of the β-lactams could be used in the design of β-lactam inhibitors of other therapeutically interesting peptidases (see Ondetti and Cushman, 1981).

Studies by Spratt and others (Spratt, 1975, 1977a,b; Curtis *et al.*, 1979a,b; Ohya *et al.*, 1979; Williamson *et al.*, 1980; Georgopapadakou and Liu, 1980a,b; Waxman *et al.*, 1981; Suzuki *et al.*, 1978; Chase *et al.*, 1981) established that, in all β-lactam sensitive organisms examined, there is a multiplicity (5–9) of membrane-bound proteins (PBP's) with molecular weights ranging from 25 000 to 140 000 daltons, that specifically form covalent complexes with β-lactam antibiotics (Fig. 14). The degree of binding of a particular β-lactam to individual PBP's depends on the β-lactam, as do the half-lives of the complexes formed (Ghuysen, 1980; Spratt, 1977a). In the case of *E. coli*, seven major PBP's have been identified (Matsuhashi *et al.*, 1979, 1981) but large differences occur with respect to the number of individual PBP molecules per cell, ranging from 20 for PBP 2 to 1800 for PBP 5 (Spratt, 1977b). Most of the PBP's have now been isolated and characterized as β-lactam sensitive enzymes of PSE's (Matsuhashi *et al.*, 1981). A surprising feature, however, is that at least five types of enzymic activity can be demonstrated; D,D-transpeptidase, D,D- and D,L-carboxypeptidase, D,D-endopeptidase and transglycosylase with most of the PBP's each being able to catalyse a number of these reactions depending on the assay conditions. Particularly interesting is the

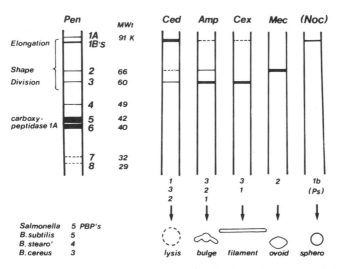

Fig. 14 Penicillin-binding proteins (*Escherichia coli*) (Cephaloridine, Ced; Ampicillin, Amp; Cephalexin, Cex; Mecillinam, Mec; Nocardicin, Noc).

recent finding that PBP's IA, IB and 3 are bifunctional with both transpeptidase and transglycosylase activities (Ishino *et al.*, 1980). Although most of the peptidase activities are inhibited to different degrees by different β-lactams, the transglycosylase activity is only significantly inhibited by the phosphorus-containing glycolipids, moenomycin or macarbomycin (van Heijenoort *et al.*, 1978; van Heijenoort and van Heijenoort, 1980; Matsuhashi *et al.*, 1981). There is also a D,D-endopeptidase in *E. coli* that is not sensitive to β-lactams (Keck and Schwarz, 1979).

The different morphological and lytic effects shown by different β-lactams can, however, be largely interpreted in terms of their relative affinity profile for the high molecular weight PBP's 1A, 1B, 2 and 3 (Spratt, 1975, 1977a; Curtis *et al.*, 1979a), with the lethal target for *E. coli* probably being 1B (Spratt, 1980; Tamaki *et al.*, 1977) (see Fig. 14). These target enzymes clearly play a vital role in controlling cell division and growth (Tamura *et al.*, 1980).

E. coli PBP 3 is involved in septum formation (Spratt, 1977a) and has both transpeptidase and transglycosylase activities (Botta and Park, 1981; Ishino and Matsuhashi, 1981). PBP 3 transpeptidase is selectively inhibited by cephalexin and furazlocillin (Schmidt *et al.*, 1981). PBP 2 is involved in shape and initiation of elongation and is selectively blocked by mecillinam (Spratt, 1977b; Curtis and Strominger, 1981). PBP 1A and the 3 PBP 1B's are blocked by cefsulodin, are involved in cell elongation and are also bifunctional for transpeptidase and transglycosylase (Ishino *et al.*, 1980; Nakagawa *et al.*, 1979). PBP 4 functions as a D,D-carboxy-, endo- and transpeptidase and is probably involved in a secondary phase of crosslinking (Mirelman, 1979; De Pedro *et al.*, 1980), which is blocked by piperacillin. PBP's 5 and 6 have D,D-carboxypeptidase activity but their role in the cell cycle is uncertain (De Pedro *et al.*, 1980). Most of the recent so-called third generation cephalosporins, such as cefotaxime, bind first to PBP's 3 and 1A followed by 1B (Chase *et al.*, 1981).

Because of the difficulty in isolating and working with these very hydrophobic multifunctional enzymes, much of the enzyme kinetics has been carried out using soluble enzymes from *Streptomyces* species

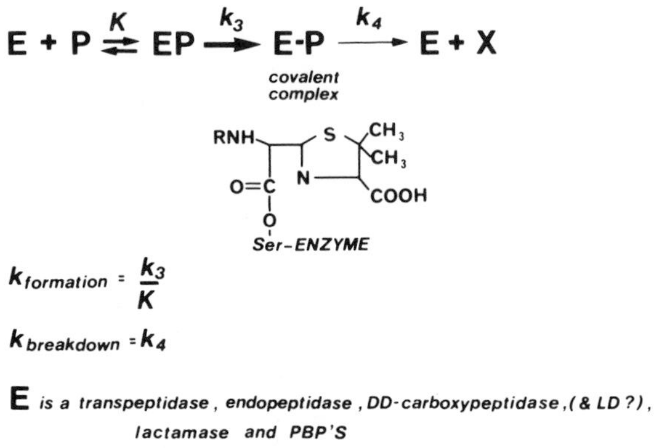

$$E + P \underset{}{\overset{K}{\rightleftharpoons}} EP \xrightarrow{k_3} E\text{-}P \xrightarrow{k_4} E + X$$

covalent
complex

RNH $\diagdown$ S $\diagup$ CH$_3$
$\diagdown$ CH$_3$
O=C N $\diagdown$ COOH
O
Ser-ENZYME

$k_{formation} = \dfrac{k_3}{K}$

$k_{breakdown} = k_4$

E is a transpeptidase, endopeptidase, DD-carboxypeptidase, (& LD?), lactamase and PBP'S

Fig. 15 Enzyme kinetics of β-lactam interaction with target hydrolases.

(Ghuysen *et al.*, 1979; Ghuysen, 1980; Charlier *et al.*, 1981). Based on work with the serine R61 and R39 D,D-carboxypeptidases as model enzymes, Ghuysen (1980) proposed a 3-site hypothesis for the interaction of β-lactams and the substrate with the enzyme active centre (see Fig. 15). First there is low affinity and low specificity initial non-covalent binding of the C-terminal D-Ala-D-Ala moiety of the natural substrate (i.e. muramyl-peptide) or the bicyclic ring system of the β-lactam (Fig. 16). This site I binding is reversible and almost certainly involves the terminal carboxyl group. The spacing of the carboxyl from the peptide bond to be cleaved is also important. Additional features are probably the two chiral centres and a preference for a *cis*–amide bond.

Second, there is interaction of the third L-amino acid residue of the peptide substrate (lysine or diaminopimelic acid) with site II, which induces a conformational change in the enzyme thus activating site I. The

a.

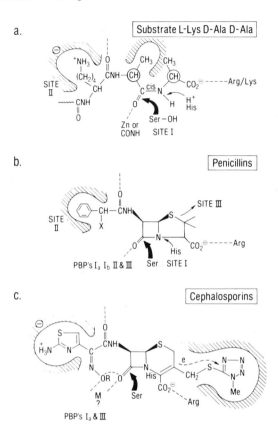

Fig. 16 Schematic interaction of the cell wall peptide and β-lactam molecules with the active site of a penicillin-sensitive enzyme.

acyl moiety on the 6- or 7-amino group of penicillins or cephalosporins is believed to carry out a similar function in terms of activating site-I.

The peptide bond is cleaved by nucleophilic attack of an activated site-I serine-residue to give a labile acylated enzyme which is subsequently rapidly hydrolysed (i.e. k_4 is high, carboxypeptidase) or attacked with another peptide amino agroup (i.e. transpeptidase). It is. interesting, however, that eukaryotic serine-peptidases only act hydrolytically. The β-lactam ring is likewise cleaved and the enzyme acylated, but this time the acyl-enzyme complex is stabilized by the interaction of the monocyclic thiazolidine or dihydrothiazine rings with a third site (site III) on the enzyme. For as long as this acyl enzyme complex remains intact the

enzyme is inactive. Reactivation of the enzyme is not just simple hydrolysis, however, as occurs with β-lactamases, fragmentation of the thiazolidine or dihydrothiazine rings also needs to occur. The effectiveness of
β-lactams as antimicrobial agents depends to a large extent on their ability
to acylate the appropriate PBP rapidly (k_3 high) giving a covalent complex
with a long half life (k_4 low). A good β-lactam should consequently have a
$k_{3/k}$ value in the region of $10^3 \, \text{M}^{-1} \text{s}^{-1}$ and a k_4 value of 10^{-4}s^{-1} or less, i.e.
the half life for the acyl enzyme is 80 min or more (Fig. 15).

The mechanism of β-lactam enzyme inhibition is therefore irreversible
but highly selective, with the inhibitor molecule initially needing to act as a
false substrate. The term "irreversible", however, refers to the inhibitor
molecule, which is chemically destroyed during its reaction with the
enzyme. The enzyme may, however, be theoretically regarded as being
reversibly inhibited since the inactive acylated enzyme has a finite lifetime.
However, in terms of bacterial generation times, the target enzyme
remains inactivated.

In part confirmation of Ghuysen's 3 site model it has been shown that
radiolabelled benzyl-penicillin binds to a serine at the active site of the R61
enzyme (Frère *et al.*, 1976) and that the site of interaction can be visualized
as a 22 Å segment using a 4·5 Å resolution Fourier map of carboxypeptidase crystals (De Lucia *et al.*, 1980). A conformational change in the
enzyme is also detected when *ortho*-iodo-phenylpenicillin is diffused into
enzyme crystals, i.e. consistent with the model site II predictions. Yocum
et al. (1979, 1980) have also shown by using Ac_2-Lys-D-Ala-D-lactate,
instead of the standard artificial substrate tripeptide Ac_2-Lys-D-Ala-D-Ala,
that the acylated enzyme intermediate accumulates. This is the result of the
rate constant k_3 being markedly increased due to cleavage of an ester
rather than amide bond. k_4 is now rate limiting instead of k_3. The
Ac_2-Lys-D-Ala and penicilloyl moieties are covalently bound to the same
serine residue for the 38 000-dalton-R61 enzyme and the 40 000-dalton
bacillus D,D-carboxypeptidase (Waxman *et al.*, 1980).

X-ray crystallographic studies are now being carried out with a number
of target and model D,D-carboxypeptidases, so that it will soon be possible
to identify precisely the ways in which different β-lactams interact with the
enzyme active sites. The Zn-containing penicillin insensitive D,D-carboxy-
peptidase G from *Streptococcus albus* and the thiol D,D-carboxypeptidase
from *Strep. faecalis* are also under investigation (Ghuysen *et al.*, 1981).

Based on the 3 site model, certain conclusions may be drawn about
β-lactam design aspects. The first is that despite various arguments
suggesting that β-lactams are transition-state analogues of the natural
D-Ala-D-Ala peptide substrate (cf. the *cis*–amide bond), the kinetics of
site-I binding indicate a weak association which is inconsistent with

transition-state theory (see Andrews, 1979; Ghuysen, 1980; Boyd, 1977). The resemblance of part of the β-lactam molecule to the D-Ala-D-Ala dipeptide and the spacing of the terminal acidic group is, however, important (Tipper and Strominger, 1965; Lee, 1971; Virudachalam and Rao, 1977; Benedetti *et al.*, 1981; Vasudevan and Rao, 1981).

Site II recognition of the β-lactam *N*-acyl moiety is clearly important for activating the enzyme and initiating nucleophilic attack on the β-lactam ring. C-3 substituents of Δ³-cephalosporins facilitate acylation of the PSE by electron delocalization outside the β-lactam ring (Boyd and Lunn, 1979a,b; Boyd *et al.*, 1980) but still the C-7 *N*-acyl group interaction is needed as a trigger. Carbapenems and penems, however, are intrinsically more reactive β-lactams due to increased ring strain and greater pyramidality of the β-lactam-*N* (Woodward, 1980; Glidewell and Mollison, 1981). The need for site II interaction for these compounds is therefore less, e.g. thienamycin has a 1-hydroxyethyl and PS-5 has only an ethyl substituent on C-6. The selectivity of acylation, however, may in these cases also be decreased since the *N*-acyl group can help specifically "direct" the inhibitor to particular target enzymes (the PSE's). The PBP profile is clearly influenced by the group in the C-6 (C-7) position. It is interesting that for *E. coli*, PBP 2 usually has the greatest affinity for β-lactams with "non-classical" groups in the 6-position, e.g. mecillinam, clavulanic acid, thienamycin (Spratt *et al.*, 1977; Spratt, 1977a) (see Fig. 17). Therefore, although most PNP's (PSE's) seem to have a similar site I specificity, there would appear to be major differences in the specificities of different site II's.

Site III is essential if the β-lactam is not to act as a substrate, i.e. the inhibitor acyl-enzyme complex must be stable to hydrolysis and k_4 is low. It

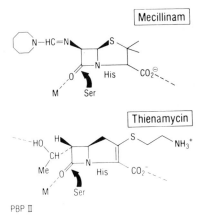

Fig. 17 Nucleophilic attack on the mecillinam and thienamycin molecules.

would be interesting to develop a true suicide inhibitor of a D,D-carboxy-peptidase which on forming the acyl enzyme intermediate would rearrange to give a reactive species (e.g. a Michael acceptor) and hence form a second covalent bond at the active site due to a further nucleophilic attack (see Mak *et al.*, 1982). This type of mechanism is already described for inhibitors of β-lactamase, e.g. clavulanic acid, sulbactam, olivanic acids, etc. (see Fisher *et al.*, 1980; Fisher and Knowles, 1980; Charnas and Knowles, 1981) and since β-lactamases and D,D-carboxypeptidases are mechanistically and possibly genetically related (Waxman and Stominger,. 1980) this type of approach is probably feasible.

The structure of active β-lactam inhibitors have in recent years moved more and more away from the classical pencillins and cephalosporins to the penems, carbapenems and monocyclic β-lactams, e.g. nocardicin and the monobactams (Brown, 1981; Sykes *et al.*, 1981). These molecules either lack site II or site III interactive moieties.

The mechanism of β-lactam inhibition of D,D-carboxypeptidases described above in the 3 site model is, however, very much idealized. It is known for some PSE's that β-lactam inhibition is non-competitive, i.e. the inhibitor binds to a site different from that of the substrate. This second site is probably normally involved in regulation. Other enzymes show reversible kinetics, i.e. the k_3 value is too low, and the β-lactam competes for site I binding with the substrate but does not acylate (see Spector and Hajian, 1981; Spector and Cleland, 1981). Inhibition in fact does not need to be irreversible to be effective. Very tight binding of the type described for the thiol-byproduct mimetic-inhibitors of Zn-containing carboxypeptidases A and B (Ondetti *et al.*, 1979) or the inverse substrate-analogues of serine-peptidases (Fujioka *et al.*, 1981) can produce very effective inhibition without covalent bonding. Ac-Gly-D-Ala-D-Glu and Ac-D,D-cyclo-diaminoadipic acid both bind to the R61 enzyme and, since they are not substrates, inhibit activity (Ghuysen, 1980). Attempts at designing other peptide inhibitors lacking the β-lactam ring have had only limited success so far (Perkins *et al.*, 1981), but with more knowledge as to the molecular details of active-site interaction coming from X-ray crystal structures of isolated PBP's, it may be possible in the future to follow some of the success described for the enzyme dipeptidyl-carboxypeptidase involved in controlling blood pressure (Ondetti and Cushman, 1981; Patchett *et al.*, 1980).

Designing inhibitors of one specific enzyme, however, is relatively easy compared with the complexities of rationalizing structure-activity relationships for the battery of PBP enzymes which have different specificities and are in most cases polyfunctional with maybe two active sites (Oka *et al.*, 1980; Noguchi *et al.*, 1979; Christensen, 1981). The design of selective inhibitors for the transglycosylase site has not yet been reported. (However, see Marshall *et al.*, 1981; Müller *et al.*, 1980.) Any potential inhibitor needs also to conform to the different porin specificities, be β-lactamase resistant and have the appropriate pharmacokinetics (Richmond, 1978; Curtis and Ross, 1981). Additional activities for β-lactams or related cell wall inhibitor compounds may be exploited in the future such as "autolysin triggering" (Tomasz, 1979; Tomasz and Höltje, 1977) and effects on the host immune system, in particular phagocytosis (Nishida *et al.*, 1978).

It will be interesting, therefore, to see whether new generations of polyfunctional non-β-lactam cell wall inhibitors emerge and whether suitably modified β-lactam-containing inhibitors can be used against other therapeutically interesting enzymes (Aoyagi *et al.*, 1977; Powers *et al.*, 1975).

2. Vancomycin

The mechanism of action of vancomycin is probably the most selective and unusual of all the inhibitors described in this review. It is also the one understood in greatest detail at a molecular level (Williams *et al.*, 1980; Pfeiffer, 1981). The vancomycin peptide binds specifically to the peptidoglycan D-Ala-D-Ala terminal dipeptide and thus blocks translocation and incorporation of the muramyl pentapeptide monomer into the growing cell wall matrix (Gale *et al.*, 1981; Perkins, 1969; Nieto and Perkins, 1971a; Perkins and Nieto, 1974; Hammes and Neuhaus, 1974). The substrate for D,D-transpeptidase and D,D-carboxypeptidases is therefore also prevented from being bound by the enzyme (Leyh-Boiulle *et al.*, 1970). Despite this almost ideal mechanism of action, the molecular weight of vancomycin and related antibiotics (ristocetin, ristomycin, actinoidin, avoparcin and A35512B) is in the range 1500–2000 daltons, i.e. too large to be able to use the Gram-negative porin channels. The spectrum of activity is therefore limited to Gram-positive organisms, in particular *S. aureus*, for which there is a growing clinical interest in vancomycin therapy owing to the lack of resistance development (see Griffith, 1981; Watanakunakorn, 1981).

The detailed molecular interaction of vancomycin with its ubiquitous acyl-D-Ala-D-Ala target peptide was first elucidated as a result of combined X-ray and NMR studies into the antibiotic's 3-dimensional structure (Williams and Kalman, 1977; Sheldrick *et al.*, 1978). Vancomycin is composed of a heptapeptide arranged in a tricyclic structure as a result of three coupled substituted phenols (see Fig. 18). Attached to the central substituted phenol is a disaccharide which does not seem important for activity. The specificity of binding to the D-Ala-D-Ala moiety is largely due to the positioning of its two methyl groups with respect to (i) bulky chlorine

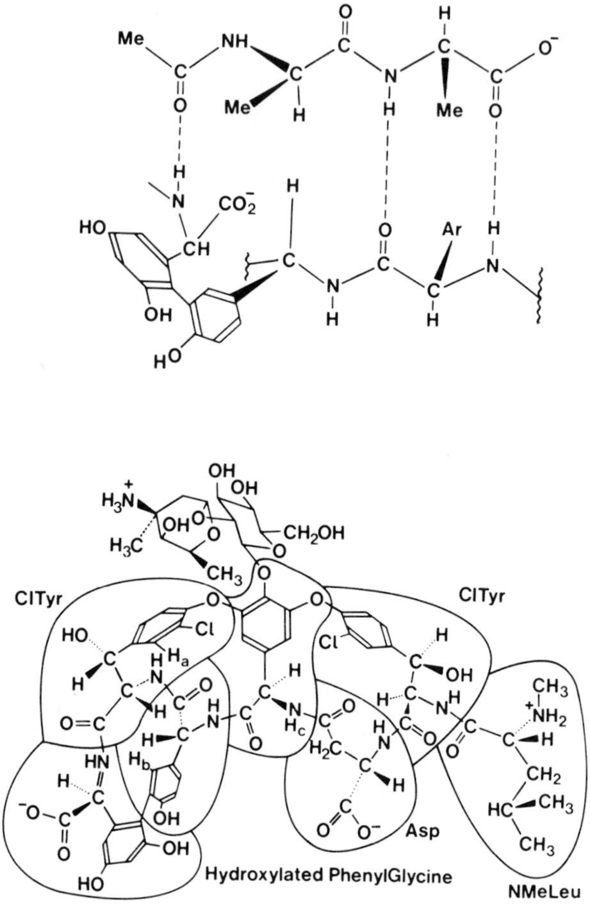

Fig. 18 Tertiary structure of vancomycin and its interaction with the peptidoglycan D-Ala-D-Ala sequence. (Reprinted by permission from *Nature* **271**, pp 223–225. Copyright © 1978 Macmillan Journals Ltd.)

groups on the central trioxygenated benzene ring and (ii) the biphenyl ring, both situated in a hydrophobic cleft in the vancomycin molecule. The *C*-terminal D-Ala methyl group fits over the face of the central benzene ring in between the two chlorine atoms. Vancomycin is thus intolerant of L-ala and of groups larger than methyl on D-amino acids in this position. The second D-Ala methyl group forms a hydrophobic bond with the biphenyl ring system. The complete complex is therefore composed of two hydrophobic bonds, one ionic bond and three hydrogen bonds (Fig. 18). More recent studies (Williams and Butcher, 1981), also indicate a major conformational change of the vancomycin molecule which allows a further two hydrogen bonds and a salt bridge to be formed.

The related glycopeptide ristocetin A has a similar heptapeptide but this time it is tetracyclic with six sugar units attached (Williams *et al.*, 1979, 1980). Binding to the target peptide is much stronger and more tolerant (Nieto and Perkins, 1971b). There are believed to be five hydrogen bonds, and because the two chlorine atoms of vancomycin are not present, hydrophobic bonding to the *C*-terminal methyl group is less specific (Williams *et al.*, 1980).

Structural modifications to the vancomycin or ristocetin aglycone have so far been very limited, but in terms of rational design these molecules would seem to be ideal candidates. Not only should the new technology of "interactive computerized molecular graphics" (Langridge *et al.*, 1981) be able to design smaller molecular weight D-Ala-D-Ala-binding polycyclic peptide mimetics that are active against Gram-negative organisms, but also be able to facilitate the design of molecules that specifically bind to other short peptide sequences of biological and therapeutic interest.

D. Lipoprotein biosynthesis, globomycin and bicyclomycin

In addition to the design approaches already described for LPS and peptidoglycan biosynthesis, it is worth briefly mentioning two other types of inhibitor mechanism that concern the biosynthesis and assembly of the major lipoprotein of the Gram-negative envelope.

Braun's lipoprotein (BLP) is a 58 amino acid major outer-membrane protein first described by Braun and co-workers (see Inouye, 1979; Braun and Sieglin, 1970; Hantke and Braun, 1973). It has an unusual but characteristic attachment at its *N*-terminus to a diglyceride via thioether glyceryl-cysteine link, which anchors BLP to the outer membrane. In addition a large proportion of lipoprotein molecules is covalently linked by a *C*-terminal lysine to the peptidoglycan diaminopimelic acid residue. BLP thus functions as both an anchor for peptidoglycan to the outer membrane and a stabilizing factor for porin trimers which are surrounded by nine BLP molecules (Di Rienzo *et al.*, 1978). Porins do, however, function in the absence of lipoprotein (Nikaido *et al.*, 1977). There would now also appear to be a number of related minor lipoproteins in *E. coli* (MLP's) and the higher molecular weight peptidoglycan-associated lipoprotein (PAL) in addition to BLP (Ichihara *et al.*, 1981; Gmeiner, 1981).

The two inhibitor mechanisms involve the multi-stage post-translation sequential modification of BLP from prolipoprotein to give the cleaved apolipoprotein, which is acylated, linked to the diglyceride and finally incorporated into the outer membrane with attachment to the peptidoglycan (Halegoua and Inouye, 1979). Recent evidence, however, now suggests that peptidase cleavage may occur after attachment of the diglyceride (Ichihara *et al.*, 1981).

1. Globomycin

The first mechanism concerns globomycin, a cyclic hexa-depsipeptide (Nakajima *et al.*, 1978) that induces spheroplast formation and was first suggested to inhibit selectively the signal peptidase involved in the

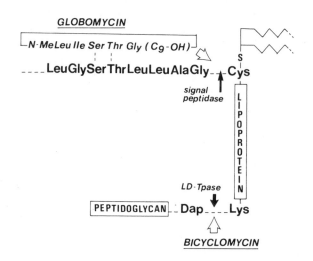

Fig. 19 Interference of globomycin and bicyclomycin with bacterial lipoprotein processing.

lipoprotein export process (Inukai *et al.*, 1978; Halegoua and Inouye, 1979). The processing of BLP prolipoprotein is particularly inhibited, as is the cleavage of the minor lipoproteins (Hussain *et al.*, 1980; Ichihara *et al.*, 1981). Other membrane proteins are not affected by globomycin, suggesting that the inhibited signal peptidase is specific for lipoproteins. Globomycin also interferes with the "processing" of *Bacillus* membrane-bound β-lactamase, but in this case not by inhibiting signal peptidase but by blocking incorporation of glycerol and fatty acids (Nielsen *et al.*, 1981). It is interesting to note that the amino acid sequence immediately prior to the signal peptidase cleavage point (Emr *et al.*, 1980) is analogous to part of the globomycin structure (Fig. 19) (Inukai *et al.*, 1978). Other more potent analogues of globomycin have also been reported (Omoto *et al.*, 1979).

2. Bicyclomycin

The second mechanism relates to bicyclomycin which has been reported to inhibit the biosynthesis of the peptidoglycan-bound form of lipoprotein (Tanaka *et al.*, 1976). About one in 10–12 BLP molecules is covalently linked to peptidoglycan using an L,D-transpeptidase. It is this stage that may be blocked by bicyclomycin. Bicyclomycin also forms covalent complexes with seven inner membrane-binding proteins from *E. coli* which are distinct from the PBP's (Someya *et al.*, 1978). From the structure of bicyclomycin it seems likely that enzyme-induced formation of a Michael acceptor precedes alkylation of an enzyme active thiol (Fig. 20) (Someya *et al.*, 1979). Attempts to improve the activity of this compound have so far

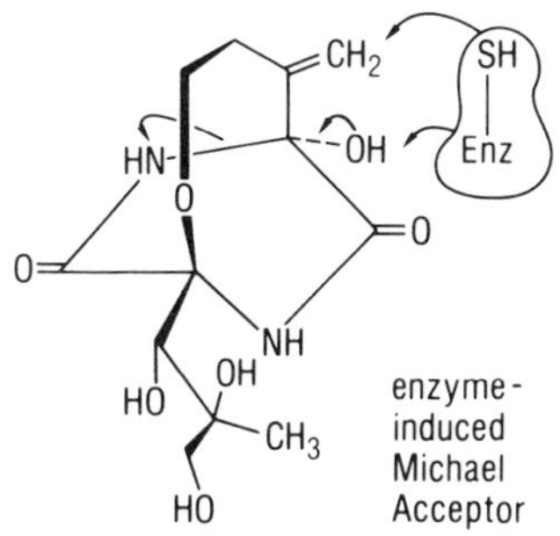

Fig. 20 Proposed enzyme-mediated nucleophilic attack on the bicyclomycin molecule.

not been successful (Müller *et al.*, 1979). The L,D-transpeptidase may, however, also be involved in the mechanism of action of nocardicin and thienamycin (Hammes and Seidel, 1978).

Of these two mechanisms, a selective inhibitor of the vital signal peptidases would seem to be the most interesting in terms of designing new inhibitors (Emr *et al.*, 1980). Such a compound would ideally block the export of all outer membrane proteins (see Wanner *et al.*, 1979) since the peptide sequence cleaved by bacterial signal peptidases is probably similar for many proteins of this type (Halegoua and Inouye, 1979; Emr *et al.*, 1980). The possibility of interfering with related mammalian signal peptidases would, however, need to be avoided.

IV. CONCLUSIONS

Despite many years of successful exploitation of the bacterial cell envelope as a target for chemotherapy, there would still seem to be many exciting challenges and possibilities left in the molecular design of new agents. Use of the envelope not only as an ultimate target of antibiotic action but also as a selective means of facilitating drug uptake have been discussed. Rational design of specific enzyme inhibitors often leads to compounds either inactive against intact organisms or with a restricted spectrum. The general concept of carrier-warhead systems, however, may offer the possibility of overcoming such problems of transport. The future of "rational" chemotherapy is now tending more towards attempts to interfere with envelope-mediated mechanisms of pathogenicity rather than direct destruction of the bacteria (e.g. LPS, Fe-uptake, adhesion, enzyme secretion). To this end, however, the same two basic questions arise, first how to identify the important molecular features of the target site or enzyme and secondly how to selectively direct the inhibitor molecule to its target. The additional possibility of further exploiting the environmentally induced plasticity of the envelope in terms of relative importance of target sites and the induction of transport systems is equally intriguing and challenging.

REFERENCES

Abeles, R. H. (1980). *Pure App. Chem.* **53**, 149–160.

Abraham, E. P., Callow, D. and Gilliver, K. (1946). *Nature* **158**, 818–821.

Adibi, S. and Morse, E. (1977). *J. Clin. Invest.* **60**, 1008–1016.

Allen, J. G., Atherton, F. R., Hall, M. J., Hassall, C. H., Holmes, S. W., Lambert, R. W., Nisbet, L. J. and Ringrose, P. S. (1978). *Nature* **272**, 56–58.

Allen, J. G., Atherton, F. R., Hall, M. J., Hassall, C. H., Holmes, S. W., Lambert, R. W., Nisbet, L. J. and Ringrose, P. S. (1979). *Antimicrob. Ag. Chemother.* **15**, 684–685.

Alper, M. D. and Ames, B. N. (1978). *J. Bacteriol.* **133**, 149–157.

Amanuma, H. and Strominger, J. L. (1981). *In* "β-Lactam Antibiotics" (S. Mitsuhashi, ed.). Springer-Verlag, New York.

Ames, B. N., Ames, G. F.-L., Young, J. D., Tsuchiya, D. and Lecocq, J. (1973). *Proc. Nat. Acad. Sci. USA* **70**, 456–458.

Ammer, J., Brennenstuhl, J. M., Schindler, M., Höltje, J. V. and Zähner, H. (1979). *Antimicrob. Ag. Chemother.* **16**, 801–807.

Andrews, P. R. (1979). In "Computer-assisted Drug Design" (E. C. Olson and R. E. Christoffersen, eds), *Amer. Chem. Soc. Symp. Series 112.* Amer. Chem. Soc., Washington.

Anraku, Y. (1978). *In* "Bacterial Transport" (B. P. Rosen, ed.). Marcel Dekker, New York.

Aoyagi, T., Ishizuka, M., Takeuchi, T. and Umezawa, H. (1977). *J. Antibiot.* **30**, Suppl., 121–132.

Atherton, F. R., Hall, M. J. Hassall, C. H., Lambert, R. W. and Ringrose, P. S. (1979a). *Antimicrob. Ag. Chemother.* **15**, 677–683.

Atherton, F. R., Hall, M. J., Hassall, C. H. Lambert, R. W., Lloyd, W. J. and Ringrose, P. S. (1979b). *Antimicrob. Ag. Chemother.* **15**, 696–705.

Atherton, F. R., Hall, M. J., Hassell, C. H., Holmes, S. W., Lambert, R. W., Lloyd, W. J. and Ringrose, P. S. (1980). *Antimicrob. Ag. Chemother.* **18,** 897–905.

Atherton, F. R., Hall, M. J., Hassall, C. H., Holmes, S. W., Lambert, R. W., Lloyd, W. J., Nisbet, L. J. Ringrose, P. S. and Westmacott. D. (1981). *Antimicrob. Ag. Chemother.* **20,** 470–476.

Atherton, F. R., Hall, M. J., Hassall, C. H., Lambert, R. W., Lloyd, W. J., Ringrose P. S. and Westmacott D. (1982). *Antimicrob. Ag. Chemother.* **22,** 571–578.

Atsumi, K., Oiwa, R. and Omura, S. (1975). *J. Antibiot.* **28,** 77–78.

Baddiley, J. and Abraham, E. P. (1980). *Phil. Trans. Roy. Soc. London. Series B.* **289,** 165–378.

Barak, Z. and Gilvarg, C. (1974). *J. Biol. Chem.* **249,** 143–148.

Barak, Z. and Gilvarg, C. (1975). *J. Bacteriol* **122,** 1200–1207.

Benedetti, E., Di Blasio, B., Pavone, V., Pedone, C., Toniolo, C. and Bonora, G. M. (1981). *J. Biol. Chem.* **256,** 9229–9234.

Bisswanger, H. (1980). *Biochem. Biophys. Res. Commun.* **95,** 513–519.

Botsford, J. L. (1981). *Microbiol. Rev.* **45,** 620–642.

Botta, G. A. and Park, J. T. (1981). *J. Bacteriol.* **145,** 333–340.

Boyd, D. B. (1977). *Proc. Natl. Acad. Sci. USA.* **74,** 5239–5243.

Boyd, D. B. and Lunn, W. H. W. (1979a). *J. Antibiot.* **32,** 855–856.

Boyd, D. B. and Lunn, W. H. W. (1979b). *J. Med. Chem.* **22,** 778–784.

Boyd, D. B., Herron, D. K., Lunn, W. H. W. and Spitzer, W. A. (1980). *J. Am. Chem. Soc.* **102,** 1812–1814.

Braun, V. and Hantke, K. (1981a). *In* "Organisation of prokaryotic cell membranes" (B. K. Ghosh, ed.), Vol. 2, pp. 1–74. CRC Press, Florida.

Braun, V. and Hantke, K. (1981b). *In* "The Future of Antibiotherapy and Antibiotic Research" (L. Ninet, P. E. Bost, D. H. Bouanchaud and J. Florent, ed), pp. 285–296. Academic Press, New York and London.

Braun, V. and Sieglin, U. (1970). *Eur. J. Biochem.* **13,** 336–346.

Braun, V., Hancock, R. E. W., Hantke, K. and Hartman, A. (1976). *J. Supramol. Struct.* **5,** 37–58.

Brodbeck, U. (ed.) (1980). "Enzyme Inhibitors". Proceedings of a meeting held in Basel, Switzerland, 20, 21 March, 1980. Verlag Chemie, Basle.

Brown, A. G. (1981). *J. Antimicrob. Chemother.* **7,** 15–48.

Chabanon, G. (1981). *In* "The Future of Antibiotherapy and Antibiotic Research" (L. Ninet, P. E. Bost, D. H. Bouanchaud and J. Florent, eds), pp. 309–325. Academic Press, London and New York.

Charlier, P., Coyett, J., Dideberg, O., Duez, C., Dusart, J., Frère, J. M., Ghuysen, J. M., Joris, B., Leyh-bouille, M. and Nguyen-Distèche, M. (1981). *In* "Recent Advances in the Chemistry of β-Lactam Antibiotics" (G. I. Gregory, ed.), pp. 184–202. Royal. Soc. Chem., London.

Charnas, R. L. and Knowles, J. R. (1981). *Biochemistry* **20,** 2732–2737.

Chase, H. A., Fuller, C. and Reynolds, P. E. (1981). *Eur. J. Biochem.* **117,** 301–310.

Chmara, H., Smulkowski, M. and Borowski, E. (1980). *Drugs Exptl. Clin. Res.* **6,** 7–14.

Chmara, H., Woynarowska, B. and Borowski, E. (1981). *J. Antibiot.* **34,** 1608–1612.

Chopra, I. and Ball, P. (1982). *Adv. Microb. Physiol.* **23,** 183–240.

Chopra, I. and Howe, T. G. B. (1978). *Microbiol. Rev.* **42**, 707–724.

Christensen, B. G. (1981). *In* "β-Lactam Antibiotics" (M. R. J. Salton and G. D Shockman, eds.), pp. 101–122. Academic Press, New York and London.

Christensen, B. G., Leanza, W. J., Beattie, T. R., Patchett, A. A., Arison, B. H., Ormond, R. E., Kuehl, F. A., Albert-Schonberg, G. and Jardetzky, O. (1969). *Science* **166**, 123–125.

Cooper, R. D. G. (1980). *In* "Topics in Antibiotic Chemistry" (P. G. Sammes, Ed.), Vol. 3, pp. 39–200. Ellis Horwood, Chichester.

Cordaro, J. C., Melton, T., Stratis, J. Pl., Atagün, M., Gladding, C., Hartman, P. E. and Roseman, S. (1976). *J. Bacteriol.* **128**, 785–793.

Cowell, J. L. (1974). *J. Bacteriol.* **120**, 139–146.

Curtis, N. A. C. and Ross, G. W. (1981). *In* "Recent Advances in the Chemistry of β-Lactam Antibiotics" (G. I. Gregory, ed.), pp. 203–216. Roy. Soc. Chem., London.

Curtis, N. A. C., Orr, D., Ross, G. W. and Boulton, M. G. (1979a). *Antimicrob. Ag. Chemother.* **16**, 325–328.

Curtis, N. A. C., Orr, D., Ross, G. W. and Boulton, M. G. (1979b). *Antimicrob. Ag. Chemother.* **16**, 533–539.

Curtis, S. J. and Strominger, J. L. (1981). *J. Bacteriol.* **145**, 398–403.

Dahlback, B., Hermansson, M., Kjelleberg, S. and Norkrans, B. (1981). *Arch. Microbiol.* **128**, 267–270.

De Graff, F. K. (1979). *Zbl. Bakt. Hyg., I. Abt. Orig. A*, **244**, 121–134.

De Lucia, M. L., Kelly, J. A., Mangion, M. M., Moews, P. C. and Knox, J. R. (1980). *Phil. Trans. Roy. Soc. London. Series B* **289**, 374–376.

De Pedro, M. A., Schwarz, U., Nishimura, Y. and Hirota, Y. (1980). *FEMS Microbiol. Lett.* **9**, 219–221.

Diddens, H., Zähner, H., Kraas, E., Göhring, W. and Jung, G. (1976). *Eur. J. Biochem.* **66**, 11–23.

Diddens, H., Dorgerloh, M. and Zähner, H. (1979). *J. Antibiot.* **32**, 87–90.

Dills, S. S., Apperson, A., Schmidt, M. R. and Saier, M. H. Jr. (1980). *Microbiol. Rev.* **44**, 385–418.

Di Masi, D. R., White, J. C., Schnaitman, C. A. and Bradbeer, C. (1973). *J. Bacteriol.* **115**, 506–513.

Di Rienzo, J. M., Nakamura, K. and Inouye, M. (1978). *Ann. Rev. Biochem.* **47**, 481–532.

Dulaney, E. L. and Ruby, C. L. (1977). *J. Antibiot.* **30**, 252–261.

Emr, S. D., Hall, M. N. and Silhavy, T. J. (1980). *J. Cell. Biol.* **86**, 701–711.

Fickel, T. E. and Gilvarg, C. (1973). *Nature* **241**, 161–163.

Fischer, E. and Braun, V. (1981). *Immun. Infekt.* **9**, 78–87.

Fisher, J. F. and Knowles, J. R. (1980). *In* "Enzyme Inhibitors as Drugs" (M. Sandler, ed.) pp. 209–218. Macmillan, London.

Fisher, J., Belasco, J. G., Charnas, R. L., Khosla, S. and Knowles, J. R. (1980). *Phil. Trans. Roy. Soc. London, Series B*, **289**, 309–319.

Formanek, H. and Weidner, H. (1981). *Z. Naturforsch.* **36c**, 71–80.

Franklin, T. J. (1973). *Critical Rev. Microbiol.* **2**, 253–272.

Franklin, T. J. (1974). *Indust. Asp. Biochem.* **30**, 549–577.

Frère, J. M., Duez, C., Ghuysen, J. M. and Vanderkerckhove, J. (1976). *FEBS Lett.* **70**, 257–260.

Fujioka, T., Tanizawa, K. and Kanaoka, Y. (1981). *J. Biochem.* **89**, 637–643.

Gale, E. F., Cundliffe, E., Reynolds, P. E., Richmond, M. H. and Waring, M. J.

(1981). "The Molecular Basis of Antibiotic Action", 2nd ed. John Wiley & Sons, London.

Gale, G. R. and Smith, A. B. (1973). *J. Bacteriol.* **114**, 460–461.

Georgopapadakou, N. H. and Liu, F. Y. (1980a). *Antimicrob. Ag. Chemother.* **18**, 148–157.

Georgopapadakou, N. H. and Liu, F. Y. (1980b). *Antimicrob. Ag. Chemother.* **18**, 834–836.

Ghuysen, J. M. (1977). *In* "The Bacterial DD-carboxypeptidase-transpeptidase Enzyme System: A New Insight into the Mode of Action of Penicillin," pp. 43–112. E. R. Squibb Lectures on Chemistry of Microbial Products. University of Tokyo Press.

Ghuysen, J. M. (1980). *In* "Antibiotics and Peptidoglycan Metabolism" (P G. Sammes, ed.), Topics in Antibiotic Chemistry, Vol. 5, pp. 9–117. Ellis Horwood, Chichester.

Ghuysen, J. M., Frère, J. M., Leyh-Bouille, M. Coyette, J., Dusart J. and Nguyen-Distèche, M. (1979). *Ann. Rev. Biochem.* **48**, 73–101.

Ghuysen, J. M., Frère, J. M., Leyh-Bouille, M., Coyette, J., Duez, C., Joris, B., Dusart, J., Nguysen-Distèche, M., Dideberg, O., Charlier, P., Knox, J. R., Kelly, J. A., Moews, P. C. and De Lucia, M. L. (1981). *In* "Beta-Lactam Antibiotics" (S. Mitsuhashi, ed.) pp. 185–201. Springer-Verlag, New York.

Gilvarg, C. (1981). *In* "The Future of Antibiotherapy and Antibiotic Research" (L. Ninet, P. E. Bost, D. H. Bouanchaud and J. Florent, eds) pp. 351–361. Academic Press, London and New York.

Glidewell, C. and Mollison, G. S. M. (1981). *J. Mol. Struct.* **72**, 203–208.

Gmeiner, J. (1981). *Arch. Microbiol.* **128**, 299–302.

Griffith, R. S. (1981). *Rev. Inf. Dis.* **3**, Suppl., 200–204.

Gronowitz, S., Dahlgren, T., Namtvedt, J., Roos, C., Sjöberg, B. and Forsgren, U. (1971). *Acta Pharm. Suecia.* **8**, 377–390.

Halegoua, S. and Inouye, M. (1979). *In* "Bacterial Outer Membranes" (M. Inouye, ed.) pp. 67–113. John Wiley & Sons, New York.

Hammes, W. P. and Neuhaus, F. C. (1974). *Antimicrob. Ag. Chemother.* **6**, 722–728.

Hammes, W. P. and Seidel, H. (1978). *Eur. J. Biochem.* **91**, 509–515.

Hancock, R. E. W. (1981a). *J. Antimicrob. Chemother.* **8**, 249–276.

Hancock, R. E. W. (1981b). *J. Antimicrob. Chemother.* **8**, 429–445.

Hantke, K. (1976). *FEBS Lett.* **70**, 109–112.

Hantke, K. and Braun, V. (1973). *Eur. J. Biochem.* **34**, 284–296.

Hartmann, A., Fielder, H. P. and Braun, V. (1979). *Eur. J Biochem.* **99**, 517–524.

Hashimoto, M., Hemmi, K., Takeno, H. and Kamiya, T. (1980). *Tetrahedron Lett.* **21**, 99–102.

Hays, J. B. (1978). *In* "Bacterial Transport" (B. P. Rosen, ed.) pp. 43–102. Marcel Dekker, New York.

Hendlin, D., Stapley, E. O., Jackson M., Wallick, H., Miller, A. K., Wolf, F. J., Miller, T. W., Chiet, L., Kahan, F. M., Foltz, E. L., Woodruff, H. B., Mata, J. M., Hernandez, S. and Mochales, S. (1969). *Science.* **166**, 122–123.

Hermsdorf, C. L. and Simmonds, S. (1980). *In* "Microorganisms and Nitrogen Sources" (J. W. Payne, ed.) pp. 301–334. John Wiley & Sons, Chichester.

Högenauer, G. and Woisetschläger, M. (1981). *Nature* **293**, 662–664.

Höltje, J. V. (1978). *Eur. J. Biochem.* **86**, 345–351.

Höltje, J. V. (1979a). *J. Bacteriol.* **137**, 661–663.

Höltje, J. V. (1979b). *Antimicrob. Ag. Chemother.* **15**, 117–181.

Huber, J. W., Gilmore, W. F. and Robertson, L. W. (1975). *J. Med. Chem.* **18**, 106–108.

Hunkapiller, M. W., Forgac, M. D. and Richards, J. H. (1976). *Biochemistry* **15**, 5581–5588.

Hussain, M., Ichihara, S., Mizushima, S. (1980). *J. Biol. Chem.* **255**, 3707–3712.

Ichihara, S., Hussain M. and Mizushima, S. (1981). *J. Biol. Chem.* **256**, 3125–3129.

Iguchi, E., Okuhara, M., Kohsaka, M., Aoki, H. and Imanaka, H. (1980). *J. Antibiot.* **33**, 18–23.

Inouye, M. (1979). *In* "Biomembranes" (L. A. Manson, ed.), Vol. 10, pp. 141–208. Plenum Press, New York.

Inukai, M., Takeuchi, M., Shimizu, K. and Arai, M. (1978). *J. Antibiot.* **31**, 1203–1205.

Ishino, F. and Matsuhashi, M. (1981). *Biochem. Biophys. Res. Comm.* **101**, 905–911.

Ishino, F., Mitsui, K., Tamaki, S. and Matsuhashi, M. (1980). *Biochem. Biophys. Res. Comm.* **97**, 287–293.

Jensen, N. P., Friedman, J. J., Kropp, H. and Kahan. F. M. (1980). *J. Med. Chem.* **23**, 6–8.

Jung, F. A., Pilgrim, W. R., Poyser, J. P. and Siret, P. J. (1980). *In* "Topics in Antibiotic Chemistry" (P. G. Sammes, ed.), Vol. 4. Ellis Horwood, Chichester.

Kaczorowski, G., Shaw, L., Laura, R. and Walsh, C. (1975). *J. Biol. Chem.* **250**, 8921–8930.

Kadner, R. J. (1978). *In* "Bacterial Transport" (B. P. Rosen, ed.) pp. 495–558. Marcel Dekker, New York.

Kadner, R. and Winkler, H. H. (1973). *J. Bacteriol.* **113**, 895–900.

Kahan, F. M. and Kropp, H. (1975). Abstract 100, 15th Interscience Conference on Antimicrobial Agents and Chemotherapy, Washington D.C.

Kahan, F. M., Kahan, J. S., Cassidy, P. J. and Kropp, H. (1974). *Ann. N.Y. Acad. Sci.*, **235**, 364–386.

Kametania, T., Kigasawa, K., Hiiragi, M., Wakisaka, K., Haga, S., Sugi, H., Tanigawa, K., Suzuki, Y., Fukawa, K., Irino, O., Saita, O. and Yamabe, S. (1981). *Heterocycles.* **16**, 1205–1242.

Kametani, T., Suzuki, Y., Kigasawa, K., Hiiragi, M., Wakisaka, K., Sugi, H., Tanigawa, K., Fukawa, K., Irini, O., Saika, O. and Yamabe, S. (1982). *Heterocycles.* **18**, 295–319.

Kaminski, K. and Sokolowska, T. (1973). *J. Antibiot.* **26**, 184–185.

Kamiya, T., Hemmi, K., Takeno, H. and Hashimoto, M. (1980). *Tetrahedron Lett.* **21**, 95–98.

Kander, R. J., Bassford, P. J. Jr. and Pugsley, A. P. (1979). *Zbl. Bakt. Hyg., I. Abt. Orig. A.* **244**, 90–104.

Keck, W. and Schwarz, U. (1979). *J. Bacteriol.* **139**, 770–774.

Kenig, M. and Abraham, E. P. (1976). *J. Gen. Microbiol.* **94**, 37–45.

Kenig, M., Vandamme, E. and Abraham, E. P. (1976). *J. Gen. Microbiol.* **94**, 46–54.

Knüsel, F. and Zimmermann, W. (1975). *In* "Antibiotics III. Mechanism of Action of Antimicrobial and Antitumor Agents" (J. W. Corcoran and F. E. Hahn, eds) pp. 653–667. Springer Verlag, New York.

Koch, A. L. (1971). *Adv. Microb. Physiol.* **6**, 147–217.

Kojo, H., Shigi, Y. and Nishida, M. (1980). *J. Antibiot.* **33**, 44–48.

Kollonitsch, J., Barash, L., Kahan, F. M. and Kropp, H. (1973). *Nature* **243**, 346–347.

Kollonitsch, J., Barash, L., Jensen, N. P., Kahan, F. M., Marburg, S., Perkins, L., Miller, S. M. and Shen, T. Y. (1975). Abstract 102, 15th Interscience Conference on Antimicrobial Agents and Chemotherapy. Washington, D.C.

Komatsu, Y. and Tanaka, K. (1972). *Biochim. Biophys. Acta.* **288**, 390–403.

Konisky, J. (1978). *In* "The Bacteria", Vol. VI, pp. 71–136. Academic Press, New York and London.

Konisky, J. (1979). *In* "Bacterial Outer Membranes" (M. Inouye, ed.) pp. 319–359. John Wiley & Sons, New York.

Konisky, J. and Tokuda, H. (1979). *Zbl. Bakt. Hyg. I. Abt. Orig. A.* **244**, 105–120.

Krieger-Brauer, H. J. and Braun, V. (1980). *Arch. Microbiol.* **124**, 233–242.

Kuroda, Y., Okuhara, M., Goto, T., Okamoto, M., Terano, H., Kohsaka, M., Aoki, H. and Imanaka, H. (1980). *J. Antibiot.* **33**, 29–35.

Lambert, M. P. and Neuhaus, F. C. (1972). *J. Bacteriol.* **110**, 978–987.

Langridge, R., Ferrin, T. E., Kuntz, I. D. and Connolly, M. L. (1981). *Science* **211**, 661–666.

Lee, B. (1971). *J. Mol. Biol.* **61**, 463–469.

Lengeler, J. (1979). *FEMS Microbiol. Lett.* **5**, 417–419.

Lengeler, J. (1980). *Arch. Microbiol.* **12**, 196–203.

Leon, J., Garcia-Lobo, J. M. and Ortiz, J. M. (1982). *Antimicrob. Ag. Chemother.* **21**, 608–612.

Leonard, J. E., Lee, C. A., Apperson, A. J., Dills, S. S. and Saier, M. H. Jr. (1981). *In* "Organization of prokaryotic cell membranes" (B. K. Ghosh, ed.), Vol. I, pp. 1–52. CRC Press, Florida.

Leung, L. S. and Frey, P. A. (1978). *Biochem. Biophys. Res. Commun.* **81**, 274–279.

Leyh-Bouille, M., Ghuysen, J. M., Bonaly, R., Nieto, M., Perkins, H. R., Schleifer, K. H. and Kandler, O. (1970). *Biochemistry* **9**, 2971–2975.

Liu, W. C., Fisher, S. M., Wells, J. S. Jr., Ricca, C. S., Principe, P. A., Trejo, W. H., Bonner, D. P., Gougoutos, J. Z., Toeplitz, B. K. and Sykes, R. B. (1981). *J. Antibiot.* **34**, 791–799.

Lo, T. C. Y. (1979). *Canad. J. Biochem.* **57**, 289–301.

Lüderitz, O., Galanos, C., Lehmann, V., Mayer, H., Rietschel, E. T. and Weckesser, J. (1978). *Naturwissenschaften.* **65**, 578–585.

Maehr, H. (1971). *Pure Appl. Chem.* **28**, 603–636.

Mak, C. P., Turnowsky, F., Hildebrandt, J., Wenzel, A., Ringrose, P. S., Fliri, H. and Stütz, P. (1982). Abstract, North Amer. Med. Chem. Symp. Toronto.

Manning, J. M. and Soper, T. (1978). *In* "Enzyme-activated Irreversible Inhibitors" (N. Siler, M. J. Jung and J. Koch-Weser, eds), Proceedings of the International Symposium on Substrate Induced Irreversible Inhibition of Enzymes, Stockholm, 1978, pp. 163–176. Elsevier/North Holland Biochemical Press, Amsterdam.

Manning, J. M., Merrifield, N. E., Jones, W. M. and Gotschlich, E. C. (1974). *Proc. Natl. Acad. Sci. USA.* **71**, 417–421.

Marshall, P. J., Sinnott, M. L., Smith, P. J. and Widdows, D. (1981). *J. Chem. Soc. Perkin I.* 1981, 366–376.

Maruyama, H. B., Arisawa M. and Sawada, T. (1979). *Antimicrob. Ag. Chemother.* **16**, 444–451.

Matsuhashi, M., Tamaki, S., Nakajima, S., Nakagawa, J., Tomoika, S. and

Takagaki, Y. (1979). *In* "Microbial Drug Resistance" (S. Mitsuhashi, ed.), Vol. 2, pp. 389–404. University Park.

Matsuhashi, M., Nakagawa, J., Ishino, F., Nakajima-Iijima, S., Tomioka, S., Dor, M. and Tamaki, S. (1981). *In* "Beta-Lactam Antibiotics" (S. Mitsuhashi, ed.), pp. 203–223. Springer-Verlag, New York.

Matthews, D. M. and Payne, J. W. (1975). *In* "Peptide transport in protein nutrition (D. M. Matthews and J. W. Payne, eds), Frontiers of Biology, Vol. 37, pp. 428–429. North-Holland/Elsevier, Oxford.

McCullough, W. G. and Merkal, R. S. (1979). *J. Bacteriol.* **137**, 243–247.

Mine, Y., Kamimura, T., Nonoyama, S., Nishida, M., Goto, S. and Kuwahara, S. (1980). *J. Antibiot,* **33**, 36–43.

Mirelman, D. (1979). *In* "Bacterial Outer Membranes: Biogenesis and Function" (M. Inouye, ed.), pp. 115–166. John Wiley & Sons, New York.

Mora, J. and Snell, E. E. (1963). *Biochemistry.* **2**, 136–141.

Müller, B. W., Zak, O., Kump, W., Tosch, W. and Wacker, O. (1979). *J. Antibiot.* **32**, 689–705.

Müller, L., Junge, B., Frommer, W., Schmidt, D. and Truscheit, E. (1980). *In* "Enzyme Inhibitors" (U. Brodbeck, ed.) pp. 109–122. Verlag Chemie, Basle.

Munch-Petersen, A., Mygind, B., Nicolaisen, A. and Phil, N. J. (1979). *J. Biol. Chem.* **245**, 3730–3737.

Murakawa, T., Sakamoto, H., Fukada, S., Konishi, T. and Nishida, M. (1982). *Antimicrob. Ag. Chemother.* **21**, 224–230.

Naider, F. and Becker, J. M. (1975). *J. Bacteriol.* **122**, 1208–1215.

Nakagawa, J., Tamaki, S. and Matsuhashi, M. (1979). *Agric. Biol. Chem.* **43**, 1379–1380.

Nakajima, M., Inukai, M., Haneishi, T., Terahara, A., Arai, M., Konoshita, T. and Tamura, C. (1978). *J. Antibiot.* **31**, 426–432.

Neuhaus, F. C. (1968). *Antimicrob. Ag. Chemother.* **1967**, 304–313.

Neuhaus, F. C. and Hammes, W. P. (1981). *Pharmac. Ther.* **14**, 265–319.

Neuhaus, F. C., Goyer, S. and Neuhaus, D. W. (1977). *Antimicrob. Ag. Chemother.* **11**, 638–644.

Neuss, N., Molloy, B. B., Shah, R. and De La Higuera, N. (1970). *Biochem. J.* **118**, 571–575.

Nielsen, J. B. K., Caulfield, M. P. and Lampen, J. O. (1981). *Proc. Natl. Acad. Sci. USA* **78**, 3511–3515.

Nieto, M. and Perkins, H. R. (1971a). *Biochem. J.* **123**, 789–803.

Nieto, M. and Perkins, H. R. (1971b). *Biochem. J.* **124**, 845–852.

Nieto, M., Perkins, H. R., Leyh-Bouille, M., Frere, J. M. and Ghuysen, J. M. (1973). *Biochem. J.* **131**, 163–171.

Nikaido, H (1973). *In* "Bacterial Membranes and Wall" (L. Leive, ed.) pp. 131–207. Marcel Dekker, New York.

Nikaido, H. (1981). *In* "β-Lactam Antibiotics: Mode of Action, New Developments and Future Prospects" (M. R. J. Salton and G. D. Shockman, eds) pp. 249–260. Academic Press, New York.

Nikaido, H. and Nakae, T. (1979). *Adv. Microbial. Phys.* **20**, 163–250.

Nikaido, H. and Rosenberg, E. Y. (1981). *J. Gen. Physiol.* **77**, 121–135.

Nikaido, H., Bavoil, P. and Hirota, Y. (1977). *J. Bacteriol.* **132**, 1045–1047.

Nishida, M., Mine, Y. and Nonoyama, S. (1978). *J. Antibiot.* **31**, 719–724.

Noguchi, H., Matsuhashi, M., Nikaido, T., Itoh, J., Matsubara, N., Takaoka, M.

and Mitshuhashi, S. (1979). *In* "Microbial Drug Resistance" (S. Mitsuhashi, ed.) pp. 361–387. Univ. Park Press, Baltimore.

Ohya, S., Yamazaki, M., Sugawara, S. and Matsuhashi, M. (1979). *J. Bacteriol.* **137**, 474–479.

Oka, T., Hashizume, K. and Fujita, H. (1980). *J. Antibiot.* **33**, 1357–1362.

Okada, Y., Tani, S., Yawatari, Y. and Yagyu, M. (1976). *Chem. Pharm. Bull.* **24**, 1925–1927.

Okada, Y., Iguchi, S., Mimura, M. and Yagyu, M. (1980). *Chem. Pharm. Bull.* **28**, 1320–1323.

Okuhara, M., Kuroda, Y., Goto, T., Okamoto, M., Terano, H. Kohsaka, M., Aoki, H. and Imanaka, H. (1980a). *J. Antibiot.* **33**, 13–17.

Okuhara, M., Kuroda, Y., Goto, T., Okamoto, M., Terano, H., Kohsaka, M., Aoki, H. and Imanaka, H. (1980b). *J. Antibiot.* **33**, 24–28.

Omoto, S., Suzuki, H. and Inouye, S. (1979). *J. Antibiot.* **32**, 83–86.

Ondetti, M. A. and Cushman, D. W. (1981). *Biopolymers.* **20**, 2001–2010.

Ondetti, M. A., Condon, M. E., Reid, J., Sabo, E. F., Cheung, H. S. and Cushman, D. W. (1979). *Biochemistry.* **18**, 1427–1430.

Osborn, M. J. (1979). *In* "Bacterial Outer Membranes: Biogenesis and Functions" (M. Inouye, ed.) pp. 15–34. John Wiley & Sons, New York.

Osborn, M. J., Rick, P. D. and Rasmussen, N. S. (1980). *J. Biol. Chem.* **255**, 4246–4251.

Oxender, D. L., Quay, S. C. and Anderson, J. J. (1980). *In* "Microorganisms and Nitrogen Sources" (J. W. Payne, ed.) pp. 153–169. John Wiley & Sons, Chichester.

Patchett, A. A., Harris, E., Tristram, E. W., Wyvratt, M. J., Wu, M. T., Taub, D., Peterson, E. R., Ikeler, T. J., ten Broeke, J., Payne, L. G., Ondeyka, D. L., Thorsett, E. D., Greenlee, W. J., Lohr, N. S., Hoffsommer, R. D., Joshua, H., Ruyel, W. V., Rothrock, J. W., Aster, S. D., Maycock, A. L., Robinson, F. M., Hirschmann, R., Sweet, C. S., Ulm, E. H., Gross, D. M., Vassil, T. C. and Stone, C. A. (1980). *Nature.* **288**, 280–283.

Payne, J. W. (1968). *J. Biol. Chem.* **243**, 3395–3403.

Payne, J. W. (1972). *J. Gen. Microbiol.* **71**, 281–291.

Payne, J. W. (1980a). *In* "Microorganisms and Nitrogen Sources" (J. W. Payne, ed.) pp. 211–256. J. Wiley & Sons, Chichester.

Payne, J. W. (1980b). *In* "Microorganisms and Nitrogen Sources" (J. W. Payne, ed.) pp. 335–358. J. Wiley & Sons, Chichester.

Payne, J. W. (1980c). *In* "Microorganisms and Nitrogen Sources", (J. W. Payne, ed.) pp. 359–377. J. Wiley & Sons, Chichester.

Payne, R. A. and Stammer, C. H. (1968). *J. Org. Chem.* **33**, 2421–2425.

Perkins, H. R. (1969). *Biochem. J.* **111**, 195–205.

Perkins, H. R. and Nieto, M. (1974). *Ann. N.Y. Acad. Sci.* **235**, 348–363.

Perkins, H. R., Frère, J.-M. and Ghuysen, J.-M. (1981). *FEBS Lett.* **123**, 75–78.

Perry, D. (1981) *J. Gen. Microbiol.* **124**, 425–428.

Perry, D. and Abraham, E. P. (1979). *J. Gen. Microbiol.* **115**, 213–221.

Pfeiffer, R. R. (1981). *Rev. Inf. Dis.* **3**, Suppl. 205–209.

Plankunov, V. K. (1973). *Antibiotiki* (Moscow) **18**, 1069–1073.

Powers, J. C., Carroll, D. L. and Tuhy, P. M. (1975). *N.Y. Acad. Sci.* **256**, 420–425.

Rando, R. (1975). *Accounts Chem. Res.* **8**, 281–288.

Ray, P. H. (1980). *J. Bacteriol.* **141**, 635–644.

Ray, P. H. and Benedict, C. D. (1980). *J. Bacteriol.* **142,** 60–68.

Reitz, R. H., Slade, H. D. and Neuhaus, F. C. (1967) *Biochemistry* **6,** 2561–2570.

Richards, R. W., Rodwell, J. L. and Schmalzl. K. J. (1977). *J. Chem. Soc. Commun.* **23,** 849–850.

Richmond, M. H. (1978). *J. Antimicrob. Chemother.* **4** (Suppl.), 1–14.

Rick, P. D. and Osborn, M. J. (1977). *J. Biol. Chem.* **252,** 4895–4903.

Rick, P. D., Fung, L. W.-M., Ho, C. and Osborn, M. J. (1977). *J. Biol. Chem.* **252,** 4904–4912.

Ringrose, P. S. (1980) *In* "Microorganisms and Nitrogen Sources" (J. W. Payne, ed.) pp. 641–692 and 805–807. John Wiley & Sons, Chichester.

Ringrose, P. S. and Lloyd, W. J. (1979). 11th International Congress Biochem. Toronto, Abs. 06-8-R69.

Ringrose, P. S., Atherton, F. R., Hall, M. J., Hassall, C. H., Lambert, R. W., Lloyd, W. J. and Nisbet, L. J. (1977). 10th International Congress of Chemotherapy, Zurich, Abs. 367.

Roantree, R. J., Kuo, T. T. and MacPhee, D. G. (1977). *J. Gen. Microbiol.* **103,** 223–224.

Roze, U. and Strominger, J. L. (1966). *Mol. Pharmacol.* **2,** 92–94.

Saier, Jr. M. H. (1979). *In* "The Bacteria" (J. R. Sokatsch and L. N. Ornston, eds) Vol. VII, pp. 167–225. Academic Press, New York and London.

Saier, Jr. M. H. and Moczydlowski, E. G. (1978). *In* "Bacterial Transport" (B. P. Rosen, ed.) pp. 103–125. Marcel Dekker, New York.

Saier, Jr. M. H., Keeler, D. K. and Feucht, B. U. (1982). *J. Biol. Chem.* **257,** 2509–2517.

Salton, M. R. J. and Shockman, G. D. (eds) (1981). "β-Lactam Antibiotics: Mode of Action, New Developments and Future Prospects." Academic Press, New York and London.

Sanderson, K. E., MacAlister, T. J., Costerton, J. W. and Cheng, K. J. (1974). *Can. J. Microbiol.* **20,** 1135–1145.

Sandler, M. (ed.) (1980). "Enzyme Inhibitors as Drugs." Report of symposium, London, 9–10 April, 1979. Macmillan, London.

Scannel, J. P. and Pruess, D. L. (1974). *In* "Chemistry and Biochemistry of Amino Acids, Peptides and Proteins" (B. Weinstein, ed.), Vol. 3., pp. 189–244. Marcel Dekker, New York.

Schindler, M. and Osborn, M. J. (1979). *Biochemistry* **18,** 4425–4430.

Schindler, M., Osborn, M. J. and Koppel, D. E. (1980a). *Nature* **283,** 346–350.

Schindler, M., Osborn, M. J and Koppel, D. E. (1980b). *Nature* **285,** 261–263.

Schmidt, L. D., Botta, G. and Park, J. T. (1981). *J. Bacteriol.* **145,** 632–637.

Shah, R., Neuss, N., Gorman, M. and Boeck, L. D. (1970). *J. Antibiot.* **23,** 613–617.

Sheldrick, G. M., Jones, P. G., Kennard, O., Williams, D. H. and Smith, G. A. (1978). *Nature* **271,** 223–225.

Shiba, T., Miyoshi, K. and Kusumoto, S. (1977). *Bull. Chem. Soc. Japan.* **50,** 254–257.

Silverman, R. B. and Abeles, R. H. (1976). *Biochemistry* **15,** 4718–4723.

Smissman, E. E., Terada, A. and El-Antably, S. (1976). *J. Med. Chem.* **19,** 165–167.

Someya, A., Iseki, M. and Tanaka, N. (1978). *J. Antibiot.* **31,** 712–718.

Someya, A., Iseki, M. and Tanaka, N. (1979). *J. Antibiot.* **32,** 402–407.

Soper, T. S. and Manning, J. M. (1978). *Biochemistry* **17,** 3377–3384.

Spector, T. and Cleland, W. W. (1981). *Biochem. Pharmacol.* **30**, 1–7.
Spector, T. and Hajian, G. (1981). *Anal. Biochem.* **115**, 403–409.
Spratt, B. G. (1975). *Proc. Natl. Acad. Sci. USA.* **72**, 2999–3003.
Spratt, B. G. (1977a). *Eur. J. Biochem.* **72**, 341–352.
Spratt, B. G. (1977b). *In* "Microbiology 1977". (D. Schlessinger, ed.) pp. 182–190. Am. Soc. Microbiol, Washington.
Spratt, B. G. (1980). *Phil. Trans. Roy. Soc. London. Series B* **289**, 273–283.
Spratt, B. G., Jobanputra, V. and Zimmermann, W. (1977). *Antimicrob. Ag. Chemother.* **12**, 406–409.
Staros, J. V. and Knowles, J. R. (1978). *J. Amer. Chem. Soc.* **17**, 3321–3325.
Sterkenburg, A. and Wouters. J. T. M. (1981). *J. Gen. Microbiol.* **124**, 29–34.
Suzuki, H., Nishimura, Y. and Hirota, Y. (1978). *Proc. Natl. Acad. Sci. USA* **75**, 664–668.
Sykes, R. B., Bonner, D. P., Bush, K., Georgopapadakou, N. K. and Wells, J. S. (1981). *J. Antimicrob. Chemother.* **8**, Suppl. E, 1–16.
Tamaki, S. and Matsuhashi, M. (1973). *J. Bacteriol.* **114**, 453–454.
Tamaki, S., Nakajima, S. and Matsuhashi, M. (1977). *Proc. Natl. Acad. Sci. USA* **74**, 5472–5476.
Tamura, T., Suzuki, H., Nishimura, Y., Mizoguchi, J. and Hirota, Y. (1980). *Proc. Natl. Acad. Sci. USA* **77**, 4499–4503.
Tanaka, N., Iseki, M., Miyoshi, T., Aoki, H. and Imanaka, H. (1976). *J. Antibiot.* **29**, 155–168.
Taylor, P. W., Messner, P. and Parton, R. (1981). *J. Med. Microbiol.* **14**, 9–19.
Tipper, D. J. and Strominger, J. L. (1965). *Proc. Natl. Acad. Sci. USA* **54**, 1133–1141.
Tomasz, A. (1979). *Rev. Infect. Dis.* **1**, 434–467.
Tomasz, A. and Höltje, J. V. (1977). *In* "Microbiology 1977" (D. Schlessinger, ed.) pp. 209–215. Amer. Soc. Microbiol., Washington.
Tsuruoka, T. and Yamada, Y. (1975). *J. Antibiot.* **28**, 906–911.
Tsuruoka, T., Miyata, A. and Yamada, Y. (1978). *J. Antibiot.* **31**, 192–201.
Unger, F. M. (1981). *Adv. Carbohyd. Chem. Biochem.* **38**, 323–377.
Unger, F. M., Stix, D., Moderndorfer, E. and Hammerschmid. F. (1978). *Carbohyd. Res.* **67**, 349–356.
van Heijenoort, Y. and van Heijenoort, J. (1980). *FEBS. Lett.* **110**, 241–244.
van Heijenoort, Y., Derrien, M. and van Heijenoort, J. (1978). *FEBS. Lett.* **89**, 141–144.
van Oss, C. J. (1978). *Ann. Rev. Microbiol.* **32**, 19–39.
Vasudevan, T. K. and Rao, V. S. R. (1981). *Biopolymers* **20**, 865–877.
Venkateswaren, P. S. and Wu, H. C. (1972). *J. Bacteriol.* **110**, 935–944.
Virudachalam, R. and Rao, V. S. R. (1977). *Int. J. Pept. Protein. Res.* **10**, 51–59.
Walenga, R. W. and Osborn, M. J. (1980a). *J. Biol. Chem.* **255**, 4252–4256.
Walenga, R. W. and Osborn, M. J. (1980b). *J. Biol. Chem.* **255**, 4257–4263.
Walker, J. E. and Abraham, E. P. (1970). *Biochem. J.* **118**, 563–570.
Walsh, C. (1977). *Horizons Biochem. Biophys.* **3**, 36–81.
Walsh, C. (1978a). "Enzymatic Reaction Mechanisms". W. H. Freeman & Co., San Francisco.
Walsh, C. T. (1978b). *Ann. Rev. Biochem.* **47**, 881–931.
Wang, E. A. and Walsh, C. (1978). *Biochemistry* **17**, 1313–1321.
Wang, E. A. and Walsh, C. (1981). *Biochemistry* **20**, 7539–7546.
Wanner, B. L., Sarthy, A. and Beckwith, J. (1979). *J. Bacteriol.* **140**, 229–239.

Wargel, R. J., Shadur, C. A. and Neuhaus, F. C. (1970). *J. Bacteriol.* **103,** 778–788.

Wargel, R. J., Shadur, C. A. and Neuhaus, F. C. (1971). *J. Bacteriol.* **105,** 1028–1035.

Watanakunakorn, C. (1981). *Rev. Inf. Dis.* **3,** Suppl., 210–215.

Watson, D. H. and Sherratt, D. J. (1979). *Nature* **278,** 362–364.

Waxman, D. J. and Strominger, J. L. (1980). *J. Biol. Chem.* **255,** 3964–3976.

Waxman, D. J., Yocum, R. R. and Strominger, J. L. (1980). *Trans Roy. Soc. London, Series B* **289,** 257–271.

Waxman, D. J., Lindgren, D. M. and Strominger, J. L. (1981). *J. Bacteriol.* **148,** 950–955.

Whitney, J. G. and Funderburk, S. S. (1970). 10th Int. Congress for Microbiology, Mexico City. Abs., p. 101.

Williams, D. H. and Butcher, D. W. (1981). *J. Amer. Chem. Soc.* **103,** 5697–5700.

Williams, D. H. and Kalman, J. R. (1977). *J. Amer. Chem. Soc.* **99,** 2768–2774.

Williams, D. H., Rajandanda, V. and Kalman, J. R. (1979). *J. Chem. Soc. Perkin I.* 1979, 782–792.

Williams, D. H., Rajananda, V., Williamson,.M. P. and Bojesen, G. (1980). *In* "Topics in Antibiotic Chemistry" (P. G. Sammes, ed.), Vol. 5, pp. 121–158. Ellis Horwood, Chichester.

Williamson, R., Hakenbeck, R. and Tomasz, A. (1980). *Antimicrob. Ag. Chemother.* **18,** 629–637.

Wise, E. M. and Park, J. T. (1965). *Proc. Natl. Acad. Sci. USA* **54,** 75–81.

Woodruff, H. B., Mata, J. M., Hernandez, S., Mochales, S., Rodriguez, A., Stapley, E. O., Wallick, H., Miller, A. K. and Hendlin, D. (1977). *Chemotherapy* **23,** Suppl 1, 1–22.

Woodruff, W. W. and Wolfenden, R. (1979). *J. Biol. Chem.* **254,** 5866–5867.

Woodward, R. B. (1980). *Phil. Trans. Roy. Soc. London. Series B* **289,** 239–250.

Wu, J. C. and Venkateswaren, P. S. (1974). *Ann. NY. Acad. Sci.* **235,** 587–592.

Yocum, R. R., Waxman, D. J., Rasmussen, J. R. and Strominger, J. L. (1979). *Proc. Natl. Acad. Sci. USA* **76,** 2730–2734.

Yocum, R. R., Rasmussen, J. R. and Strominger, J. L. (1980). *J. Biol. Chem.* **255,** 3977–3986.

Yokota, Y., Murakawa, T. and Nishida, M. (1981). *J. Antibiot.* **34,** 876–883.

Zähner, H., Diddens, H., Keller-Schierlein, W. and Naegeli, H. U. (1977). *Jap. J. Antibiot.* **30,** Suppl., 201–206.

Zimmermann, S. B., Stapley, E. O., Wallick, H. and Baldwin, R. (1970). *Antimicrob. Ag. Chemother.* **1969,** 303–309.

9 Exploitation of the bacterial envelope: rational design of vaccines

PETER HAMBLETON and JACK MELLING

I. INTRODUCTION

Any attempt towards the rational design of a vaccine against microbial infection must depend on a good understanding of the mechanisms involved in the pathogenesis of that disease. Fortunately, the vast majority of microorganisms are harmless to man and animals—indeed, many are of great benefit—but a few do have the property of pathogenicity, or virulence, and these pathogenic microbes must possess biochemical characteristics which distinguish them from the harmless non-pathogens.

Broadly speaking, in order to produce disease, bacteria must first enter the host by surviving on, or penetrating, mucous membranes or surviving within wounds. Subsequently, the organism must multiply in the host tissue and produce damage either directly at sites of infection and replication or at some distance by means of exported toxic substances. In addition, the organisms must in some way interfere with humoral and cell mediated host defence mechanisms. The biochemical characteristics of microorganisms enabling these disease processes are referred to as *virulence determinants* (Smith, 1972). In general, virulent organisms must possess several virulence determinants to establish disease in a susceptible host and loss of even one of the determinants may result in avirulence or attenuation. For example, virulent strains of *Bacillus anthracis* possess a capsular component, poly-D-glutamic acid, that inhibits host defence mechanisms and excretes a lethal toxin. Strains that produce either the capsular component or the toxin, but not both, are avirulent. Thus, successful prophylaxis or

MEDICAL MICROBIOLOGY, 3
ISBN 0 12 228003 3

therapy of infectious disease must depend on the effective neutralization of one or more virulence determinants.

Although chemotherapy has proved to be effective in controlling many bacterial diseases, the stimulation of the host's own immune defences by vaccination has been equally effective and with the increasing emergence of antibiotic resistant strains immune prophylaxis and therapy may take on increasing importance. Concern at the possibility that individuals might suffer damaging side effects as a result of active immunization has led to the realization that new or improved vaccines should contain a minimum of unwanted components that might be of doubtful immunological benefit and could even be harmful to the recipient.

The study and recognition of bacterial determinants of pathogenicity could lead to the development of vaccines designed to neutralize specifically one or more such determinants and so interfere with the pathogenesis of disease. Since pathogenicity may result from several virulence factors and virulence can only really be expressed *in vivo*, the recognition of determinants is difficult. Initial studies must be made in diseased hosts, subsequent investigations may be performed in isolated organ or cell cultures. *In vitro* tests can then be relevant to the known behaviour and characteristics of the microorganism *in vivo*.

The initial interaction between a pathogen and its host will involve components of the bacterial envelope and the host cell membrane, so the investigation of bacterial envelope constituents that may have virulence functions is an obvious point to start in the choice of components for rationally designed vaccines. It has been clearly shown that the ability of enteropathogenic bacteria to adhere to host intestinal epithelium resides with specific envelope components, for example, the K88 adhesion antigen of enteropathogenic *Escherichia coli*. Indeed, other antigens may even discriminate between different regions of the intestine. In other instances, although adhesion is clearly an important virulence factor, the components responsible for adhesion are unknown. Thus, for *in vitro* cultured gonococci, the presence of pili on virulent strains promotes adhesion to tissue culture cells, whereas non-pilated avirulent strains do not adhere; both strains, however, will adhere to human fallopian tube and endocervix epithelium. The recognition of bacterial components involved in other aspects of virulence, such as the ability to survive and replicate in the host, to counter host defence mechanisms and to cause damage to host tissues, might further indicate candidates for possible inclusion in highly specific vaccines. In the case of cholera, for example, an increasing understanding at the molecular level of mechanism of pathogenesis has led to the development of vaccines having components designed to prevent microbial adhesion to the intestinal wall and to neutralize the ability of the toxin to bind to its specific site. In contrast, much less is known of the determinants of pathogenesis in whooping cough with the result that hitherto relatively crude vaccines have been used that contain many unwanted bacterial components of unknown or doubtful immunological benefit, that may also be harmful to the recipient.

Generally, vaccination against bacterial infections is given by injection which does not mimic natural routes of infection. This may result in a low or even inadequate level of topical immunity at the site of natural infection. Consequently, interest in mimicking normal routes of infection could lead to improved protection from vaccines.

With the exception of exotoxins (and enzymes) the bacterial components responsible for pathogenicity are most likely to reside on or near the surface of the bacterial cell envelope. It is beyond the scope of this article to give a detailed account of current knowledge concerning bacterial envelope structure—for this, the reader is referred to an excellent review by Ward and Berkeley (1980). However, it is relevant to consider the major features of the surfaces of Gram-negative and Gram-positive bacteria and their possible roles as somatic antigens.

All bacteria (except Archaebacteria) contain peptidoglycan as the main structural component of their envelope. In Gram-positives this may constitute up to 80% of the dry weight of the envelope; in Gram-negatives the polymer is generally only a minor proportion of the wall. The polymer consists of alternating residues of muramic acid and glutosamine, usually *N*-acetylated, in β1–4 linkage; the carboxyl groups of muramic acid are substituted with short peptides of L and D amino acids. In Gram-negatives the peptide chains have the same basic structure (L-Ala-D-isoGlu-meso-diaminopimelic acid-D-Ala) but Gram-positives may contain a greater variety of peptides. In Gram-negative bacteria, peptidoglycan is located within the outer membrane and is unlikely to function antigenically. In contrast, the polymer is exposed at the surface of Gram-positive organisms and antibodies to the polymer are raised.

Gram-positive envelopes also contain other polymers such as the teichoic and teichuronic acids and some polysaccharides. These components function antigenically; many as group specific antigens. Proteins that function as type specific antigens are also found on the outer surfaces of some Gram-positive bacteria.

A. The Gram-negative outer membrane

Gram-negative envelopes are more complex than those of Gram-positive organisms containing protein, lipid and complex polysaccharide in addition to the peptidoglycan. The envelope itself is composed of several layers; the peptidoglycan exists as a dense layer external to the cytoplasmic membrane and external to this is the outer membrane. The outer membrane is of interest since it carries the lipopolysaccharide (LPS) which carries the O specific antigen of many bacterial species, is responsible for endotoxic activity and acts as a receptor site for some bacteriophages. In addition, numerous proteins are located in the outer membrane, some serving as specific binding sites for a wide range of molecules, others being involved in transport functions; those exposed on the surface of the membrane could stimulate antibody production.

B.   Other envelope-associated components

Both Gram-positive and Gram-negative bacteria may possess capsules; in general, these are polysaccharides that form a viscous coat surrounding the bacterium.

Members of the genus *Bacillus* may form capsules of poly-D-glutamic acid. Some polysaccharide capsules are homopolymers, but the majority are made of more than one sugar residue. The capsules are antigenic, an exception being the hyaluronic acid capsules of the group A and C streptococci. In general, the presence of a capsule does not prevent the formation of antibody against envelope components inferior to the capsule.

Many bacteria also have surface appendages which extend into the surrounding medium. Pili (fimbriae) are commonly found on enteric bacteria and many other Gram-negatives, some organisms may possess up to several hundred. They are 5–25 nm in diameter, but up to 2 μm in length, almost entirely proteinaceous. Bacterial flagellae are primarily associated with the property of motility and may carry somatic antigens, e.g. the H antigens of enterobacteria.

The role of envelope components in pathogenesis is of importance in the design of vaccines. LPS endotoxin may induce a range of systemic effects in a host, but other components may be relevant to the virulence factors, in particular adhesion. Changed polymers on bacterial surfaces may be involved in non-specific interactions that enable more specific binding to occur.

Capsules and slimes are frequently thought to be involved in the adhesion of bacteria to host cell surfaces, but it is the pili which have been most clearly implicated in adhesion.

II. CHOLERA/ENTEROPATHOGENIC BACTERIA

Diarrhoeal disease caused by enteropathogenic bacteria constitutes a major worldwide health problem, especially in young children; in 1975, some 17–18 million deaths were attributed to this cause (Finkelstein, 1980). Cholera represents a relatively small proportion of the diarrhoeal diseases, but an understanding of this disease and the development of approaches to immunoprophylaxis are relevant since it appears that up to half the "non-specific" diarrhoeal diseases are attributable to enteric bacteria that produce enterotoxins which are structurally, functionally and antigenically related to the cholera enterotoxin.

Cholera, caused by *Vibrio cholerae*, is characterized by an excessive fluid-loss diarrhoea that results from the action of an exotoxin elaborated by the microorganism on the epithelium of the intestine (De, 1959; Dutta *et al.*, 1959). The toxin, a protein, itself comprises two non-covalently linked subunits. The heavy (H or A) toxin has a molecular weight of about 28 000 daltons and is responsible for the biological activity of the toxin, viz. stimulation of the adenylcyclase system, giving enhanced levels of cAMP which causes a major shift in the sodium–potassium pump of the epithelial cells with a resultant outpouring of fluid. To affect epithelial cells of the small bowel, however, requires the A toxin to be associated with the B region which itself consists of 5 or 6 non-covalently associated light (L) polypeptides of about 11 500 MW. The B region is essentially non-toxic, but is required for the binding of the complete toxin (holotoxin) to host cell membrane receptors containing the GM1 ganglioside, which in turn facilitates entry of the A subunit into the target cell and subsequent activating of adenylcyclase (Holmgren and Svennerholm, 1977; Finkelstein, 1980).

Early cholera vaccines were relatively unsophisticated, consisting of killed whole organisms or lipopolysaccharide, and were of poor effectiveness in field trials, giving only limited short-term immunity that was restricted to relatively immune adults in areas where cholera is an endemic paediatric disease (DasGupta *et al.*, 1967; Mosley *et al.*, 1969; Finkelstein, 1973, 1980); it appeared doubtful as to whether effective immunity against cholera was, in fact, possible. The problem of inducing protective immunity was undoubtedly a consequence of the non-invasive nature of the microorganism, which is limited to the lumen and the epithelial surface of the small intestine (Gangarosu *et al.*, 1960); protection is only likely if specific antibody against organism or toxin is present in, or at the surface of, the small intestine. However, the disease itself is immunogenic as shown by the resistance of convalescent volunteers to rechallenge (Cash *et al.*, 1974). The inadequacy of the early killed vaccines may be related to their inability to induce antibody active at the site of infection.

Toxoids are frequently effective against diseases caused by toxigenic organisms, but cholera toxoids have not yielded the levels of protection hoped for. Formalized cholera toxoids induced variable immunity against homologous and heterologous challenge in animals (Finkelstein and Hollingsworth, 1970; Northrup and Chisari, 1972) and even in humans (Verwey *et al.*, 1972), but there was reversion of toxoid to toxin *in vivo* that resulted in severe localized reaction after subcutaneous injection. Although a glutaraldehyde-inactivated toxoid was stable (Rappaport *et al.*, 1974) it had a low efficacy in field trials (Curlin *et al.*, 1976).

In addition to having different sizes and biological activity, the H and L components of cholera toxin are immunologically distinct with the B region being immundominant; antisera react most strongly with the latter component and the anti-L subunit antibodies have a higher capacity to neutralize toxin than anti-H antibodies (Holmgren and Svennerholm, 1977). Since immunological protection against cholera toxin appeared to result from prevention of toxin binding to the GM1 ganglioside, Holmgren *et al.* (1977) developed a vaccine consisting of toxoided purified L suburits; such a vaccine should be incapable of reversion to a toxic state. The vaccine afforded protection in rabbits, but was more effective when used in conjunction with conventional cholera LPS vaccine, the two components acting synergistically (Table 1). Holmgren *et al.* (1977) considered that this synergism resulted from interference by antibody in separate pathogenic mechanisms. Synergism between toxoid-whole cell vaccine combinations was reported by Peterson (1979) to be effective against experimental cholera in rabbits.

Although the pathogenesis of cholera is primarily a consequence of toxin production, motility appears also to be a virulence factor (Guentzel and Berry, 1975; Yancey *et al.*, 1978) and consequently the use of crude flagellae (CF) from *V. cholerae* in vaccines has been studied. CF vaccines were found to be effective in preventing experimental cholera in mice (Eubanks *et al.*, 1977) and rabbits (Yancey *et al.*, 1979) and the levels of protection afforded exceed those obtained with toxoid or killed whole cell vaccines. Since it is highly likely that anti-flagellar immunity and anti-toxin immunity neutralize different virulence determinants, Resnick *et al.* (1980) prepared a combined CF-toxoid vaccine. The CF-toxoid vaccine gave improved protection against cholera in rabbits compared with single vaccines and a killed whole cell vaccine, although whether this improvement was additive or synergistic was not clear. The concept of combined vaccines was extended by Rappaport and Bonde (1981) who proposed the development of a single vaccine to confer protection against cholera and

Table 1 Protection of rabbits against challenge with live *Vibrio cholerae* afforded by combinations of *V. cholerae* somatic antigen and L-subunit toxoid[b]

Vaccine	Relative protection against live vibrio challenge[a]	Serum antibody titre 21 days post-vaccination	
		against LPS	against toxin
Purified lipopolysaccharide (LPS; 1·25 mg)	4		
Cholera vaccine (2 × 10⁸ killed vibrios)	5		
Cholera vaccine (4 × 10⁸ killed vibrios)	15	300 000	<500
L-subunit toxoid (10 μg)	7	<500	200 000
L-subunit toxoid (30 μg)	14–25		
Cholera vaccine (4 × 10⁹ killed vibrios) plus L-subunit toxoid (10 μg)	105	500 000	600 000
Cholera vaccine (2 × 10⁸ killed vibrios) plus L-subunit toxoid (30 μg)	134		
LPS (1·25 mg) + L-subunit toxoid (30 μg)	390		

[a] ED_{50} for immunized rabbits/ED_{50} for non-vaccinated controls.
[b] Data abstracted from Holmgren *et al.*, 1977.

some *E. coli* diarrhoeal disease. This arises from the ability of cholera antitoxin to neutralize cholera and *E. coli* heat labile toxins and the apparent adjuvant effect of killed whole *E. coli* on cholera toxoids. In their experiments, a combination of killed whole *E. coli* and cholera toxoid was more effective in affording protection against either *V. cholerae* or *E. coli* experimental infections than cholera toxoid, *V. cholerae* whole cell vaccine or *E. coli* whole cell vaccine given singly or in other combinations. It is now conceivable that a single vaccine will eventually be available to protect against a range of diarrhoeal disease organisms.

In contrast to the idea of vaccines against specific virulence factors, Honda and Finkelstein (1979) and Finkelstein (1980) have reasoned that since cholera is, in effect, a form of local immunization presenting to the host a variety of surface antigens and enterotoxin as immunogens, an ideal vaccine could be an oral live attenuated vaccine. To this end they have selected for and assessed mutants of *V. cholerae* lacking the A(ADP-ribosylating) portion of the cholera enterotoxin. Such tox⁻ mutants when tested in animals have been capable of colonization of the intestine whilst remaining innocuous. In volunteer studies, immunity against cholera challenge was induced, but this was less than the immunity observed on convalescence from the disease itself. One factor that could weigh against the use of such mutants is the observation that mutants appeared to be unstable and a reversion to toxin production occurred.

A further possibility is for live oral vaccines such as *E. coli* or a non-toxigenic *V. cholerae* containing DNA coding for the B toxin subunits (Kaper and Levine, 1981; Gennaro *et al.*, 1982). Such a live *V. cholerae* vaccine would possess all the required somatic antigens and would elaborate relatively large amounts of the highly immunogenic but non-toxic B subunits.

A genetically engineered vaccine against scours, a severe diarrhoeal disease of cattle and pigs caused by enteropathogenic *E. coli*, has recently become available commercially (*New Scientist*, 6 May 1982). The vaccine comprises a genetically engineered non-pathogenic (toxigenic) *E. coli* capable of producing relatively large amounts of the protective K88 and K99 protective antigens and is claimed to be superior to previous tradition-al whole killed vaccines and toxoids. It seems likely that human vaccines of this nature will soon be available.

III. PERTUSSIS

Pertussis (whooping cough) is naturally a disease only of man that can give rise to severe sequelae in infants. Infection is spread from person to person via the respiratory route, usually from patients with early or catarrhal infections or possibly carriers. Once a common disease pertussis was a scourge of young children, but the disease has apparently been brought under control in development countries by widespread vaccination pro-grammes.

The mechanisms of infection and immunity are not well understood. For example, it is not known why children recover naturally from pertussis nor which antigens may be involved in evoking a protective immunological response and as a consequence design of vaccines is not easy. Natural infections and immunization give rise to various antibody types in animals and man, but no one class of antibody nor any specific antibody action correlates well with protection or recovery (Aftandelians and Connor, 1973). Despite this lack of knowledge, the proper use of vaccination seems to afford the best means of controlling the disease, since chemotherapy is of limited use, except perhaps in the control of secondary bacterial infection (Manclark, 1981).

The current vaccines in use against pertussis consist of killed whole cells; they appear to be effective (McKendrick *et al.*, 1980) but have raised more controversy than any other vaccine because of doubts held by some as to what they consider to be a high risk-to-benefit ratio. Indeed, many doubt that the vaccines afford sufficient protection to justify use, in view of possible adverse reactions (Grady and Wetterlow, 1978). However, the assessment of complications arising from pertussis vaccination is not easy; the boundary between toxicity and potency is poorly defined and there are limitations on methods to define these parameters. An association between pertussis vaccination and some neurological illness is clear (Miller *et al.*, 1981), though cases are few and in most instances recovery is complete. The National Childhood Encephalopathy Study showed that the estimated risk of serious neurological disorders occurring within seven days after immunization with diphtheria, tetanus and pertussis vaccine in previously normal children is 1 in 110 000 injections and the risk of neurological sequelae persistence for one year post-vaccination is 1 in 310 000 (Miller *et al.*, 1981). However, as Miller *et al.* (1981) point out, because of broad assumptions made in calculating these risk figures and their wide confidence limits, they cannot be regarded as precise measures and extreme caution should be taken in interpreting these data. There appears to be general agreement that new vaccines are required that give maximum protection for minimum risk and·such development will depend on a good understanding of mechanisms of pathogenicity and immunity in the disease.

The plasticity of the Gram-negative envelope is an important factor in the context of achieving an appropriate mixture of antigenic material to afford protection. It is now well established that changes in growth environment can induce marked changes in the composition of bacterial envelopes and *Bordetella pertussis* is no exception. Leslie and Gardner (1931) described a phase variation whereby a series of mutational changes give rise to the so-called phase IV organisms, which are avirulent and lack the protective antigen (PA), HSF and agglutinogen characteristic of freshly isolated, virulent phase I organisms. Lacey (1960) first observed a process of phenotypic modulation whereby growth in a high magnesium, low sodium medium (C-medium) yields C-mode bacteria which lack some of the biologically active components of conventionally grown (X-mode) bacteria, such as PA, LPF, HSF, etc.; these changes are freely reversible by alteration of growth conditions. Cultivation in a high nicotinic acid medium induces similar reversible variation (Wardlaw *et al.*, 1976). The loss of these various biological activities in phase IV and C-mode organisms appears to correlate with a deficiency of two major components of the pertussis envelope having molecular weights of 28 000 and 30 000 (Wardlaw and Parton, 1978). This propensity of *B. pertussis* for antigenic modulation is an important factor to be considered in optimizing yields of protective antigens and vaccine production.

B. pertussis is not an invasive organism, it produces only a localized infection and has a wide range of biologically active components (Table 2),

Table 2 Biological components of *Bordetella pertussis*

Protective antigens
Histamine sensitizing factor
Lymphocytosis promoting factor (LPF) ⎫ Pertussigen
Islets activating protein ⎬
Filamentous haemagglutinin ⎭
Lipopolysaccharide
Agglutinogens
22 S Antigen
Adenyl cyclase
Heat labile toxin

but the nature of the organisms pathogenic determinants are not known. Clearly, an important step is the attachment of the organism to epithelial cells of the respiratory tract and the so-called filamentous haemagglutinin (FHA) may be involved in this process, but might function more as a proximity factor than a specific binding component (Jones, 1977). FHA was generally believed to be derived from fimbriae, but recent work by Ashworth *et al.* (1982b) showed that fimbriae do not bind antibody to FHA but do bind antibody to serotype-specific agglutinogen.

The effects of infection may well be due to toxic components acting both at the site of infection and/or systemically. A component of particular interest is the so-called pertussigen to which have been ascribed many of the biological activities observed in mice given pertussis vaccine, such as, histamine-sensitizing factor (HSF), Islet activating protein (IAP), late-appearing toxic factor, mouse protective antigen and lymphocytosis pro-moting factor (LPF) (Munoz and Bergmann, 1977, 1979) although not all investigators agree that these substances are identical. Lymphocytosis promoting factor (LPF) (Morse and Morse, 1976), dermonecrotic toxin (DNT), tracheal cytotoxin (TCT), which causes ciliostasis and pathological changes in epithelial cells (Manclark, 1981) and polymorphonuclear leuko-cyte-inhibitory factor (PIF) (Utsumi *et al.*, 1978) are all toxins isolated from *B. pertussis* that could be virulence factors. Although the presence of pertussigen in extracts of *B. pertussis* usually correlates with protective activity in mice, purified pertussigen itself is toxic and non-protective unless detoxified with glutaraldehyde (Munoz *et al.*, 1981a; Robinson *et al.*, 1982).

Glutaraldehyde inactivated pertussigen has been claimed to be the most important protective antigen using the mouse intracerebral challenge (i.c.) test (Munoz *et al.*, 1981b). Robinson *et al.* (1982), however, reported that native pertussigen did not express any protective activity, but their material did exhibit an adjuvant effect (Table 3). Thus, removal of

Table 3 Protective potencies of various *Bordetella pertussis* preparations in the mouse intracerebral challenge test in the presence and absence of lymphocytosis promoting factor (LPF; 0·2 or 0·5 μg/mouse)

Preparation	PD_{50} (μg protein)	
	No LPF	plus LPF
Outer membrane protein (OMP)	3·0	—
OMP-Haptoglobin	24·6	1·6
Glutaraldehyde-OMP	16·7	1·2
SDS-OMP	112.·0	1·5
Fimbrial haemagglutinin (solid grown)	17·8	1·6
C-mode OMP	29·1	1·2
Phase IV OMP	NP (>50)	1·0
22 S Antigen	NP (>73)	8·0
LPF	NP (>4)	—

NP = Not protective.
Data kindly provided by Dr A. Robinson.

pertussigen from outer membrane protein preparations of *B. pertussis* reduced the i.c. protective potency of the latter, which could be restored by re-addition of purified pertussigen. In addition, envelope protein preparations of *Bordetella bronchiseptica*, *Bordetella parapertussis*, or phase IV (avirulent) strains of *B. pertussis* which had no protective potency were made highly protective against mouse, i.c. challenge with *B. pertussis* by adding small amounts of native pertussigen, but such synergism was not shown with other organisms such as *E. coli* or *Neisseria gonnorhoeae* (Table 4).

The nature of this potentiation by pertussigen is unclear, but may result from an alteration in the mouse blood–brain barrier that allows access of antigen and/or antibodies to the site of infection (Robinson *et al.*, 1982). These workers consider that the i.c. protection test may be so dependent on the adjuvant effect of pertussigen that highly purified antigens might be inactive in this particular challenge test, but might still be highly protective against, for example, respiratory challenge. Because of doubts about the interpretation of results from the mouse i.c. test (Preston *et al.*, 1980), any putative subunit pertussis vaccine would thus need to be assessed in a respiratory infection model. However, the potentiating activity of pertussigen might still be included in a vaccine if the pharmacological toxicity of the material could be chemically inactivated without destroying its antigenicity (Robinson *et al.*, 1982).

Table 4 Effect of LPF (0·2 or 0·5 μg per mouse) on the protective potencies of non-pertussis preparations against *Bordetella pertussis* challenge

Preparation	PD_{50} (μg protein)	+LPF PD_{50} (μg protein)
Bordetella bronchiseptica FHA	20	2·7
Bordetella bronchiseptica OMP	>50	2·1
Bordetella parapertussis OMP	>50 (NP)	1·1
Escherichia coli OMP	>50 (NP)	>50 (NP)
Neisseria gonorrhoeae OMP	>50 (NP)	>50 (NP)

NP = Not protective.
Data kindly provided by Dr A. Robinson.

Considerable effort has been made to isolate and characterize possible protective antigens of *B. pertussis*, in particular the FHA and LPF components. Because of their possible roles in virulence and immunological significance they are candidate components for inclusion in putative acellular vaccines. Japanese workers have, in fact, developed a new component vaccine containing FHA together with some detoxified LPF that has some adjuvant effect (Manclark, 1981); this vaccine meets WHO requirements for pertussis vaccine (Cameron, 1980). Over one million doses of this vaccine were administered to children aged 2–4 years and there was very low local or febrile reactivity. Antibodies against LPF and FHA were induced together with an adequate agglutinin response. However, the effectiveness and low reactogenicity of this vaccine in 3-month-old infants has yet to be confirmed.

The need to consider outer membrane proteins as constituents of an acellular pertussis vaccine in addition to purified FHA and toxoided LPF has been demonstrated in recent work of Robinson and Hawkins (in press). Detergent extracts of *B. pertussis* outer membrane proteins were found to be highly immunogenic with presence of LPF using the mouse i.c. test (Table 2).

It appears, then, that the technological advances made since the introduction of whole cell pertussis vaccine some three decades ago may finally yield an acellular pertussis vaccine designed to give maximum protection with minimum risk of adverse reaction.

IV. HAEMOPHILUS INFLUENZAE

The problem of endemic bacterial meningitis in infants is now recognized as being one for which the development of effective vaccine prophylaxis seems appropriate. The incidence of the disease in the USA is now such that for each 1000 births, 1–2 will develop neonatal meningitis with nearly 4 more acquiring *H. influenzae* type b (Hib) meningitis in the first 5 years of life (Gotschich *et al.*, 1978). Indeed, *H. influenzae* type b is the most important cause of endemic bacterial meningitis in the USA (CDC, 1979), Finland and Sweden (Gotschlich *et al.*, 1978); in addition, this organism may cause epiglottitis, arthritis and pneumonitis. Despite antibiotic therapy, the mortality rate remains at about 10% and, unfortunately, one-third to one-half of those who contract Hib meningitis and survive suffer permanent severe neurological sequelae, including blindness, deafness, convulsions and mental retardation (Michaels, 1971; Sell *et al.*, 1972). The appearance of plasmid-mediated antibiotic resistance in hospital isolates (Gotschlich *et al.*, 1978) emphasizes the appositeness of developing an effective vaccine.

In many ways, the attempts to find an effective vaccine against Hib exemplifies attempts to introduce rationality into the vaccine design. Early studies on the pathogenesis of systemic Hib disease indicated that the polysaccharide capsule (phosphoribosylribitolphosphate, PRRP) elaborated by the organism plays a critical role (Chandler, Fothergill and Dingle, 1937; Weller *et al.*, 1977) and the development of anticapsular antibody is a marked feature of host resistance to Hib infection (Weller *et al.*, 1978). Consequently, Hib capsular material has been used in a human vaccine (Anderson *et al.*, 1972; Schneerson *et al.*, 1971; Rodrigues *et al.*, 1971), but evidence suggests that although humoral antibody can be induced by capsular immunization in adults and children over 2 years old and older children may be significantly protected, purified PRRP vaccine is not effective in children under 2 years old (Lynn *et al.*, 1977; Hanson *et al.*, 1981). Unfortunately, it is this group which contracts about 70% of all serious infections. Evidence suggests that antibody directed against non-capsular antigens may also be important in immunity against Hib disease, since preadsorbtion of human sera with PRRP did not totally remove bactericidal and opsonizing antibody activities (Anderson *et al.*, 1972; Norden, 1972). The role of Hib capsular polysaccharide in vaccines is still under investigation and recent works suggests that when complexed with traces of protein and LPS, this material may have enhanced protective capability. For example, Schneerson *et al.* (1980) activated Hib polysaccharide with cyanogen bromide and reacted this with adipic hydrazide derivatives of various proteins. Whereas purified Hib polysaccharide was poorly immunogenic, covalent linking of the capsular material with immunogenic carriers such as serum albumen appeared to result in a satisfactory immune response to subcutaneous vaccination. More recently, Anderson *et al.* (1982) investigated the vaccine potential of PRPP extracted from Hib culture supernatants using the cationic detergent cetrimide (Cetavlon). Such preparations contained protein complexed to the carbohydrate and were highly immunogenic in infant children. SDS-PAGE analysis suggested that the complexed protein components closely resembled protein found in crude membrane preparations. This suggests that an effective Hib vaccine might be based on covalent complexes of PRRP with protective outer membrane proteins.

A.   Ribosomal and outer membrane protein vaccines

Since the observation by Youmans and Youmans (1965) that ribosomal fractions of an avirulent *Mycobacterium tuberculosis* were capable of inducing high levels of immunity in mice against a virulent challenge, attention has been drawn to the possible immunogenic properties of ribosomal fractions from many other bacterial species. Ribosomal fractions of *Salmonella typhimurium* (Eisenstein, 1975), *Pseudomonas aeruginosa* (Smith *et al.*, 1974), *Staphylococcus aureus* (Winston and Berry, 1970), *V. cholerae* (Jensen et al., 1972), *Streptococcus pneumoniae* (Thompson and Snyder, 1971), *Francisella tularensis* (Hambleton *et al.*, 1974), *N. gonorrhoeae* (Cooper *et al.*, 1980) and *H. influenzae* (Lynn *et al.*, 1977) have all been found to function as protective antigens. Some, indeed, appear to have advantages over conventional whole cell vaccines, for example the pneumococcal ribosomal vaccine confers cross-serotype protection (Einstein, 1978).

The immunoprotective activity of ribosomes from *H. influenzae* type b has been investigated by Solotorovsky and his co-workers. Washed ribosomes that sedimented as a single peak on sucrose density gradients and contained 25% protein and 75% RNA induced protective immunity in mice comparable to that obtained after sublethal infection. Immunodiffusion tests showed the ribosomes to be free of contamination with capsular material, indeed ribosomes from a non-capsulated strain were as immunogenic as those from a virulent capsulated one (Lynn *et al.*, 1977). It was subsequently shown (Tewari *et al.*, 1978) that the major immunoprotective antigen associated with the ribosomes was proteinaceous. Treatment of ribosomes with ribonuclease did not affect their immunogenicity whereas proteolytic enzymes diminished their protective capacity (Table 5). Protein extracted from ribosomes with 2-chloroethanol induced immunity comparable to that elicited by whole ribosomes and the low levels of protection afforded by phenol-extracted RNA related to the degree of protein contamination.

Table 5 Immunoprotective activity in mice of components of *Haemophilus influenzae* type b.

Component	Dose (i.p. infection)	Survival (%) 7 days post-challenge with 500 LD_{50} live *H. influenzae* type b
Live cells	5×10^3	70–85
Killed whole cells + FIA	2×10^8	40
Ribosomes + FIA	50 μg[a]	75–90
Ribosomal protein + FIA	100 μg	60
Ribosomal RNA (3 × phenol extracted)	200 μg	70
Ribosomal RNA (7 × phenol extracted)	200 μg	35
Ribosomal RNA (7 × phenol extracted, Pronase treated)	200 μg	0
OMP + FIA	100 μg	90–100
OMP + FIA	50 μg	60–90
IMP + FIA	100 μg	60–90
IMP + FIA	50 μg	40–45

[a] = Expressed as protein content.
FIA = Freund's incomplete adjuvant.
OMP = Outer membrane protein.
IMP = Inner membrane protein.
Data kindly provided by Professor M. Solotorovsky.

The nature of the protective antigens in ribosomal preparations of Hib and other bacteria is, as yet, unclear; ribosomal proteins, RNA and contaminating O antigens have been suggested as possible protective antigens in such preparations (Smith and Bigley, 1972; Venneman *et al.*, 1970; Eisenstein, 1975). It is difficult to conceive how intracellular components can be effective in raising antibody effective against intact organisms and it seems most likely that in fact non-ribosomal antigens become associated with ribosomal fractions during their preparation; the true ribosomal components may well exert some adjuvant effect (Eisenstein, 1978; Hoops *et al.*, 1976; Cooper *et al.*, 1980; Gongrijp *et al.*, 1980).

By absorbing immune sera from vaccinated mice Gongrijp *et al.* (1980) showed that the protective antigenicity of a pseudomonas ribosomal vaccine appeared to be due to contaminating cell envelope antigens, in particular LPS; antibodies to ribosomal antigens were not protective and RNA appeared to exert only an adjuvant effect, which was nullified by ribonuclease treatment.

If the protective activity of *Haemophilus* ribosomes (Lynn *et al.*, 1977; Tewari *et al.*, 1978) is due to contamination with non-ribosomal protective antigens, then the observation that ribosomes from capsulated strains are equally protective as those from uncapsulated strains suggests that non-capsular surface antigens common to both types may be the true protective antigens. In fact, outer membrane preparations prepared by Solotorovsky's team (personal communication, see Table 4) are proving effective immunogens in mice. Similarly, Hansen *et al.* (1981) identified several different immunogenic outer membrane proteins of Hib to which infant rats mounted a detectable antibody response, although individual animals were found to vary in the quality and quantity of their immune response to these proteins. Nevertheless, antibody against non-capsular somatic antigens does protect infant rats against experimental Hib infection (Lam *et al.*, 1980). Loeb and Smith (1982) have identified at least three outer membrane proteins which appear common to some 50 strains of Hib. These are of particular interest since, if shown to be protective, these might form the basis of a rationally designed vaccine capable of protecting against all Hib disease.

V. GRAM-NEGATIVE OPPORTUNISTIC PATHOGENS

Infections due to Gram-negative bacteria of the enterobacteriaceae and pseudomonadaceae are an increasing problem in hospitals particularly with patients undergoing immunosuppression or with respiratory damage, renal or hepatic disease or compromised by burns, neutropenia or surgical invasion being especially vulnerable. Chemotherapy is certainly of immense value in controlling such infections, but the increasing frequency of antibiotic resistance, often plasmid-borne, amongst hospital isolates and the presence of residual endotoxin, during and after chemotherapy, mean that vaccine prophylaxis and therapy could have an important role in combatting these so-called opportunistic pathogens. Unfortunately, because of the antigenic diversity of the organisms in these groups, effective vaccines need either to be derived from cross-protective antigens or comprise a mixture of protective antigens from individual strains. It has frequently been suggested that a broad spectrum Gram-negative bacterial vaccine could be prepared from components common to the envelopes of Gram-negative organisms, however, such a goal has not yet been achieved. Rather, more diverse multicomponent vaccines have been found to be effective.

Lipopolysaccharide (LPS) is a particularly immunogenic component, common to the envelopes of all Gram-negative bacteria. As such, LPS could form the basis of a broad spectrum Gram-negative vaccine, except that LPS is synonymous with endotoxin and is toxic to man and animals, causing a range of systemic effects including intravascular coagulation, low blood pressure, renal cortical necrosis and lethal endotoxic shock (Braude *et al.*, 1973). However, serum endotoxin neutralizing antibodies from animals tolerant to LPS from one species of bacteria will passively immunize non-tolerant animals against LPS from another bacterial species (Freedman, 1959). Luderitz *et al.* (1966) explained this phenomenon with the discovery of the similarity of the toxic glycolipid "core" region of the LPS from O-somatic antigenically correlated bacteria (see Fig. 1).

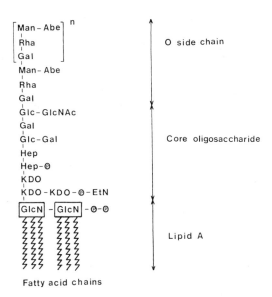

Fig. 1 Diagrammatic representation of lipopolysaccharide molecule of *Salmonella typhimurium*. The molecule consists of three regions: O side chain, core oligosaccharide and Lipid A. (Abe, abequose; Man, mannose; Rha, L-rhamnose; Gal, galactose; Glc, glucose, GlcNAc, *N*-acetyl glucosamine; Hep, heptulose; KDO, 2-keto-3-deoxyoctonate; EtN, ethanolamine; GlcN, glucosamine; ℗, phosphate).

Antisera against core glycolipid protect against endotoxin (Tate *et al.*, 1966) and Gram-negative bacterial challenge (Chedid *et al.*, 1968). McCabe *et al.* (1977) found that core glycolipid from a mutant of *Salmonella minnesota* that contained only 2-keto-3-deoxyoctonate and lipid A protected against klebsiella, proteus and salmonella challenge whereas the lipid A alone gave no protection.

Although antibody to core glycolipid is effective in counteracting endotoxin challenge it may be less effective against live bacterial challenge than type-specific antibody (McCabe *et al.*, 1977); nevertheless, in clinical trials treatment of human Gram-negative bacteraemia with antiserum against core glycolipid was deemed effective (Ziegler *et al.*, 1981). In addition to being used to provide human antiserum for therapy for Gram-negative bacteraemia and endotoxin shock, core glycolipid vaccines could prove of value for prophylaxis with hospital patients identified as being at risk to Gram-negative infection. Prevention of *P. aeruginosa* infection is of concern with burn patients as well as cases of cystic fibrosis and therefore development of a vaccine is of particular relevance.

Early attempts to protect mice against a lethal *P. aeruginosa* challenge with whole killed organisms were described by Markley and Smallman (1968) who also demonstrated that culture filtrates had a protective effect. Carney and Jones (1968) and later Jones (1969) demonstrated that protection could be achieved against not only a homologous serotype, but by using culture filtrates from several serotypes heterologous protection was achieved. From this early work, a successful polyvalent *P. aeruginosa* vaccine was developed (Miller *et al.*, 1977), which has been used with some success in clinical trials to combat *P. aeruginosa* infections in burn patients (Jones *et al.*, 1976; Jones *et al.*, 1980). This vaccine is a formol-inactivated EDTA-extract of whole organisms and undoubtedly contains a mixture of LPS and outer envelope antigens, although its composition is not known in detail at present.

More recently, Pavlovskis *et al.* (1981) described the immunization of mice with a chemically inactivated *P. aeruginosa* exotoxin A. In the presence of a synthetic adjuvant (N-acetylmuramyl-L-alanyl-D-isogluta-mine) high levels of anti-exotoxin antibody were induced that afforded protection to burned and infected mice. Immunization with toxoid alone did not induce antitoxin. Another recent report (Fernandes *et al.*, 1981) described attempts to develop a vaccine based on outer membrane proteins common to all serotypes of *P. aeruginosa*, but purified, free of LPS and hence of endotoxin activity. These workers identified a 58 500 dalton envelope protein as being the only immunogenic protein that was access-ible to the immune system when whole, fixed cells were used to immunize. However, these serum antibodies did not protect cystic fibrosis patients against further lung infection with *P. aeruginosa*. Although such attempts to produce vaccines of defined composition having minimum toxicity and wide protective activity may, in due course, be successful, it must be borne in mind how much success has been achieved using rather more empirical approaches to the problem (Jones, 1969; Miler *et al.*, 1977; Jones *et al.*, 1980).

A. Capsular vaccines

The potential value of capsular polysaccharide vaccines for preventing disease caused by encapsulated bacteria is being investigated widely (Gotschlich *et al.*, 1978) and in particular a pneumococcal polysaccharide vaccine has been extensively studied (see *Reviews of Infectious Diseases* (1981) Vol. 3 suppl.). As mentioned earlier, there is considerable evidence that the PRPP capsule of *H. influenzae* type b is an important virulence factor in systemic Hib disease (Weller *et al.*, 1977) and anticapsular antibody may have an important protective role (Weller *et al.*, 1978; Gotschlich *et al.*, 1978). *E. coli* K1 and group B meningococci have a chemically identical polysaccharide and it might seem that a common vaccine is possible, however the immune response to these polysaccharide antigens has proved disappointing in humans (Gotschlich *et al.*, 1978). Nevertheless, since polysaccharide capsular antigens are shared by many species of bacteria (*E. coli, Klebsiella aerogenes* and *Strep. pneumoniae*) and antibodies against these antigens act as opsonins (Young and Stevens, 1977), this is still an interesting line of investigation. At least 12 of the 15 antigens present in contemporary pneumococcal vaccines are similar to capsular antigens of *K. aerogenes* and of *E. coli* (Heidelberger and Nimmich, 1976); such similarities support the concept outlined earlier of vaccines possibly effective against a broad spectrum of Gram-negative organisms.

VI. ANIMAL MODELS

Although the success of any vaccine resides in its ability to prevent the natural disease in humans, successful development may be a function of the availability of an animal model with which to assess the vaccine experimentally. Ideally, an animal model should mimic the essential features of the natural disease and enable the effects of vaccination to be readily assessed.

It could be argued that one reason for the abundance of work on developing vaccines against cholera and other enteropathogenic bacteria is the excellence of the available animal model; the ligated rabbit ileal loop test which was described in 1953 by De and Chatterje. For this, the rabbit intestine is surgically exposed and materials under test injected directly into ligated sections of ileum. After about 18 hours, the animal is sacrificed and responses measured by recording the ratio of fluid accumulation to length of loop. This model is so good because it utilizes the fundamental pathogenic feature of the enteric diseases, viz. massive fluid movement into the gut lumen, so assessments can accurately reflect the effect of a vaccine on this central feature of the disease. An additional important feature of the model is the fact that the fundamental biochemical mechanism of fluid transfer is similar among different animal species. Although suckling mice have been used to assess some enteric diseases, the relevance and effectiveness of the ligated ileal loop test remains unchallenged.

Unfortunately, such a clear situation does not exist for pertussis. The only routinely available animal test for protective potency of pertussis vaccines is the mouse intracerebral (i.c.) challenge test (Robinson *et al.*, 1982). Although this test would at first appear very relevant in view of the serious neurological sequelae that can be a feature of the disease, the test cannot be considered to mimic the natural route of infection, since *B. pertussis* is a respiratory pathogen that is essentially non-invasive. It appears also that data on vaccine potencies derived from the mouse i.c. challenge test can be misleading (Preston *et al.*, 1980; Ashworth *et al.*, 1982a) perhaps because of a potentiating effect of pertussigen that may result from some alteration in the mouse blood–brain barrier (Robinson *et al.*, 1982); as a consequence, antigens apparently non-protective in the mouse i.c. test might still protect against respiratory infections. Respiratory challenge of the rabbit by intranasal instillation (Ashworth *et al.*, 1982a) or by large droplet aerosol (Druett and MacLennan, unpublished data; Irons and MacLennan, 1979) might provide a better system for assessing protective mechanisms in the upper respiratory tract, even though the resulting colonization may be asymptomatic. Respiratory infection of the mouse (Pittman *et al.*, 1980; Sato *et al.*, 1980) is not an entirely satisfactory model, since it involves the entire respiratory tract, but this still may hold advantages over the mouse i.c. test.

Several animal models have been studied for use in evaluation of vaccines and chemotherapeutic agents against *H. influenzae* type b meningitis. In 1941, De Torregrosa and Francis used intracerebral injection of mice to determine Hib strain virulence, but this does not satisfactorily reflect the natural development of the disease (Burans *et al.*, 1981). Another model similar to the mouse mucin model involves i.p. injection of infant rats with organisms suspended in saline. Results with this model resemble those with intranasal instillation of young rats in that bacteraemia and meningitis occur, but mortality arises less frequently than in the mouse mucin test (Burans et al., 1981). Although i.p. challenge can be criticized as being an unnatural route of infection, results obtained with i.n. or i.p. challenged rats are similar and i.p. injection would not appear to invalidate an animal model (Burans et al., 1981).

Studies on immunization against Gram-negative bacteraemia caused by pseudomonadaceae or enterobacteriaceae were considerably aided by using rabbits having a neutropenia induced by nitrogen mustard (Ziegler et al., 1973). This model closely resembles the neutropenic patient who appears to be at high risk of developing Gram-negative bacteraemia. Infection of burns with pseudomonads is a common serious complication in burns patients and controlled burning of anaesthetized mice (Jones and Lawrence, 1964) was used in assessing potential protective antigens of P. aeruginosa (Carney and Jones, 1968). It is not clear with either of these models how closely the biochemical responses to the induced lesions mimic those in the human disease situations, but nevertheless they have proved valuable and effective.

For a number of Gram-negative species of interest infection can occur via the respiratory route and development of vaccines against such infections may require relevant animal respiratory challenge models. For infections of the upper respiratory tract administration of infectious agents by intranasal instillation or large droplet aerosol may be most appropriate; for example, as discussed above with petussis. In the case of infections sited deeper in the lung however, the above methods could be inappropriate since the characteristics of dispersion of the invading organism would be markedly different from that arising from inhalation of small droplet aerosols. The landing site of inhaled particles in the respiratory tract and the extent to which they are retained depends on their size (see review by Strange and Cox, 1976); from 0.5 μm diameter it decreases and from 2 to 15 μm diameter it increases at first, then falls off. In general, the larger the particle the greater the number of bacteria required to produce infection; with particles of appropriate size, infection may be caused by one organism (Hood, 1961; Tigertt et al., 1961).

Although particle size is an important factor in the establishment of respiratory infection the survival of bacteria in the airborne state is a prerequisite to their infectivity and so factors which affect bacterial survival must influence their infectivity. A wide range of factors influence survival of airborne bacteria including relative humidity, atmospheric composition, temperature, cloud age, the presence of additives to the spray fluid, method of sampling the cloud (see reviews by Anderson and Cox, 1967 and Strange and Cox, 1976) and metabolic status of the organisms (Hambleton *et al.*, 1972). These factors should be carefully controlled in any model respiratory challenge if it is to be reliable and reproducible. For example, exposure to small droplet aerosols of *Legionella pneumophila* generated and held under carefully controlled conditions facilitated the development of an acute respiratory infection in several animal species so providing the first effective model of human legionellosis (Baskerville *et al.*, 1981). This approach could readily be applied to developing animal models applicable to studying other Gram-negative bacterial respiratory diseases such as those caused by pseudomonads or klebsiella.

VII. REFERENCES

Aftandelians, R. V. and Connor, J. D. (1973). *J. Infect. Dis.* **128**, 555–558.

Anderson, J. D. and Cox, C. S. (1967). *Symp. Soc. Gen. Microbiol.* **17**, 203–226.

Anderson, P., Johnston, R. B. Jr. and Smith, D. H. (1972). *J. Clin. Invest.* **51**, 31–38.

Anderson, P., Insel, R. A. and Smith, D. H. (1982). *In* "Bacterial Vaccines" (J. B. Robbins, J. C. Hill and J. C. Sadoff, eds), Seminars Infect. Dis., Vol. IV, pp. 327–333. Thieme-Stratton, New York.

Ashworth, L. A. E., Fitzgeorge, R. B., Irons L. I., Morgan, C. P. and Robinson, A. (1982a). *J. Hyg. Camb.* **88**, 475–486.

Ashworth, L. A. E., Irons, L. I. and Dowsett, A. B. (1982b). *Infect. Immun.* **37**, 1278–1281.

Baskerville, A., Fitzgeorge, R. B., Broster, M., Hambleton, P. and Dennis, P. J. (1981). *Lancet* **ii**, 1389–1390.

Braude, A. I., Douglas, H. and David, C. E. (1973). *J. Infect. Dis.* **128**, S 5157–S 5164.

Burans, J. P., Kruszewski, F. H., Lynn, M. and Solotorovsky, M. (1981). *Brit. J. Exp. Path.* **62**, 496–503.

Cameron, J. (1980). *J. Biol. Stand.* **8**, 297–302.

Carney, S. A. and Jones, R. J. (1968). *Brit. J. Exp. Pathol.* **49**, 395–410.

Cash, R. A. Music, S. I., Libonati, J. P., Snyder, M. J., Wenzel, R. P. and Hornick, R. B. (1974). *J. Infect. Dis.* **129**, 45–52.

CDC (1979). *Morbid. Mortal. Weekly Rep.* **28**, 277–279.

Chandler, C. A., Fothergill, L. D. and Dingle, J. H. (1937). *J. Exp. Med.* **66**, 789–799.

Chedid, L., Parant, M., Parant, F. and Boyer, F. (1968). *J. Immunol.* **100**, 292–301.

Cooper, M. D., Tewari, R. P. and Bowser, D. V. (1980). *Infect. Immun.* **28**, 92–100.

Curlin, G., Levine, R., Aziz, K. M. A., Rahman, A. S. M. and Verwey, W. F. (1976). *In* "Proceedings of the 11th Joint Conference of the U.S.-Japan Co-operative Medical Science Program Symposium of Cholera", pp. 314–335. Dept. of Health, Education and Welfare, Washington, D.C.

DasGupta, A., Sinha, R., Shrivastava, D. L., De, S. P., Taneja, B. L., Rao, M. S. and Abon-Gareeb, A. H. (1967). *Bull. W.H.O.* **37**, 371–385.

De, S. N. (1959). *Nature* **183**, 1533–1534.

De, S. N. and Chatterje, D. N. (1953). *J. Pathol. Bacteriol.* **66**, 559–562.

De Torregrosa, M. V., Francis, T., Jr. (1941). *J. Infect. Dis.* **68**, 57–63.

Dutta, N. K., Panse, M. V. and Kulkarni, D. R. (1959). *J. Bacteriol.* **78**, 594–595.

Eisenstein, T. K. (1975). *Infect. Immun.* **12**, 364–377.

Eisenstein, T. K. (1978). *In* "New trends and developments in vaccines" (A. Voller and H. Friedman eds) pp. 211–222. MTP Press Ltd, Lancaster.

Eubanks, E. R., Guentzel, M. N. and Berry, L. J. (1977). *Infect. Immun.* **15**, 533–538.

Fernandes, P. B., Kim, C., Cundy, K. R. and Huang, N. N. (1981). *Infect. Immun.* **33**, 527–532.

Finkelstein, R. A. (1973). *CRC Crit. Rev. Microbiol.* **2**, 553–569.

Finkelstein, R. A. (1980). *Prog. Clin. Biol. Res.* **47**, 133–142.

Finkelstein, R. A. and Hollingsworth, R. C. (1970). *Infect. Immun.* **1**, 468–473.

Fothergill, L. D., Dingle, J. H. and Chandler, C. A. (1937). *J. Exp. Med.* **65**, 721–732.

Freedman, H. H. (1959). *Proc. Soc. Exp. Biol. Med.* **102**, 504–506.

Gangarosu, E. J., Beisel, W. R., Benyayati, C., Sprinz, H. and Pyaratu, P. (1960). *Amer. J. Trop. Med. Hyg.* **9**, 125–135.

Gennaro, M. L., Greenaway, P. J. and Broadbent, D. A. (1982). *Lancet* **i**, 1239–1240.

Gongrijp, R., Muller, W. J. H. A., Lemmens, P. J. M. R. and van Boven, C. P. A. (1980). *Infect. Immun.* **27**, 204–210.

Gotschlich, E. C., Austrian, R., Cvjetanovic, B. and Robbins, J. B. (1978). *Bull. W.H.O.* **56**, 509–518.

Grady, G. F. and Wetterlow, L. M. (1978). *N. Engl. J. Med.* **298**, 966–967.

Guentzel, M. N. and Berry, L. J. (1975). Motility as a virulence factor for *Vibrio cholerae. Infect. Immun.* **11**, 890–897.

Hambleton, P., Strange, R. E. and Benbough, J. E. (1972). *MRE (Porton Down) Report no. 62.*

Hambleton, P., Evans, C. G. T., Hood, A. M. and Strange, R. E. (1974). *Brit. J. Exp. Pathol.* **55**, 363–373.

Hansen, E. J., Frisch, C. F., McDade, R. L. Jr. and Johnston, K. H. (1981). *Infect. Immun.* **32**, 1084–1092.

Heidelberger, M. H. and Nimmich, W. (1976). *Immunochemistry* **13**, 67–80.

Holmgren, J. and Svennerholm, A. (1977). *J. Infect. Dis.* **136**, S 105–S 107.

Holmgren, J., Svennerholm, A. M., Lonnroth, I., Fall-Persson, M., Markman, B. and Lundbeck, H. (1977). *Nature* **269**, 602–604.

Honda, T. and Finkelstein, R. A. (1979). *Proc. Natl. Acad. Sci. U.S.A.* **76**, 2052–2056.

Hood, A. M. (1961). *J. Hyg. Camb.* **59**, 497–504.

Hoops, P., Prather, N. E., Berry, L. J. and Ravel, J. M. (1976). *Infect. Immun.* **13**, 1184–1192.

Irons, L. I. and MacLennan, A. P. (1979). *In* "International Symposium on Pertussis" (C. R. Manclark and J. C. Hill eds) pp. 338–349. Dept. of Health, Education and Welfare. Pubn. no. 79–1830, Washington, D.C.

Jensen, R., Gregory, B., Naylor, J. and Acton, P. (1972). *Infect. Immun.* **5**, 947–952.

Jones, G. B. (1977). *In* "Receptors and recognition microbial interactions" (J. L. Reissig ed.) series B, Vol. 3, pp. 139–176, Chapman and Hall, London.

Jones, R. J. (1969). *J. Hyg. Camb.* **67**, 241–247.

Jones, R. J. and Lawrence, J. C. (1964). *Brit. J. Exp. Pathol.* **45**, 198–206.
Jones, R. J., Roe, E. A., Lowbury, E. J. L., Miler, J. M. and Spilsbury. J. F. (1976). *J. Hyg.* **76**, 429–439.
Jones, R. J., Roe, E. A. and Gupta, J. L. (1980). *Lancet* **ii**, 1263–1265.
Kaper, J. B. and Levine, M. M. (1981). *Lancet* **ii**, 1162–1163.
Lacey, B. W. (1960). *J. Hyg. Camb.* **58**, 57–93.
Lam, J. S., Granoff, D. M., Gilsdorf, J. R. and Costerton, J. W. (1980). *Curr. Microbiol.* **3**, 359–364.
Leslie, P. H. and Gardner, A. D. (1931). *J. Hyg.· Camb.* **31**, 423–434.
Loeb, M. R. and Smith, D. H. (1982). *In* "Bacterial Vaccines" (J. B. Robbins, J. C. Hill and J. C. Sadoff, eds) Seminars Infect. Dis. Vol. IV, pp. 334–338. Thieme-Stratton, New York.
Luderitz, O., Staub, A. M. and Westphal, O. (1966). *Bact. Rev.* **30**, 192–255.
Lynn, M., Tewari, R. P. and Solotorovsky, M. (1977). *Infect. Immun.* **15**, 453–460.
Manclark, C. R. (1981). *Bull. W.H.O.* **59**, 9–15.
Markley, K. and Smallman, E. (1968). *J. Bacteriol.* **96**, 67–74.
McCabe, W. R., Bruins, S. C., Craven, D. E. and Johns, M. (1977). *J. Infect. Dis.* **128**, S 284–S 289.
McKendrick, N. W., Gully, P. R. and Geddes, A. M. (1980). *Brit. Med. J.* **281**, 1390–1391.
Michaels, R. H. (1971). *N. Engl. J. Med.* **285**, 666–667.
Miler, J. M., Spilsbury, J. F., Jones, R. J., Roe, E. A. and Lowbury, E. J. L. (1977). *J. Med. Microbiol.* **10**, 19–27.
Miller, D. L., Ross, E. M., Alderslade, R., Bellman, M. H. and Rawson, N. S. B. (1981). *Brit. Med. J.* **282**, 1595–1599.
Morse, S. I. and Morse, J. H. (1976). *J. Exp. Med.* **143**, 1483–1502.
Mosley, W. H., McCormick, W. M., Ahmed, A., Chowdhury, A. K. M. A. and Barui, R. K. (1969). *Bull. W.H.O.* **40**, 187–197.
Moxon, E. R. and Anderson, P. (1969). *J. Infect. Dis.* **140**, 471–478.
Munoz, J. J. and Bergman, R. K. (1977). *In* "*Bordetella pertussis*. Immunological and Other Biological Activities" (N. Rose ed.) Immunological series, Vol. 4, pp. 1–235. Marcel Dekker, New York.
Munoz, J. J. and Bergman, R. K. (1979). "Microbiology–1979" (D. Schlessinger, ed.) pp. 193–197. Amer. Soc. Microbiol. Washington, D.C.
Munoz, J. J., Arai, H., Bergman, R.. K. and Sadowski, P. L. (1981a). *Infect. Immun.* **33**, 820–826.
Munoz, J. J., Arai, H. and Cole, R. L. (1981b). *Infect. Immun.* **32**, 243–250.
Norden, C. W. (1972). *Proc. Soc. Exp. Biol. Med.* **139**, 59–61.
Northrup, R. S. and Chisari, F. V. (1972). *J. Infect. Dis.* **125**, 471–479.
Pavlovskis, O. R., Edman, D. C., Leppla, S. H., Wretlind, B., Lewis, L. R. and Martin, K. E. (1981). *Infect. Immun.* **32**, 681–689.
Peterson, J. W. (1979). *Infect. Immun.* **26**, 528–533.
Pittman, M., Furman, B. L. and Wardlaw, A. C. (1980). *J. Infect. Dis.* **142**, 56–65.
Preston, N. W., Timewell, R. M. and Carter, E. J. (1980). *J. Infect.* **2**, 227–235.
Rappaport, R. S. and Bonde, G. (1981). *Infect. Immun.* **32**, 534–541.
Rappaport, R. S., Bonde, G., McCann, T., Rubin, B. A. and Tint, H. (1974). *Infect. Immun.* **9**, 304–317.
Resnick, I. G., Ford, C. W., Shackleford, G. M. and Berry, L. J. (1980). *Infect. Immun.* **30**, 375–380.
Robinson, A. and Hawkins, D. C. (1982). In press.

Robinson, A., Ashworth, L. A. E. and Irons, L. I. (1982). *Lancet* **ii,** 108.
Rodrigues, L. P., Schneerson, R. and Robbins, J. B. (1971). *J. Immunol.* **107,** 1071–1080.
Sato, Y., Izumiya, K., Sato, H., Cowell, J. L. and Manclark, C. R. (1980). *Infect. Immun.* **29,** 261–266.
Sell, S. H. W., Merrill, R. E., Doyne, E. O. and Zimsky, E. P. (1972). *Paediatrics* **49,** 206–211.
Schneerson, R., Rodrigues, L. P., Parke, J. C. Jr. and Robbins, J. B. (1971). *J. Immunol.* **107,** 1081–1090.
Schneerson, R., Robbins, J. B., Barrera, O., Sutton, A., Habig, W. B., Hardegree, M. C. and Chaimovich, J. (1980). *Prog. Clin. Biol. Res.* **47,** 77–4.
Smith, H. (1972). *Symp. Soc. Gen. Microbiol.* **22,** 1–24.
Smith, R. A. and Bigley, N. J. (1972). *Infect. Immun.* **6,** 377–383.
Smith, R. L., Wysocki, J. A., Brunn, J. N., DeCourcy, S. J. Jr., Blakemore, W. S. and Mudd, S. (1974). *J. Reticuloendothelial Soc.* **15,** 22–31.
Solotorovsky, M. and Lynn, M. (1978). *CRC Crit. Rev. Microbiol.* **6,** 1–32.
Strange, R. E. and Cox, C. S. (1976). *Symp. Soc. Gen. Microbiol.* **26,** 111–154.
Tate, W. J., Douglas, H. and Braude, A. I. (1966). *Ann. N.Y. Acad. Sci.* **133,** 746–762.
Tewari, R. P., Lynn, M., Birnbaum, A. J. and Solotorovsky, M. (1978). *Infect. Immun.* **19,** 58–65.
Thompson, H. C. W. and Snyder, I. S. (1971). *Infect. Immun.* **3,** 16–23.
Tigertt, W. D., Benensen, A. S. and Gochenour, W. S. (1961). *Bact. Rev.* **25,** 285–293.
Utsumi, S., Sonoda, S., Imagawa, T. and Kanoh, H. (1978). *Biken. J. 21,* 121–135.
Venneman, N. R., Bigley, N. J. and Berry, L. J. (1970). *Infect. Immun.* **1,** 574–582.
Verwey, W., Craig, J. P., Feeley, J. C., Greenough, W. B. III., Guckian, J. C. and Pierce, N. F. (1972). *In* "Proceedings of the 7th Joint Conference, US-Japan Cooperative Medical Science Program, Cholera Panel", pp. 99–100. U.S. Dept. of State, Washington D.C.
Ward, J. B. and Berkeley, R. C. W. (1980). *In* "Microbial Adhesion to Surfaces" (R. C. W. Berkeley, J. M. Lynch, J. Melling, P. R. Rutter and B. Vincent, eds) pp. 47–66. Ellis Horwood, Chichester.
Wardlaw, A. C. and Parton, R. (1978). *In* "International Symposium on Pertussis" (C. R. Manclark and J. C. Hill eds) pp. 94–98. U.S. Dept. Health, Education, Welfare. Pub. No. (NIH) 79–1830.
Wardlaw, A. C., Parton, R. and Hooker, M. J. (1976). *J. Med. Microbiol.* **9,** 89–100.
Weller, P. F., Smith, A. L., Anderson, P. and Smith, D. H. (1977). *J. Infect. Dis.* **135,** 34–41.
Weller, P. F., Smith, A. L., Smith, D. H. and Anderson, P. (1978). *J. Infect. Dis.* **138,** 427–436.
Winston, S. H. and Berry, L. J. (1970). *J. Reticuloendothel. Soc.* **8,** 66–73.
Yancey, R. J., Willis, D. L. and Berry, L. J. (1978). *Infect. Immun.* **22,** 387–392.
Yancey, R. J., Willis, D. L. and Berry, L. J. (1979). *Infect. Immun.* **25,** 220–228.
Youmans, A. S. and Youmans, G. P. (1965). *J. Bacteriol.* **89,** 1291–1298.
Young, L. S. and Stevens, P. (1977). *J. Infect. Dis.* **136,** S 174–S 180.
Ziegler, E. J., Douglas, H., Sherman, J. E., Davis, C. E. and Braude, A. I. (1973). *J. Immunol.* **111,** 433–438.
Ziegler, E. J., McCutchan, J. A. and Braude A. I. (1981). *Clin. Res.* **29,** 576a.

Index

257